MANUAL of SMALL ANIMAL INFECTIOUS DISEASES

Edited by

Jeffrey E. Barlough, D.V.M., Ph.D.

Diplomate
American College of Veterinary Microbiologists
Lecturer
Department of Veterinary Microbiology, Immunology and
  Parasitology
New York State College of Veterinary Medicine
Cornell University
Ithaca, New York

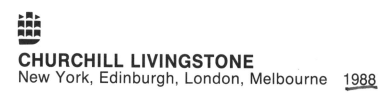

CHURCHILL LIVINGSTONE
New York, Edinburgh, London, Melbourne 1988

Library of Congress Cataloging in Publication Data

Manual of small animal infectious diseases.

Bibliography: p.
Includes index.
1. Dogs—Diseases. 2. Cats—Diseases.
3. Communicable diseases in animals. I. Barlough,
Jeffrey E.
SF991.M23 1988   636.7'08969   87-23849
ISBN 0-443-08508-0

© **Churchill Livingstone Inc.   1988**

Distributed in the United Kingdom by Churchill
Livingstone, Robert Stevenson House, 1-3 Baxter's Place,
Leith Walk, Edinburgh EH1 3AF, and by associated
companies, branches, and representatives throughout the
world.

Accurate indications, adverse reactions, and dosage
schedules for drugs are provided in this book, but it is
possible that they may change. The reader is urged to
review the package information data of the manufacturers
of the medications mentioned.

Sponsoring Editor: *Linda Panzarella*
Assistant Editor: *Nancy Terry*
Copy Editor: *Ozzievelt Owens*
Production Supervisor: *Jocelyn Eckstein*

Printed in the United States of America

First published in 1988

Domestic animals contribute to our intelligence, to our needs, their superior powers, their wonderful instincts, their ever-ready servitude, their entire substance. They are at once sources of revenue, machines, means of transport, laborers, companions, at times friends even; clothes, nourishment, docile subjects with abundant experience: what are they not to us? They partake of our labors without profiting by them; of our pleasures without enjoyment in them; of our glory even without hesitation. They live and die to serve us, and we seek but too often the secret of our own good at the very heart even of their sufferings.

Such is the object of your studies, which are endless in their variety . . . to study with patience and persistence, the formidable maladies that afflict domestic animals and that sometimes are transmitted from animal to man . . .

Veterinary science, it is necessary to say . . . is still but recent: it scarcely dates its foundation but from that of the very school we are now in, from less than a hundred years. The future holds for you many discoveries, among which, let us hope, will be found efficacious remedies for some of these horrific diseases that are yet without means of cure.

M. Merruau

Secretary General of the Prefecture of the Seine, speaking at the Distribution of Prizes and Diplomas, École Nationale Vétérinaire d'Alfort, August 29, 1852, as reported in Recueil de Médecine Vétérinaire Pratique 29:667, 1852, and The Veterinarian (London) 26:100, 1853

Assistance in translation provided by Mrs. L. Winter, Cornell University

CONTRIBUTORS

Donna Walton Angarano, D.V.M.
Diplomate, American College of Veterinary Dermatology; Associate Professor, Department of Small Animal Surgery and Medicine, Auburn University College of Veterinary Medicine, Auburn, Alabama

Max J. G. Appel, Dr. Med. Vet., Ph.D.
Professor, Department of Veterinary Microbiology, Immunology and Parasitology, James A. Baker Institute for Animal Health, New York State College of Veterinary Medicine, Cornell University, Ithaca, New York

Marie H. Attleberger, D.V.M., M.S., Ph.D.
Professor, Department of Microbiology, Auburn University College of Veterinary Medicine, Auburn, Alabama

John R. August, B. Vet. Med., M.S., M.R.C.V.S.
Diplomate, American College of Veterinary Internal Medicine; Professor and Head, Department of Small Animal Medicine and Surgery, Texas A & M University College of Veterinary Medicine, College Station, Texas

Jeffrey E. Barlough, D.V.M., Ph.D.
Diplomate, American College of Veterinary Microbiologists; Lecturer, Department of Veterinary Microbiology, Immunology and Parasitology, New York State College of Veterinary Medicine, Cornell University, Ithaca, New York

Ralph E. Barrett, D.V.M.
Diplomate, American College of Veterinary Internal Medicine; Staff Internist, Sacramento Animal Medical Group, Inc., Carmichael, California

Malcolm Bennett, B.V.Sc., Ph.D., M.R.C.V.S.
Research Associate, Department of Microbiology, University of Tennessee College of Veterinary Medicine, Knoxville, Tennessee

Dawn Merton Boothe, D.V.M., M.S.
Diplomate, American College of Veterinary Internal Medicine; Fellow, Clinical Pharmacology (Pharmacological Manufacturer's Foundation); Veterinary Clinical Associate, Department of Veterinary Physiology and Pharmacology, Texas A & M University College of Veterinary Medicine, College Station, Texas

W. S. Botha, B.V.Sc. (Hons.) M. Med. Vet. (Path.)
Consultant Veterinary Pathologist, Onderstepoort, South Africa

Ralph G. Buckner, D.V.M.
Diplomate, American College of Veterinary Internal Medicine; Emeritus Professor, Department of Medicine and Surgery, Oklahoma State University College of Veterinary Medicine, Stillwater, Oklahoma

Elizabeth C. Burgess, D.V.M., Ph.D.
Assistant Professor, Department of Medical Sciences, University of Wisconsin School of Veterinary Medicine; Director, Research Animal Resources Center Laboratory, University of Wisconsin, Madison, Wisconsin

Leland E. Carmichael, D.V.M., Ph.D.
Diplomate, American College of Veterinary Microbiologists; John M. Olin Professor of Virology, Department of Veterinary Microbiology, Immunology and Parasitology, James A. Baker Institute for Animal Health, New York State College of Veterinary Medicine, Cornell University, Ithaca, New York

Thomas M. Craig, D.V.M., Ph.D.
Professor, Department of Veterinary Microbiology and Parasitology, Texas A & M University College of Veterinary Medicine, College Station, Texas

James W. Crissman, D.V.M., Ph.D.
Diplomate, American College of Veterinary Pathologists; Veterinary Pathologist, Section of Pathology, Stuart Pharmaceuticals, Division of ICI Americas, Inc., Wilmington, Delaware

Cheryl R. Dhein, D.V.M., M.S.
Diplomate, American College of Veterinary Internal Medicine; Assistant Professor, Department of Veterinary Clinical Medicine and Surgery, Washington State University College of Veterinary Medicine, Pullman, Washington

Brian R. H. Farrow, B.V.Sc., M.R.C.V.S., Ph.D., F.A.C.V.Sc.
Associate Professor, Department of Veterinary Anatomy, University of Sydney; Consultant in Neurology, University of Sydney Veterinary Teaching Hospital, Sydney, New South Wales, Australia

James G. Fox, D.V.M., M.S.
Diplomate, American College of Laboratory Animal Medicine; Professor and Director, Division of Comparative Medicine, Massachusetts Institute of Technology, Cambridge, Massachusetts; Adjunct Professor of Comparative Medicine, Tufts University School of Veterinary Medicine, North Grafton, Massachusetts

Rosalind M. Gaskell, B.V.Sc., Ph.D., M.R.C.V.S.
Research Fellow, Department of Veterinary Pathology, University of Liverpool, Veterinary Field Station, Leahurst, Neston, Wirral, England

Craig E. Greene, D.V.M., M.S.
Diplomate, American College of Veterinary Internal Medicine; Professor, Department of Small Animal Medicine, University of Georgia College of Veterinary Medicine, Athens, Georgia

Donald P. Gustafson, D.V.M., M.S., Ph.D.
Diplomate, American College of Veterinary Microbiologists; Leo Philip Doyle Professor of Virology, Department of Veterinary Microbiology, Pathology and Public Health, Purdue University School of Veterinary Medicine, West Lafayette, Indiana

John W. Harvey, D.V.M., Ph.D.
Diplomate, American College of Veterinary Pathologists; Professor, Department of Physiological Sciences, University of Florida College of Veterinary Medicine; Chief, Clinical Pathology Service, Veterinary Medical Teaching Hospital, University of Florida, Gainesville, Florida

Cynthia J. Holland, M.S., Ph.D.
Research Associate, Department of Veterinary Pathobiology, University of Illinois College of Veterinary Medicine, Urbana, Illinois

David L. Huxsoll, D.V.M., Ph.D.
Commander, U.S. Army Medical Research Institute of Infectious Diseases, Fort Detrick, Frederick, Maryland

Donald E. Kahn, D.V.M., Ph.D.
Diplomate, American College of Veterinary Microbiologists; Director of Virological Research and Production, Pitman-Moore, Inc., Washington Crossing, New Jersey

Ann B. Kier, D.V.M., Ph.D.
Diplomate, American College of Laboratory Animal Medicine; Associate Professor, Department of Laboratory Animal Medicine, and Department of Pathology, University of Cincinnati College of Medicine, Cincinnati, Ohio

Carl E. Kirkpatrick, V.M.D., Ph.D.
Assistant Professor, Department of Veterinary Pathobiology, University of Illinois College of Veterinary Medicine, Urbana, Illinois

Joyce S. Knoll, V.M.D., Ph.D.
Instructor, Department of Pathobiological Sciences, University of Wisconsin School of Veterinary Medicine, Madison, Wisconsin

George E. Lees, D.V.M., M.S.
Diplomate, American College of Veterinary Internal Medicine; Associate Professor, Department of Small Animal Medicine and Surgery, Texas A & M University College of Veterinary Medicine, College Station, Texas

Daria N. Love, B.V.Sc., Ph.D., M.R.C. (Path.), M.A.S.M.
Associate Professor, Department of Veterinary Pathology, University of Sydney, Sydney, New South Wales, Australia

E. Gregory MacEwen, V.M.D.
Diplomate, American College of Veterinary Internal Medicine; Professor, Department of Medical Sciences; Interim Chairman, Department of Surgical Sciences; Affiliate Professor, Department of Veterinary Science, University of Wisconsin School of Veterinary

Medicine; Associate Member, Wisconsin Clinical Cancer Center, Department of Human Oncology, University of Wisconsin School of Medicine, Madison, Wisconsin

Peter S. MacWilliams, D.V.M., Ph.D.
Diplomate, American College of Veterinary Pathologists; Clinical Associate Professor, Department of Pathobiological Sciences, University of Wisconsin School of Veterinary Medicine, Madison, Wisconsin

Dennis W. Macy, D.V.M., M.S.
Diplomate, American College of Veterinary Internal Medicine; Associate Professor, Department of Clinical Sciences, Colorado State University College of Veterinary Medicine and Biomedical Sciences, Fort Collins, Colorado

George Migaki, D.V.M.
Diplomate, American College of Veterinary Pathologists; Chief Pathologist, Registry of Comparative Pathology, Armed Forces Institute of Pathology, Washington, D.C.; Clinical Professor of Pathology, Uniformed Services University of the Health Sciences; Scientist Associate, Universities Associated for Research and Education in Pathology, Inc., Bethesda, Maryland

Richard L. Ott, D.V.M.
Diplomate, American College of Veterinary Internal Medicine; Emeritus Professor, Department of Veterinary Clinical Medicine and Surgery, Washington State University College of Veterinary Medicine, Pullman, Washington; Consultant in Hematology/Oncology, Department of Medicine, University of Washington School of Medicine, Seattle, Washington

Allan J. Paul, D.V.M., M.S.
Extension Veterinarian, University of Illinois College of Veterinary Medicine, Urbana, Illinois

Roy V. H. Pollock, D.V.M., Ph.D.
Assistant Professor, Section of Epidemiology, Department of Clinical Sciences; Director, Center for Medical Informatics, New York State College of Veterinary Medicine, Cornell University, Ithaca, New York

David J. Polzin, D.V.M., Ph.D.
Diplomate, American College of Veterinary Internal Medicine; Assistant Professor, Department of Small Animal Clinical Sciences, University of Minnesota College of Veterinary Medicine, St. Paul, Minnesota

Karen Regan, D.V.M.
Teaching Associate, Department of Veterinary Pathobiology, University of Illinois College of Veterinary Medicine, Urbana, Illinois

Miodrag Ristic, D.V.M., Ph.D.
Diplomate, American College of Veterinary Microbiologists; Professor, Department of Veterinary Pathobiology, University of Illinois College of Veterinary Medicine, Urbana, Illinois

Robert C. Rosenthal, D.V.M., M.S., Ph.D.
Diplomate, American College of Veterinary Internal Medicine; Assistant Professor, Department of Medical Sciences, University of Wisconsin School of Veterinary Medicine; Associate Member, Wisconsin Clinical Cancer Center, Department of Human Oncology, University of Wisconsin School of Medicine, Madison, Wisconsin

Fredric W. Scott, D.V.M., Ph.D.
Diplomate, American College of Veterinary Microbiologists; Professor, Department of Veterinary Microbiology, Immunology and Parasitology; Director, Cornell Feline Health Center, New York State College of Veterinary Medicine, Cornell University, Ithaca, New York

John A. Shadduck, D.V.M., Ph.D.
Diplomate, American College of Veterinary Pathologists; Professor and Head, Department of Veterinary Pathobiology, University of Illinois College of Veterinary Medicine, Urbana, Illinois

Edward H. Stephenson, D.V.M., Ph.D.
Diplomate, American College of Veterinary Microbiologists; Associate Professor, Department of Veterinary Preventive Medicine, University of Maryland Virginia-Maryland Regional College of Veterinary Medicine, College Park, Maryland

Lea Stogdale, B.V.Sc., M.R.C.V.S., M.A.C.V.Sc.
Diplomate, American College of Veterinary Internal Medicine; Staff Clinician, Academy Emergency Clinic, Winnipeg, Manitoba, Canada

John P. Thilsted, D.V.M., Ph.D.
Diplomate, American College of Veterinary Pathologists; Veterinary Pathologist, Veterinary Diagnostic Services, New Mexico Department of Agriculture, Albuquerque, New Mexico

Kenneth S. Todd, Jr., Ph.D.
Professor and Assistant Head, Department of Veterinary Pathobiology, University of Illinois College of Veterinary Medicine, Urbana, Illinois

Kimberly S. Waggie, D.V.M., M.S., Ph.D.
Diplomate, American College of Laboratory Animal Medicine; Chief, Microbiology Unit, Comparative Pathology Section, Veterinary Resources Branch, Division of Research Services, National Institutes of Health, Bethesda, Maryland

Joseph E. Wagner, D.V.M., M.P.H., Ph.D.
Diplomate, American College of Laboratory Animal Medicine; Professor and Chairman, Department of Veterinary Pathology, University of Missouri College of Veterinary Medicine, Columbia, Missouri

Stephen D. White, D.V.M.
Diplomate, American College of Veterinary Dermatology; Assistant Professor, Department of Medicine, Tufts University School of Veterinary Medicine, North Grafton, Massachusetts

George T. Wilkinson, M.V.Sc., M.R.C.V.S., F.A.C.V.Sc.
Associate Professor, Department of Companion Animal Medicine and Surgery, University of Queensland School of Veterinary Science, St. Lucia, Brisbane, Queensland, Australia

Alice M. Wolf, D.V.M.
Diplomate, American College of Veterinary Internal Medicine; Associate Professor, Department of Small Animal Medicine and Surgery, Texas A & M University College of Veterinary Medicine, College Station, Texas

PREFACE

Few areas of scientific inquiry in veterinary medicine are as changeable today as are microbiology and the study of infectious diseases. In an era of rapid advancement in molecular biology and the routine manipulation of genetic elements, novelty and innovation are fleeting and "knowledge" itself becomes a relative term. Few areas in veterinary medicine seem as poorly translated into practical terms for the benefit of the veterinary practitioner—undoubtedly a result of the innate complexity of the field and the relative small number of microbiologists with a clinical veterinary orientation. One only need consider the examples of the canine viral enteritides, feline respiratory tract disease, the interpretation of feline coronaviral antibody titers, or the pros and cons of feline leukemia virus vaccination, to appreciate some of the difficulties.

In this book we have sought to present, in clear and concise form, relevant and up-to-date information for the practicing veterinarian on the infectious disease entities in dogs and cats. No attempt has been made to produce a weighty collection of exhaustive microbiological reviews; rather, the emphasis is on the clinical and practical—recognition of infectious disease signs, identification of disease agents, therapy, prophylaxis, and public health considerations where appropriate. Illustrations are included primarily as an aid in identifying etiologic agents (i.e., primarily those agents that can be routinely identified in the practitioner's laboratory). References have been kept to a minimum, and are included only as recommended readings at the end of each chapter, in order to enhance readability and flow of the text, which is prepared in an outline format. We have strived to produce a ready, readable guide to small animal infectious diseases for the busy practicing veterinarian.

I am indebted to the many contributing authors who took time from their busy clinical and academic schedules to share in this undertaking. Thanks are also due Toni Tracy and the other members of the Churchill Livingstone staff, whose patient advice and professional skill at all stages of production greatly facilitated the creation of this work. I am indebted also to you, the reader, for your interest in the field of small animal infectious diseases, and encourage your active participation, by your communicated comments and suggestions in the preparation of any subsequent edition.

Jeffrey E. Barlough, D.V.M., Ph.D.

CONTENTS

1

Feline Panleukopenia

Donald E. Kahn

ETIOLOGY

I. Feline panleukopenia is recognized to occur throughout the world. While this disease is of viral etiology, the normal intestinal microbial flora both predisposes the gut epithelial cells to infection and amplifies the clinical illness.

II. The physical properties of feline panleukopenia virus (FPLV) (small size, i.e., diameter 20 nm, or approximately 1/1,270,000 in; cubic [icosahedral] geometry; single-stranded deoxyribonucleic acid [DNA] genome; lack of a limiting envelope) confer extreme resistance to chemical and physical inactivation. FPLV is not inactivated by surfactant disinfectants. The virus will remain infectious in the environment for long periods of time, and may retain viability after more than a year's storage at room temperature.

III. Antigenicity

A. The small size of the FPLV genome codes for a single capsid protein building block.

B. There is a single serotype of FPLV. Immunity acquired through spontaneous infection or by vaccination will protect against all recognized field strains. Point mutations of the DNA genome occur relatively frequently, producing single amino acid substitutions within the capsid polypeptide. Such mutations produce antigenic diversity among FPLV isolates. While detectable in laboratory assays using appropriate monoclonal antibodies, these mutations are too small to produce biologically significant changes in antigenicity. On several occasions extensive mutations have occurred, producing more antigenically divergent progeny. Mink enteritis virus and canine parvovirus are thought to have originated from FPLV in this way.

C. Feline panleukopenia and mink enteritis viruses are closely related serologically. Feline panleukopenia virus vaccines protect dogs against canine parvovirus disease.

1

IV. The host range of feline panleukopenia virus includes
   A. Cats (Felidae), both domesticated and exotic species
   B. Mink (*Mustela vison*)
   C. Procyonids
      1. Raccoons (*Procyon lotor*)
      2. Coatimundi (*Nasua nasua*)
   V. Replication of FPLV is restricted to populations of rapidly dividing cells. Transplacental infection of the embryo and fetus occurs. Embryonic resorption or fetal death may be the only manifestation of FPLV infection of the pregnant queen. Modified-live virus vaccine strains, as well as virulent field strains, can cross the placenta and infect the unborn kittens. The thymus and cerebellum are favored targets when infection occurs perinatally. Destruction of the thymus causes immunosuppression, manifested clinically as a "fading kitten syndrome." Neuronal destruction can produce ataxia. Leukocytic stem cells in the bone marrow, lymphocytes in lymphoid tissues, and the crypt epithelium of the small intestine are involved regardless of the cat's age. Destruction of leukocytes produces panleukopenia, the most characteristic manifestation of FPLV infection. The intestinal bacterial flora maintains the high mitotic activity of the gut mucosa, predisposing to viral infection of the crypt epithelial cells. Secondary bacterial infection amplifies the enteric disease.
VI. Transmission of feline panleukopenia virus
   A. Transmission of FPLV most frequently results from direct contact between infected and susceptible cats. Large quantities of virus are present in saliva, vomitus, feces, and urine during the acute stage of the illness.
   B. Fleas and other biting insects may spread the virus mechanically after feeding on viremic hosts. Recovered cats may continue to harbor FPLV virus asymptomatically.
   C. The kidney may become chronically infected, and infectious virus has been recovered from the urine of cats more than 1 year after infection.
   D. The extreme resistance of FPLV to inactivation potentiates indirect viral transmission on fomites (feed bowls, articles of clothing, etc.).

CLINICAL SIGNS

   I. Pathogenesis
      The usual route of exposure to FPLV virus is ingestion or inhalation. Primary viral replication occurs in the oropharynx and is fol-

lowed by hematogenous spread to secondary sites such as the thymus, intestinal crypt epithelium, spleen, Peyer's patches, lymph nodes, and endothelial cells.

II. Clinical entities produced by FPLV include:
   A. Infectious enteritis
   B. Panleukopenia
   C. Feline ataxia, or cerebellar hypoplasia. Before FPLV was known to infect and destroy cerebellar neurons, this condition was classified as a genetic defect.

III. Exposure to FPLV is common. The majority of susceptible cats experience subclinical infections, but in some FPLV can induce overt illness.
   A. The disease is characterized by its sudden onset, acute course, and high morbidity and mortality. Fever, depression, inappetence, dehydration, vomition, and diarrhea are common manifestations of FPLV infection. The disease can be especially fulminant in kittens, and death may occur with few premonitory signs. Infection may precede overt signs of illness by 4–9 days.
   B. The most consistent manifestation of FPLV infection is panleukopenia. At the onset of illness peripheral blood leukocyte counts often decline to fewer than 4,000/ml[3]. Massive destruction of leukocytic stem cells may result in generalized lymphadenopathy. In nonfatal infections peripheral blood leukocyte counts increase and neutrophilia may occur during convalescence.

DIAGNOSIS

I. The prevalence of FPLV makes it logical to include panleukopenia at or near the top of the list of differential diagnoses whenever kittens or older cats with unknown vaccination histories are presented with high fever, vomition, inappetence, dehydration, and lethargy. Total and differential leukocyte counts may provide useful information.

II. Enteric feline leukemia virus (FeLV) infection may result in clinical signs very similar to FPLV-induced enteritis. The appearance of enteric disease in cats with known histories of FPLV vaccination warrants testing for FeLV. The enteric form of FeLV infection is an illness of low morbidity and is a consequence of close association with FeLV-infected cats. Other lesions of FeLV infection, such as thymic neoplasia or nonregenerative anemia, may be present in cats living in the same household.

TREATMENT

There is no specific treatment for feline panleukopenia. The therapeutic regimen should be designed to ameliorate the signs of illness.
  I. Fluid replacement therapy to reverse dehydration
 II. Broad-spectrum antibiotic therapy to lessen secondary bacterial infection of the intestinal tract
III. Forced alimentation to meet energy and nutritional needs

PREVENTION

  I. Good management practices are the key to the prevention of FPLV infections. While it often is not possible to manage catteries and breeding colonies as closed facilities, care should be taken to limit exposure of susceptible cats to FPLV.
      A. Sanitation should include use of a disinfectant viricidal for FPLV. A 1:32 dilution of sodium hypochlorite bleach is effective once the area is free of organic material.
      B. Pregnant queens and litters of kittens should be isolated from other cats.
      C. An animal about to be placed in a cattery or multiple-cat household either should have a known vaccination history or should be vaccinated and held in isolation for a week.
      D. Vaccination of kittens should be an established part of the management routine.
 II. Kittens nursing colostrum of immune queens acquire passive immunity to feline panleukopenia. The duration of this maternally derived passive protection is a function of the quantity of antibody received by the kitten. Maternal antibody can interfere with successful vaccination for as long as 3 months after birth. The queen's preparturition serum antibody titer can be determined and used to calculate the earliest appropriate age to vaccinate her kittens. If this laboratory procedure cannot be performed, the susceptibility of kittens to virulent FPLV can be lessened by repeated inoculations of vaccine. A recommended program is administration of the first dose when the kitten is 6 weeks old, with revaccination at 3- to 4-week intervals until it is 16 weeks of age. Either inactivated (killed) or modified-live virus (MLV) vaccines will be effective if used in a prophylactic program.

III. Annual revaccination usually is recommended to ensure continued protection, but for most cats this is not necessary. Revaccination of breeding females prior to queening will increase the quantity of specific antibody present in the colostrum.

    A. Either an inactivated or MLV vaccine can be used prior to breeding the queen.

    B. *Only inactivated vaccine should be administered to pregnant cats.*

IV. Hyperimmune serum formerly was available from commercial sources. Kittens were given a dose of serum when they were first presented for veterinary examination and then inoculated with FPLV vaccine at their next visit. Improvement of vaccines, imposition of more stringent regulatory requirements, and the high cost of preparing hyperimmune serum led to the withdrawal of this type of product. Some practitioners prepare serum from donor cats and administer it to kittens prophylactically. Donor cats should be checked periodically to assure freedom from FeLV, *Haemobartonella felis*, and other bloodborne pathogens. The development of monoclonal hybridoma techniques for production of specific antibodies promises to revive interest in this treatment modality. At some time in the future it would not be surprising to see the introduction of high-titered neutralizing monoclonal antibody for passive protection of kittens against FPLV.

SUGGESTED READINGS

Carlson JH, Scott FW, Duncan JR: Feline panleukopenia. I. Pathogenesis in germfree and specific pathogen-free cats. Vet Pathol 14:79, 1977

Carlson JH, Scott FW: Feline panleukopenia. II. The relationship of intestinal mucosal cell proliferation rates to viral infection and development of lesions. Vet Pathol 14:173, 1977

Csiza CK, Scott FW, DeLahunta A, et al: Pathogenesis of feline panleukopenia virus in susceptible newborn kittens. I. Clinical signs, hematology, serology, and virology. Infect Immun 3:833, 1971

Csiza CK, DeLahunta A, Scott FW, et al: Pathogenesis of feline panleukopenia virus in susceptible newborn kittens. II. Pathology and immunofluorescence. Infect. Immun 3:838, 1971

Larsen S, Flagstad A, Aalbaek B: Experimental feline panleucopenia in the conventional cat. Vet Pathol 13:216, 1976

Kahn DE: Pathogenesis of feline panleukopenia. J Am Vet Med Assoc 173:628, 1978

Schultz RD, Mendel H, Scott FW: Effect of feline panleukopenia virus infection on development of humoral and cellular immunity. Cornell Vet 66:324, 1976

Scott FW, Csiza CK, Gillespie JH: Maternally derived immunity to feline panleukopenia. J Am Vet Med Assoc 156:439, 1970

2

Canine Viral Papillomatosis

Robert C. Rosenthal

ETIOLOGY

I. Canine viral papillomatosis (CVP) is caused by the canine oral pap-illomavirus (COPV), a member of the Papovaviridae family. Papo-vaviruses are nonenveloped, double-stranded DNA viruses, which reproduce in the nucleus of infected cells and are released by cytolysis.

II. The mode of transmission in naturally occurring cases is unknown but probably involves contact between the virus and the oral mucosa. The disease has been reproduced experimentally by inoculation.

III. Canine viral papillomatosis is seen in three forms: oral, ocular, and cutaneous. The COPV grows best in the oral mucosa; ocular struc-tures and the skin are less readily involved. There is some question as to whether the viral particles seen in the cutaneous form represent COPV or another papovavirus.

CLINICAL SIGNS

I. The *oral* form of the disease is usually seen in dogs less than 2 years of age. The oral mucosa of the lip margins, hard and soft palate, tongue, pharynx, and epiglottis may be affected; the gingiva, glottis, and larynx are spared. Multiple lesions are the rule. Owners may present these young dogs after noticing the warty lesions, which are at first smooth, white, and slightly elevated and are of little clinical consequence except that they may seed the oral cavity with COPV. Later they develop roughness and take on a cauliflower-like appear-ance. The lesions may reach 2 cm in diameter, and their number may increase for the first 4–6 weeks. Owners may notice signs associated with the lesions: foul breath odor secondary to tumor necrosis, hemorrhage secondary to tumor trauma, a thick oral discharge, or reluctance to eat.

II. The *ocular* form is also seen in young dogs, most often between 6 months and 4 years of age. The lid margin, conjunctiva, or cornea may be involved, unilaterally or bilaterally. The lesions are similar in appearance to those of the oral form but may not be quite so distinctive. Differential diagnoses include sebaceous adenomas or adenocarcinomas, melanomas, squamous cell carcinomas, histiocytomas, mastocytomas, basal cell carcinomas, fibromas, and lipomas.

III. The *cutaneous* form is usually seen in dogs older than those usually presented with the other two forms. There is a predilection for males and for cocker spaniels and Kerry blue terriers. Cutaneous papillomas may be caused by virus, but this is uncertain. Lesions are often present on the head, limbs, and tail. They may be solitary or multiple and are variable in appearance. Cutaneous papillomas usually are small (less than 0.5 cm) and well circumscribed but may be either firm or soft, smooth or keratinous. A form of cutaneous papilloma noted in racing greyhounds in Australia is seen in 12-to 18-month-old dogs as solitary lesions located distal to the hock or carpus. The lesions usually undergo spontaneous regression within 9 weeks.

DIAGNOSIS

    The history and physical examination usually are sufficient to make a diagnosis. A description of the progression (and perhaps regression) of lesions in one or more young dogs is common with the oral form. Physical findings as described above are quite characteristic, especially in the oral and cutaneous forms. Histologic confirmation may be helpful and more important in the ocular form.

TREATMENT

I. The oral form generally is considered to be a self-limiting disease, with lesions regressing without treatment usually within 12 weeks. In cases marked by significant trauma to the lesions or by interference with normal function, surgical excision is indicated and may even hasten regression of other lesions. Cryosurgery and electrosurgery may limit the spread of virus during the procedure. A good prognosis is warranted. Following recovery, immunity is life-long.

   A. In the rare cases that do not regress spontaneously, chemotherapy with vincristine (Oncovin, Lilly), at 0.8 mg/m^2 IV once weekly, or cyclophosphamide (Cytoxan, Bristol-Myers Oncology), at 300 mg/m^2 IV once weekly or 50 mg/m^2 PO for 4 consecutive days each week, may be beneficial. Among these cases there may be some that do not respond at all.

   B. A case of carcinoma development has been reported in association with oral papillomatosis, but there was no virologic evidence for a causal relationship.

II. Surgery is the treatment of choice for the ocular form, especially if secondary irritation has occurred or if malignancy is suspected. Cryosurgery has the advantage of being less likely to spread virus, but some excision is necessary for histopathologic evaluation. The prognosis is good.

III. Cutaneous papillomas can be removed surgically if necessary. The prognosis is good.

IV. The usefulness of autologous vaccines is difficult to evaluate because of spontaneous remissions, but they are probably of little value. In dogs undergoing surgery autovaccination may account for the apparently hastened regression reported in certain instances.

PREVENTION

Experimentally, adjuvanted preparations of COPV, injected subcutaneously or intramuscularly, protected young dogs from challenge; however, it is important to remember that such vaccines are species-specific. In another study some dogs developed squamous cell carcinomas at the site of injection of ground oral papilloma tissue. Routine vaccination against COPV is not indicated.

PUBLIC HEALTH CONSIDERATIONS

There appears to be no significant public health risk at this time. A possible association between human papillomavirus and canine disease is not well supported.

SUGGESTED READINGS

Belkin PV: Ocular lesions in canine oral papillomatosis (a case report). Vet Med [Small Anim Clin] 74:1520, 1979

Bonney CH, Koch SA, Dice PF, et al: Papillomatosis of conjunctiva and adnexa in dogs. J Am Vet Med Assoc 176:48, 1980

Calvert CA: Canine viral and transmissible neoplasias. p. 461. In Greene CE (ed): Clinical Microbiology and Infectious Diseases of the Dog and Cat. WB Saunders, Philadelphia, 1984

Gwin RM, Gelatt KN, Williams LW: Ophthalmic neoplasms in the dog. J Am Anim Hosp Assoc 18:853, 1982

Harvey CE, O'Brien JA, Rossman LE, et al: Oral, dental, pharyngeal, and salivary gland disorders. p. 1126. In Ettinger SJ (ed): Textbook of Veterinary Internal Medicine. 2nd. Ed. Vol. 2. WB Saunders, Philadelphia, 1983

Muller GH, Kirk RW, Scott DW: Small Animal Dermatology. 3rd ed. WB Saunders, Philadelphia, 1983

Roberts SM, Severin GA, Lavach JD: Prevalence and treatment of palpebral neoplasms in the dog: 200 cases (1975–1983). J Am Vet Med Assoc 189:1355, 1986

Sundberg JP, O'Banion MK, Schmidt-Didier E, et al: Cloning and characterization of a canine oral papillomavirus. Am J Vet Res 47:1142, 1986

Watrach AM, Small E, Case MT: Canine papilloma: progression of oral papilloma to carcinoma. JNCI 45:915, 1970

3

Infectious Canine Hepatitis

David J. Polzin

ETIOLOGY

I. Infectious canine hepatitis (ICH) is caused by canine adenovirus type 1 (CAV-1). This virus is serologically homogeneous worldwide and is antigenically distinct from canine adenovirus type 2 (CAV-2), which causes respiratory disease in dogs. CAV-1 produces clinical illness in dogs, foxes, and other canids. Although vaccination procedures have largely eliminated ICH as a clinical entity among domestic canines, wild canids may serve as a reservoir of infection for susceptible domestic dogs.

II. Following exposure of susceptible dogs to CAV-1, virus may be found in all body tissues and secretions. Saliva, urine, and feces from infected dogs may be infectious for other dogs. Transmission of ICH is primarily by direct oronasal exposure; other possible modes include contact with contaminated fomites and ectoparasites. By 10–14 days postexposure the virus is cleared from other tissues and is localized to the kidneys. The virus may then be excreted in urine for at least 6–9 months after infection. Aerosol transmission of virus via urine appears to be unlikely; susceptible dogs housed 6 in away from dogs shedding virus did not become infected.

III. CAV-1 is resistant to environmental inactivation and will survive disinfection with ether, acid, formalin, and chloroform.

A. At room temperature CAV-1 can survive for 3–11 days on soiled fomites, such as wet or dry instruments and hypodermic needles. It can survive for at least 9 months at 40°C and even longer at colder temperatures. However, the virus is susceptible to heat inactivation and can be inactivated by exposure to 50–60°C for 5 minutes. Therefore, steam cleaning may be used to successfully disinfect contaminated surfaces and fomites.

B. Iodine, phenol, and sodium hydroxide may be effective as chemical disinfectants against CAV-1.

CLINICAL SIGNS

I. Following oronasal exposure CAV-1 localizes in the tonsils and spreads to regional lymph nodes and the bloodstream. Subsequent viremia results in widespread dissemination of the virus. Prime target organs include the liver and vascular endothelial cells. The kidneys, eyes, lymph nodes, and bone marrow are also susceptible to CAV-1 infection.

II. Clinical effects of CAV-1 infection are determined by the immune status of the host.
   A. Widespread centrolobular to panlobular hepatic necrosis, which is often fatal, develops in susceptible dogs with persistently low antibody titers ($<$ 1:4).
   B. Dogs with partial immunity (antibody titers of 1:16 or higher but less than 1:500) after 4–5 days of infection may develop chronic active hepatitis and hepatic fibrosis.
   C. If a sufficient immune response (antibody titer of 1:500 or greater) develops by 7 days postexposure, the virus is eliminated from blood and hepatic tissues, which limits the extent of hepatic damage.
   D. Dogs that have protective immunity (antibody titers of 1:500 or higher) on the day of exposure show little evidence of clinical disease. However, dogs immune to parenteral challenge with CAV-1 may still develop respiratory disease when exposed to aerosolized virus.

III. Clinical signs of classic ICH result from involvement of the liver (abdominal pain, gastrointestinal signs such as vomiting or diarrhea, etc.), vascular endothelium (hemorrhage), and eyes (uveitis, corneal edema). Clinical disease is most commonly seen in unvaccinated dogs less than 1 year of age.
   A. Onset of ICH may be peracute, with death occurring within hours. In such cases owners often believe the animal has been poisoned. Clinical signs may include vomiting, abdominal pain, depression, diarrhea, and, occasionally, seizures. Hemorrhage may or may not be evident.
   B. Clinical signs occurring during acute ICH may include:
      1. Pyrexia (103–106°F)

2. Tonsillar enlargement (often accompanied by laryngitis and pharyngitis)
3. Cervical lymphadenopathy, often associated with subcutaneous edema of the head, neck, and dependent portions of the trunk
4. Abdominal pain
5. Hepatomegaly
6. Hemorrhagic diathesis, manifested by widespread ecchymotic and petechial hemorrhages, epistaxis, hematochezia or melena, and bleeding from venipuncture sites
7. Abdominal distention due to accumulation of serosanguineous modified transudate or blood
8. Central nervous system signs, such as depression, disorientation, seizures, or coma

C. Icterus is rare but may occur in dogs that survive the acute, fulminant form of the disease. In uncomplicated cases clinical signs often last about 5–7 days before improvement is seen. Persistence of signs occurs when concurrent infection exists (e.g., canine distemper), or when chronic active hepatitis develops.

D. Anterior uveitis and corneal edema ("blue eye") may develop during recovery from ICH. Ocassionally corneal opacity is the only clinical evidence of infection with CAV-1.

1. Ocular lesions occur in approximately 20 percent of spontaneously occurring cases of ICH. They may also occur in dogs injected subcutaneously with modified-live CAV-1 vaccines.
2. Within days of infection with CAV-1, the virus spreads to and replicates within the uveal tract and corneal endothelial cells. Anterior uveitis and corneal edema develop by about 7 days postexposure. Antigen-antibody complex formation with complement fixation initiates an inflammatory response, which causes disruption of intact corneal endothelium, leading to accumulation of edema fluid within the corneal stroma.
3. Uncomplicated ocular lesions are usually self-limiting, with recovery occurring in about 21 days. However, in severe cases inflammatory debris may block the filtration angle, causing glaucoma and hydrophthalmos.

IV. CAV-1 infection usually results in glomerular and renal tubulointerstitial lesions but rarely causes clinical signs referable to the urinary system.

A. Renal infection with CAV-1 results in shedding of active virus in urine for up to 6–9 months postinfection.

   B. Renal CAV-1 infections do not typically cause chronic renal failure in dogs; however, dogs with renal lesions due to CAV-1 may be predisposed to the development of pyelonephritis.

DIAGNOSIS

  I. Diagnosis of ICH is usually based on knowledge of the patient's vaccination status and probability of exposure, clinical findings, and laboratory evaluation. While these data only provide a tentative diagnosis, they are adequate in most cases for the initiation of appropriate therapy.
    A. Hematologic findings include leukopenia due to lymphopenia and neutropenia, followed several days later by neutrophilia and lymphocytosis. In addition, increased numbers of nucleated red blood cells may be seen in peripheral blood owing to endothelial damage within sinusoidal compartments of the bone marrow.
    B. Increases in serum alanine aminotransferase, aspartate aminotransferase, and alkaline phosphatase activities develop as the virus becomes localized in the liver. Activities of these enzymes usually begin to decrease after about 14 days. Persistent or recurrent elevations suggest possible chronic active hepatitis. Hyperbilirubinemia is not common in ICH because the centrolobular necrosis typical of ICH causes little intrahepatic cholestasis. Sulfobromophthalein retention at 30 minutes may be increased.
    C. A coagulation profile may reveal evidence of disseminated intravascular coagulation. Prolonged prothrombin time, activated partial thromboplastin time, thrombocytopenia, and increased blood concentrations of fibrin degradation products may be detected.
 II. The diagnosis of ICH may be confirmed by biopsy. In addition, serologic testing and virus isolation may provide confirmatory evidence; however, such diagnostic aids are rarely employed clinically.
    A. Hepatic biopsy (surgical, core, or fine-needle aspiration biopsy) may be evaluated for presence of intranuclear inclusions in Kupffer cells and viable hepatocytes.
    B. An enzyme-linked immunosorbent assay has been developed that permits accurate detection of CAV-1 antibodies. These antibodies may also be detected by indirect hemagglutination, charcoal agglutination, or complement fixation, although cross-reactivity with human adenoviruses has been found by using complement fixation.

C. CAV-1 may be isolated from the tonsils early in the disease. After viremic spread, the virus may be isolated from many tissues; however, it is difficult to isolate from the liver because hepatic arginase inhibits viral nucleic acid replication. Virus may be isolated from urine for at least 6–9 months after infection.

III. Central nervous system (CNS) signs developing in dogs with ICH may result from hepatic encephalopathy, hypoglycemia, intracranial hemorrhage, or nonsuppurative encephalitis resulting from localization of the virus in the brain. The cause of neurologic signs may be differentiated based on evaluation of cerebrospinal fluid (CSF) and blood ammonia and glucose concentrations. Increases in protein concentration and mononuclear cells in the CSF suggest viral encephalitis. Cerebrospinal fluid findings consistent with hemorrhage include: red blood cells, erythrophagocytosis, a dull red to brown coloration, xanthochromia, and increased protein concentrations. Hypoglycemia and hepatic encephalopathy are associated with normal CSF findings and must be confirmed and differentiated on the basis of blood ammonia and blood glucose concentrations.

TREATMENT

I. Clinical recovery and hepatocellular regeneration may be possible with ICH-induced centrolobular hepatic necrosis. The goals of therapy are to ameliorate clinical signs and to provide supportive care so that the patient lives long enough for hepatocellular regeneration to occur.

II. Therapy of ICH involves fluid therapy, control of hemorrhage, and treatment of hepatic encephalopathy.

A. An indwelling intravenous catheter should be placed and fluid therapy initiated with lactated Ringer's solution to which sufficient dextrose has been added to make a 5% dextrose solution (50 g/L).

1. The quantity of fluid to be administered should be based on an estimate of the patient's dehydration; however, dehydration may be difficult to detect in young, previously healthy dogs and may not be clinically apparent when losses have been very recent. If the patient does not have clinical evidence of dehydration, fluid needs may be estimated at 3 to 5% of body weight. The patient may then be serially monitored to determine if fluid therapy has been adequate. If the patient is in shock, fluids should be administered to effect (i.e., until shock is controlled) at a rate of 90 ml per kilogram of body weight per hour.

2. Hypokalemia should be avoided because it promotes renal ammoniagenesis and hyperammonemia. Hypokalemia may be controlled by administration of potassium supplements.

3. Addition of dextrose to lactated Ringer's solution is designed to minimize the development of hypoglycemia. However, blood glucose concentrations should be monitored. If hypoglycemia develops despite therapy, additional glucose supplementation may be considered.

B. Treatment for blood loss and coagulopathy may be indicated when hemorrhage is progressive and/or extensive. Fresh whole blood has been recommended for treatment of the hemorrhagic diathesis of ICH. If progressive consumption of transfused coagulation factors occurs, heparin therapy to reduce clotting may be considered. Therapy with vitamin K is of questionable value.

C. Therapy of hepatic encephalopathy involves catharsis, gut "sterilization," and reduction of protein intake.

1. Complete catharsis of the colon should be performed as soon as possible after signs of encephalopathy develop. Catharsis flushes out colonic bacteria and potentially toxic products within the colon. Enemas using acidifying agents such as dilute vinegar or lactulose (Merrell Dow) are more effective than warm water enemas in reducing blood ammonia concentrations and in improving clinical signs.

a) Vinegar should be diluted 1:10 with warm water and given as a retention enema for 20 to 30 minutes. The goals are to remove fecal material from the colon and to reduce colonic pH below 5.0 in order to trap ammonia within the lumen of the colon as ammonium.

b) Lactulose should be diluted with warm water (3 parts lactulose to 7 parts water). Approximately 20–30 ml/kg should be infused and retained for 20–30 minutes before allowing the patient to evacuate. After the enema, the evacuated colon should have a pH below 5.0. If the colonic pH is higher than 5.0, the enema should be repeated.

2. Nonabsorbable oral antibiotics such as neomycin, kanamycin, vancomycin, or paramomycin should be administered in order to reduce the population of intestinal bacteria responsible for ammonia production.

a) Neomycin is given at a dosage of 20 mg/kg qid. Neomycin (liquid) may be given per rectum to patients that will not tolerate oral medication. Rarely, neomycin may cause ototoxicity, nephrotoxicity, severe diarrhea, and malabsorption.

b) Lactulose may be used instead of or in addition to neomycin. The combination of these two medications may be superior to either used individually. Lactulose is given at a dosage of 5 to 15 ml tid, which should result in two to three soft stools daily; if diarrhea develops, the dose should be reduced. Adding viable *Lactobacillus acidophilus* organisms to the therapy may augment fermentation of lactulose and improve its efficacy.

3. All oral intake of food should cease during acute hepatoencephalic crisis until signs of CNS dysfunction abate. Cessation of protein intake eliminates exogenous sources of ammonia, aromatic amino acids, short-chain fatty acids, and toxic amines.

PREVENTION

I. Modified-live virus (MLV) vaccines containing either CAV-1 or CAV-2 are currently available for use in prophylaxis against ICH. Although CAV-1 and CAV-2 are antigenically distinct, MLV CAV-2 vaccines effectively prevent ICH.

II. MLV CAV-1 vaccines can produce long-lasting immunity with a single dose. Although highly effective, the vaccine virus has been found to localize in the kidneys and produce mild subclinical interstitial nephritis, with persistent shedding of virus. In addition, anterior uveitis occurs in approximately 0.4% of dogs after intramuscular or subcutaneous injection.

III. MLV CAV-2 vaccines do not produce ocular or renal disease when administered intramuscularly or subcutaneously. However, MLV CAV-2 vaccine virus may replicate in and be shed from the upper respiratory tract.

IV. Dogs should be vaccinated against ICH with either CAV-1 or CAV-2 vaccines beginning at 8–10 weeks of age.

A. A minimum of two injections of vaccine should be given 3–4 weeks apart, usually at 8–10 weeks and at 12–14 weeks of age. This vaccination protocol is usually performed in concert with vaccination efforts directed at canine distemper.

B. Never reduce the dose of vaccine recommended by the manufacturer.

C. Vaccines should be kept refrigerated at the appropriate temperature until used. Once a vaccine has been reconstituted, it must be used immediately.

D. Annual revaccination is recommended.

SUGGESTED READINGS

Carmichael LE: Canine adenovirus infection. p. 1303. In Kirk RW (ed): Current Veterinary Therapy. Vol. 6. WB Saunders, Philadelphia, 1977

Farrow BRH, Love DN: Bacterial, viral, and other infectious problems. p. 269. In Ettinger SJ (ed); Textbook of Veterinary Internal Medicine. Vol. 1. WB Saunders, Philadelphia, 1983

Greene CE: Infectious canine hepatitis. p. 406. In Greene CE (ed): Clinical Microbiology and Infectious Diseases of the Dog and Cat. WB Saunders, Philadelphia, 1984

Hardy RM: Hepatic diseases. p. 463. In Davis LE (ed): Handbook of Small Animal Therapeutics. Churchill Livingstone, New York, 1985

4

Canine Herpesvirus

Jeffrey E. Barlough
Leland E. Carmichael

ETIOLOGY

I. Canine herpesvirus (CHV), or canid herpesvirus 1, is a member of
the Alphaherpesvirinae subfamily of herpesviruses. It has a restricted
host range in that infections appear to be limited exclusively to canids.
Severe disease is recognized primarily in puppies less than 3–4 weeks
of age, with fatalities in those less than 1–2 weeks of age. However,
occasional cases have been observed in dogs as old as 4 months.
Herpesvirus infection has only rarely been found to be the cause of
puppy deaths within the first 3 days of life. Mild rhinitis and/or va-
ginitis/balanoposthitis have been observed in older dogs infected with
the virus, but the primary importance of CHV as a pathogen appears
to be related to its effects on pups.

II. The virus can be recovered from the respiratory tract of normal adult
dogs as well as from some with upper respiratory tract disease, and
there is circumstantial evidence that it may be involved in some cases
of tracheobronchitis. It is believed that CHV in adult and adolescent
dogs is transmitted primarily by the oronasal route. The virus is capable of persisting in infected dogs in a latent or inapparent state,
with recrudescence of virus shedding manifested during periods of
stress. Similar features probably apply to infection of the genital tract,
in which case viral recrudescence may provide an additional important means by which neonates can become exposed. In utero infections have also been reported. Venereal transmission between adult
dogs may also be of importance in spread of the agent.

III. Serologic studies indicate that CHV infections are widespread in the
canine population, although the frequency of infection varies with the
particular population under study. The virus appears to have a worldwide distribution.

IV. As is the case with many other herpesviruses, CHV is relatively unstable once outside its natural host and is rapidly inactivated by most common household detergent and disinfectant preparations.

CLINICAL SIGNS

I. Neonatal infection
   A. The infection is initiated in cells of the nasal epithelium and pharyngeal tonsils, whence it spreads via a cell-associated (leukocyte) viremia to other tissues of the body. Secondary viral replication then occurs at these distant sites—kidneys, liver, lungs, gastrointestinal tract, spleen, adrenal glands, brain, lymph nodes—producing characteristic multifocal lesions of hemorrhage and necrosis. Virtually all tissues eventually contain infectious virus. In young puppies (those less than 1–2 weeks of age), the infection frequently terminates in death.
   B. The clinical course is characterized by the sudden death of apparently healthy puppies after a brief period of illness that usually lasts no longer than 24–48 hours. Affected pups appear depressed and lethargic, stop nursing, and pass a soft, odorless, yellow-green stool. They cry persistently and demonstrate abdominal pain and tenderness upon palpation. A nasal discharge and/or an erythematous ventral abdominal rash, characterized by the presence of papules and pustules, may also be present. There is no fever. Terminally, puppies may develop neurologic signs (seizures, opisthotonos) or may die from systemic effects of the infection before neurologic abnormalities become apparent. Animals that survive frequently demonstrate neurologic sequelae, including blindness, ataxia, and cerebellar vestibular deficits.
   C. Body temperature and its regulation are important in the pathogenesis of CHV infection in pups. The optimal temperature range for CHV replication has been shown to vary between 35 and 36°C, with a dramatic inhibition of growth beyond either end of this range. Although the normal core body temperature of the dog exceeds this range, pups in the immediate postnatal period are not yet capable of properly controlled temperature regulation, having a core body temperature that frequently coincides with that for optimal CHV replication. This temperature sensitivity may help to explain in part the marked age resistance of dogs to CHV disease.

D. Pups with maternal antibody are readily infected by CHV; however, there is no clinical illness because the infection remains localized. Neutralizing antibodies develop after infection and can persist at low levels for years.

II. Adult infection

A. The disease in older dogs is largely confined to the respiratory and genital tracts. A mild or inapparent upper respiratory tract infection caused by CHV has been demonstrated, while genital localization may result in vesicular lesions on the vaginal mucosa or on the prepuce and base of the penis. In males there may also be a serous preputial discharge.

B. Infections are latent, and viral recrudescence at various times postinfection is recognized to occur. Virus appears to be shed from the genital region only when the characteristic lesions are present.

C. British researchers in the early 1970s associated a herpesvirus with abortions, stillbirths, and infertility problems in a kennel of Alsatians. The virus isolated from the genital tract of affected dogs was antigenically indistinguishable from CHV; however, certain cultural differences were apparent. Unfortunately, the genital isolate was lost and is no longer available for study.

D. Bitches that have given birth to an affected litter will passively immunize subsequent litters, which still may become infected with the virus but generally will show few clinical signs or remain asymptomatic.

III. Pathologic lesions

A. Pathologic lesions in fatal cases are usually quite characteristic, consisting of disseminated multifocal hemorrhage and necrosis. The lesions may be found in virtually any organ. Especially characteristic are the subcapsular hemorrhages in the kidneys, which appear grossly as a network of bright red spots on a gray background of necrotic cortex ("speckled kidneys") (Figure 4-1). Focal necrosis and hemorrhage are also commonly found in the lungs, liver, gastrointestinal tract, and adrenal glands. The lungs are usually diffusely pneumonic. Splenomegaly and generalized lymphadenopathy are consistently seen. Meningoencephalitic lesions often are present, even in cases in which terminal neurologic signs are not observed. Ocular lesions (panuveitis, keratitis) may also occur.

B. Histologically, single basophilic intranuclear inclusion bodies typical of herpesviruses can be found in some infected cells, especially in the kidneys and liver.

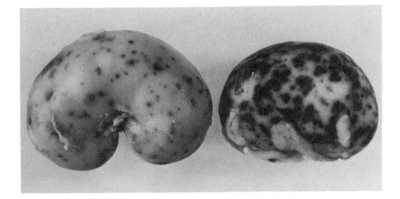

Fig. 4-1. Canine herpesvirus: systemic neonatal disease with necrosis and focal hemorrhages, producing the characteristic mottled or "speckled" appearance of the kidneys. The hyperemic and hemorrhagic areas are sharply demarcated from the surrounding cortical tissue. (Carmichael LE, Squire RA, Krook L: Clinical and pathologic features of a fatal viral disease of newborn pups. Am J Vet Res 26:803, 1965.)

DIAGNOSIS

   I. A presumptive diagnosis of CHV infection in neonates can be made on the basis of the history, physical examination, and characteristic pathologic alterations. Isolation of virus from affected tissues (especially kidneys, adrenal glands, lungs, liver, or spleen) will provide a confirmatory diagnosis.

  II. In pups that survive, the history, physical examination, and presence of virus-neutralizing antibodies in serum samples from the bitch and pup(s) will provide a fairly firm diagnosis.

 III. In older animals the disease may pass unnoticed. In symptomatic animals virus isolation from the oropharynx or from genital lesions will provide definitive evidence. Serologic titers may or may not be of assistance in diagnosis of the infection in these animals, owing to the probable latent carrier state.

TREATMENT

I. Because of the rapidly fatal evolution of the disease in neonates, treatment of affected pups, even if a definitive diagnosis has been reached, is generally unsuccessful. In addition, pups that do survive frequently have residual lesions and are latently infected carriers of the virus.

II. Despite extensive coverage of the topic in the relevant literature, there is little evidence to support the idea that artificially raising the body temperature of affected pups (by use of heating pads, heat lamps, etc.) will ameliorate the CHV disease process.

III. A single intraperitoneal injection of 1–2 ml of CHV hyperimmune serum may be useful in order to passively immunize seronegative pups at birth. Pooled sera from animals known to have been exposed to the virus (e.g., bitches that have given birth to an infected litter) may be used.

PREVENTION

I. Because of the sporadic nature of the disease and the generally poor immunogenicity of CHV, there has been little medical or financial incentive to market a prophylactic vaccine. However, several experimental inactivated and modified-live virus vaccines have been developed, each with varying shades of efficacy.

II. Care should be taken to see that the ambient temperature is sufficient for healthy pups at risk to maintain a core body temperature above that which is optimal for CHV replication. This is also good puppy management, regardless of the chances of exposure to CHV.

III. Prophylactic protection via hyperimmune antiserum may be useful in protecting unaffected puppies in a kennel with an existing CHV problem.

IV. It has been recognized for some time that surviving puppies excrete large amounts of virus for several weeks following recovery. Adequate disinfective and hygienic measures should be undertaken in order to destroy residual virus in the environment and to minimize its spread by fomite transmission. Infected bitches and their litters should be isolated from other dogs.

V. Eradication of the virus from the canine population is not within the realm of reality at the present time.

SUGGESTED READINGS

Carmichael LE: Canine herpesvirus: a recently discovered cause of death of young pups. Gaines Vet Symp 15:24, 1965

Carmichael LE: Herpesvirus canis: aspects of pathogenesis and immune response. J Am Vet Med Assoc 156:1714, 1970

Carmichael LE: Canine herpesvirus infection in puppies. p. 1296. In Kirk RW (ed): Current Veterinary Therapy. Vol. 6. WB Saunders, Philadelphia, 1977

Carmichael LE, Barnes FD, Percy DH: Temperature as a factor in resistance of young puppies to canine herpesvirus. J Infect Dis 120:669, 1969

Carmichael LE, Squire RA, Krook L: Clinical and pathologic features of a fatal viral disease of newborn pups. Am J Vet Res 26:803, 1965

Carmichael LE, Strandberg JD, Barnes FD: Identification of a cytopathogenic agent infectious for puppies as a canine herpesvirus. Proc Soc Exp Biol Med 120:644, 1965

Cornwell HJC, Wright NG: Neonatal canine herpesvirus infection: a review of present knowledge. Vet Rec 84:2, 1969

Greene CE, Kakuk TJ: Canine herpesvirus infection. p. 419. In Greene CE (ed): Clinical Microbiology and Infectious Diseases of the Dog and Cat. WB Saunders, Philadelphia, 1984

Hashimoto A, Hirai K, Yamaguchi T, et al: Experimental transplacental infection of pregnant dogs with canine herpesvirus. Am J Vet Res 43:844, 1982

Hill H, Mare CJ: Genital disease in dogs caused by canine herpesvirus. Am J Vet Res 35:669, 1974

Kraft S, Evermann JF, McKeirnan AJ, et al: The role of neonatal canine herpesvirus infection in mixed infections in older dogs. Compend Contin Ed Pract Vet 8:688, 1986

Krakowka S: Canine herpesvirus-1. p. 137. In Olsen RG, Krakowka S, Blakeslee JR (eds): Comparative Pathobiology of Viral Diseases. Vol. I. CRC Press, Boca Raton, 1985

Poste G, King N: Isolation of a herpesvirus from the canine genital tract: association with infertility, abortion and stillbirths. Vet Rec 88:229, 1971

Wright NG, Thompson H, Cornwell HJC, et al: Canine respiratory virus infections. J Small Anim Pract 15:27, 1974

5

Pseudorabies

Donald P. Gustafson

ETIOLOGY

I. Pseudorabies, also known as *Aujeszky's disease*, is caused by a herpesvirus. The core of the pseudorabies virus (PrV) virion (the complete infectious particle) contains a single molecule of double-stranded DNA. The capsid encompassing the core is composed of proteins arranged into 162 capsomeres in icosahedral symmetry, forming a dodecahedron. Covering the capsid is an envelope containing structural lipids and about 40% of the total protein of the virus.

II. There are four principal antigenic proteins of the virus and they are glycosylated. It is important to note that the antigenic proteins—those important in eliciting antibody responses—are present in the envelope, which also contains structural lipids. The envelope surface is marked with chemical configurations required for attachment of the virus to receptor sites on susceptible cells. If these attachment sites are destroyed or denatured, the virus is rendered noninfectious (see VIII below).

III. The Herpesviridae family contains approximately 70 viruses. There are three subfamilies, with PrV belonging to the subfamily Alphaherpesvirinae. Members of this subfamily have a short (less than 24-hour) replication cycle, and latent infections in sensory nerve ganglia frequently occur. These viruses are generally highly cytopathogenic in cell culture, producing rapid lysis of susceptible cells.

IV. The cycle of infection, from attachment of the virus to cessation of replication and lysis of the host cell, requires about 15–19 hours. A single replicative cycle for virus within a cell takes 6–9 hours. After attachment and penetration the virus is uncoated and its DNA moves (or is moved) from the cytoplasm directly to the nucleus, where it takes control of cellular metabolic processes. Thereafter, viral mRNAs are released into the cytoplasm and translated by ribosomes into viral proteins or their precursors. The viral nucleic acid is replicated in the nucleus. The viral proteins produced in the cytoplasm move to the nucleus, where viral assembly occurs. The envelope is added during subsequent passage of virions through virally altered, chemically modified areas of the nuclear membrane. Most of the virus is released from infected cells through lysis of the cell membrane.

V. Transmission of pseudorabies to dogs or cats is almost always a direct result of the ingestion of virus-contaminated material. However, accidental parenteral inoculation is also possible, and experimental aerosol infections have been accomplished under heroic conditions. As might be expected, dogs and cats on swine production enterprises are at greatest risk. However, there have been occasional reports of pseudorabies in dogs used for hunting feral swine. Other, rather urban, infections have been effected through feeding of raw abattoir-derived pork to dogs in commercial kennels.

VI. Pseudorabies is considered to be primarily a disease of swine, which are much more resistant than other susceptible species (with the possible exception of horses and birds), and are the most productive reservoir for the virus. Most mammals, except for human beings and tailless apes, are susceptible to PrV infection. Pseudorabies in dogs and cats is invariably fatal; hence these cases represent dead-end infections because they do not serve to propagate the disease in nature through continued release of virus. Occasionally a dog that has eaten material containing a significant quantity of infectious virus remains asymptomatic; in every case tested, the animal has been found to be fully susceptible to infection by parenteral administration of virus. Reports of lateral or vertical transmission of PrV in dogs and cats have not been found in the available literature.

VII. The virus is found in all parts of the world where significant populations of swine subject to international commerce are present, with the possible exception of Australia and mainland China. In addition, the disease has occurred in geographic locations where swine-producing farms are absent but where raw pork scraps have been fed to mink or foxes being raised for fur. Infections have also been reported in cattle and sheep living on small islands off a mainland coast where there are no swine, without satisfactory explanation.

VIII. The virus is inactivated by lipid solvents such as ethyl ether, acetone, sodium deoxycholate, and chloroform. These agents denature the structural lipids of the viral envelope. Disinfectants such as 0.5% sodium hydroxide, 1% quaternary ammonium bases, 1% chlorinated lime ($CaOCl_2$), 1% phenolic derivatives, and 10% Lugol's solution probably denature the entire virion.

IX. Once an affected animal has died and been disposed of, questions arise regarding survival of the virus in the environment. Survival is related to the effects of temperature, drying, ultraviolet light (sunlight), and pH on the quantity of virus to be inactivated. Optimal conditions for virus denaturation are: temperatures of 40°C and above; drying conditions; exposure to ultraviolet light (commercial lamp at 15 in for 1 hour); and pH values of 9 and 10.

CLINICAL SIGNS

I. Pseudorabies in dogs develops after the virus has invaded sensory nerve endings in the naso-oropharynx and traveled in the epineural lymph to the ganglia. As ganglioneuritis ensues, viral invasion of the brainstem, cerebrum, and cerebellum results in panencephalitis and meningitis. Infection of respiratory epithelium occurs at about the same time, resulting in inflammation of the trachea, bronchial tree, and alveolar sacs. In most cases, a syndrome leading to death becomes apparent approximately 36 hours following ingestion of infectious material. Uneasiness is expressed by restlessness and a look of anxiety, sometimes followed by vomiting of a bile-colored viscous fluid. Within a few hours a copious flow of stringy saliva becomes evident.

Often there is an intense pruritus; the dog may respond by biting the affected area until it is mutilated or may rub against a hard, secure surface until the area is raw, bleeding, and often edematous. It must be kept in mind, however, that pruritus and self-mutilation may not occur, with profound depression being the dominant clinical sign. Aggressive behavior towards humans or other animals has not been observed nor reports of it found. Anorexia develops, and fever may reach 105°F. As central nervous system involvement progresses, depression deepens and dyspnea becomes more pronounced. Coma and death follow shortly. The syndrome lasts a relatively short time (usually about 36 hours) but in rare cases may last for as long as 10 days. Time between exposure to virus and death is therefore typically about 72 hours.

II. The usual clinical syndrome in cats generally parallels the canine syndrome but is less consistent. The excitement phase is somewhat different in that cats first appear to be sluggish and then become agitated. Their movements suggest discomfort just prior to the onset of salivation, which in turn signals the approach of a variety of signs.

At about this time the fur becomes matted with saliva, and vomiting may occur. Spasms of facial muscles and paralysis of an eyelid or lower lip may be seen. Cats develop anisocoria in about 10% of naturally occurring cases. Labored breathing appears late in the syndrome, and the pulse may climb to 130–140 per minute. Reduced food and water consumption leads to dehydration and hemoconcentration. However, qualitative red and white cell counts remain in the normal range. When the cat is picked up, often it will void urine immediately from a full bladder. Priapism is frequently present. The abdomen may be slightly distended owing to intestinal gas. Mewing of a low timbre is frequent and seems to deepen as depression becomes more pronounced. Eventually balance is lost and is followed shortly by terminal coma. There is widespread belief that PrV-infected cats nearly always develop an intense pruritis at a site on the head, leading to self-mutilation. Actually about 40 percent of naturally infected cats do *not* develop pruritis. In cases with pruritis, it may be that a break in the integument has become infected or perhaps the cat perceives centrally that an irritant is present at the site. This may be a result of the diminution of functional capacity of the brain to analyze information or an alteration in esthetic sensitivity of the skin.

III. Less commonly, the course of disease is one of rapidly developing depression, accompanied by anorexia and copious salivation and followed by weakness. It becomes apparent that swallowing is difficult. In this expression of the disease, the head is held low while the cat is in a crouched position, its tail moving laterally back and forth. Other signs are essentially absent. Death follows in 24–36 hours.

IV. Experimental infections range in duration from 4 to 9 days. Those animals that survive exposure (i.e., are asymptomatic) have been found to be fully susceptible when a larger dose of virus is subsequently given.

V. Pseudorabies is ultimately a neurologic disease. Because essentially all infections occur following ingestion of contaminated material, initial viral invasion and replication occur in cells of the pharyngeal mucosa and the epithelium of the tonsils. The virus invades endings of the trigeminal (V), glossopharyngeal (IX), and vagus (X) nerves in the oropharynx, and travels in the epineural lymph to the respective nerve ganglia, spreading to the rest of the brain and to the meninges. Virus may be found in the cervical spinal cord as early as 24 hours after exposure and in the thoracic cord by 72 hours. Virus may also be isolated from pharyngeal lymph nodes, salivary glands, lungs, mesenteric lymph nodes, and adrenal glands but has not been isolated from the gut or its contents.

DIAGNOSIS

I. Most often the diagnosis of pseudorabies in dogs and cats is reached through an interpretation of clinical signs and patient history. The presence of the virus in tissues may be detected by immunofluorescence, by inoculation of cell cultures with tissue extracts, or by inoculation of laboratory animals (rabbit, mouse, or day-old chick) with tissue extracts. If there is even a small amount of virus present in the tissue, these animals will show signs and die within 4–5 days. Tissue extracts may be prepared by grinding the tissue to a pulp and mixing one part of tissue with nine parts of water or saline. A common procedure is to inoculate 0.2 ml into a rabbit subcutaneously; or into a mouse intraperitoneally; or 0.05 ml into a day-old chick intracranially. Chicken embryos at 10 days of incubation may be inoculated with 0.1 ml of tissue extract into the allantoic sac for isolation of the virus and therefore diagnosis.

TREATMENT AND PREVENTION

I. Once signs of the disease have appeared in dogs or cats, death has been the only outcome reported. Much experimentation in treatment regimens involving both prodromal and late stages of the disease has been reported without success. The use of heterologous antisera, antibiotics, cortisone preparations, or cholinesterase inhibitors has failed. Two reports of success in putative cases occurring under natural conditions lack substantial data for diagnosis and consequently are suspect.

II. In recent experiments it has been found that human recombinant interferon is efficacious in preventing the syndrome if it is applied at the proper moment. Those interested should be aware of this development and make inquiry if an animal is thought to be at risk. One has a period of perhaps 24 hours in which to act.

III. Most recently cats have been found to be resistant to live thymidine kinase-deficient strains of PrV, which are used in vaccines for swine. However, such cats remain fully susceptible to standard virulent virus. Currently available inactivated PrV vaccines will not protect cats against virulent PrV. As stated above, heterologous antiserum has likewise been found to be of no benefit. This may be due to the neurotropism involved. Tests for viremia indicate that a low level of virus is found intermittently in the blood.

IV. The most effective method of prevention is avoidance. Cats and dogs should not be fed raw pig flesh; lung, brain, throat, and spinal cord are to be especially avoided. When the disease is present in swine or other livestock in a swine-raising enterprise, cats and dogs should be sequestered in a virus-free environment until all affected animals have been removed from the premises and until the contaminated environment has been cleaned.

PUBLIC HEALTH CONSIDERATIONS

I. It is becoming clear that human beings are refractory to PrV. Some 45 years ago it was reported that a transient pruritus had occurred as a result of a laboratory accident. Further reports in the literature have not been found. Indeed, all efforts to find evidence of the susceptibility of tailless apes or human beings have been fruitless. In 25 years PrV has not resulted in infection in our laboratory as evidenced by a lack of neutralizing antibodies in the sera of all people tested, nor did any of 16 swine producers develop antibodies following episodes of pseudorabies in their animals. It is safe to believe that human beings are refractory to the virus by the common methods of exposure: aerosols, animal bites, contamination of wounds, ingestion, and ocular exposures. However, certain nonhuman primates *are* susceptible and therefore the virus deserves cautious respect.

SUGGESTED READINGS

Davies EB, Beran GW: Influence of environmental factors upon the survival of Aujeszky's disease virus. Res Vet Sci 31:32, 1981

Gustafson DP: Herpesvirus diseases of mammals and birds: comparative aspects and diagnosis. p. 205. In Kurstak E, Kurstak C (eds): Comparative Diagnosis of Viral Diseases. Vol. III, Part A. Academic Press, New York, 1981

Gustafson DP: Pseudorabies (Aujeszky's disease, mad itch, infectious bulbar paralysis). p. 242. In Holzworth J (ed): Diseases of the Cat. Vol. I. WB Saunders, Philadelphia, 1987

Horváth Z, Papp L: Clinical manifestations of Aujeszky's disease in the cat. Acta Vet Acad Sci Hung 17:49, 1967; Abst 4188, Vet Bull 37:739, 1967

Howard DR: Pseudorabies in dogs and cats. p. 1071. In Kirk RW (ed): Current Veterinary Therapy IX. WB Saunders, Philadelphia, 1986

Roizman B, Batterson W: Herpesviruses and their replication. p. 497. In Fields B (ed): Virology. Raven Press, New York, 1985

Vandevelde M: Pseudorabies. p. 381. In Greene CE (ed): Clinical Microbiology and Infectious Diseases of the Dog and Cat. WB Saunders, Philadelphia, 1984

6

Feline Poxvirus Infection

Malcolm Bennett
Rosalind M. Gaskell

ETIOLOGY

I. Feline poxvirus infection is an increasingly recognized disease entity characterized by widespread skin lesions, which are occasionally accompanied by mild systemic signs, and, rarely, by severe illness and death.

II. The cause of all cases of poxvirus infection in domestic cats thus far investigated has been shown to be cowpox virus. Cowpox virus is a member of the genus *Orthopoxvirus* and as such is closely related to the viruses of vaccinia, smallpox, ectromelia (mousepox), and raccoonpox.

III. Other viruses closely related to traditional cowpox virus (the so-called cowpox-like viruses) also exist and have been isolated from big cats and from other zoo animals. The precise classification of the cowpox-like viruses is uncertain. Some workers regard them as true cowpox virus, whereas others emphasize their differences from traditional cowpox virus strains. A better understanding of the relationships of these viruses is obviously necessary if their epizootiology is to be properly studied.

IV. Occasional anecdotal accounts of feline orf (a *Parapoxvirus*) are also sometimes encountered, but these have yet to be virologically confirmed.

V. The epizootiology of cowpox virus is not fully understood. Although traditionally considered to be enzootic in cattle, bovine cowpox virus infection is, in fact, very rare; the cat is now the most frequently recognized host of cowpox virus. Cowpox virus and the closely related cowpox-like viruses have a wide host range, having also been isolated from big cats, elephants, rhinoceroses, okapis, and anteaters in European zoos. Human infection, although uncommon, can also occur.

VI. It is now generally believed that cowpox virus and the cowpox-like viruses circulate in small wild mammal—probably rodent—populations, and that cats become infected while hunting.

VII. Cowpox and the cowpox-like viruses are geographically limited to Europe. Feline poxvirus infection has been reported from Great Britain, Austria, and the Netherlands.

VIII. Cat-to-cat and cat-to-human transmission can occur but are uncommon. Cat-to-cat transmission often produces only subclinical infection, but cat-to-human transmission results in typical cowpox disease.

IX. Although the domestic cat is by far the most commonly recognized host of cowpox virus, the precise incidence of the disease in cats is not yet known. Increasing numbers of cases are diagnosed each year, but this probably reflects simply an increasing awareness of the condition among veterinarians, rather than a true increase in incidence.

X. Most infected cats come from rural environments, although urban cats may also become infected. Most cases are recognized in the autumn, possibly as a result of increasing contact between cats and the reservoir host. There is no recognized sex or age predilection.

XI. Poxviruses are relatively hardy, and dried scabs may remain infective for long periods if kept in a dry, cool environment. However, clinical infection of both cats and humans probably requires inoculation into a skin wound; thus environmental contamination is probably of little epizootiologic significance.

XII. Disinfection of premises can be achieved with hypochlorite or detergents.

CLINICAL SIGNS

I. Pathogenesis

The pathogenesis of feline cowpox infection appears to resemble the pathogenesis of other generalized *Orthopoxvirus* infections. The usual route of virus entry is probably via the skin, although oronasal infection is also possible. Following the development of a primary (usually skin) lesion, virus spreads to and replicates in the local lymph nodes. A white cell-associated viremia develops that, in turn, gives rise to generalization and the development of secondary skin lesions.

II. Clinical history

   A. Most cats (about 70%) have a history of a single recent skin lesion (the primary lesion), invariably on the head, on the neck, or on a forelimb.

   B. The primary lesion can vary in character from a small scab to a large abscess or extensive cellulitis but is often described as having originated as a "bite-like" wound.

   C. Widespread secondary skin lesions develop about 10 days later. The onset of secondary lesion development may be accompanied by mild systemic illness. It is at this stage that most cats are presented for veterinary attention.

III. Physical examination

   A. The clinical signs observed will vary according to the stage of the disease at which the cat is presented. Some owners may seek advice when only a primary lesion is present. Because these can be so variable in character, it is unlikely that cowpox would be suspected at this stage.

   B. Most cats are presented during development of secondary skin lesions. Secondary lesions first appear as widespread, small (approximately 1-mm-diameter) epithelial nodules, which enlarge over 2–4 days to become discrete, 1- or 2-cm scabbed ulcers. Almost all cats develop more than 5 secondary lesions; most (more than 70%) develop more than 10.

   C. Vesicle formation is rarely seen macroscopically; however, occasional vesicles may be found on the inner pinna of the ear. These soon ulcerate and scab over.

   D. Fresh secondary lesions usually continue to appear for only 2–4 days, although this period may be extended if the cat is treated with corticosteroids.

   E. Secondary bacterial infection of both primary and secondary skin lesions commonly occurs but usually can be readily controlled with broad-spectrum antibiotics.

   F. Some cats may show pruritus, usually in association with the primary lesion or with healing secondary lesions.

   G. Buccal ulceration may also be seen in approximately 20% of cases.

   H. Cats examined just prior to or during early development of secondary skin lesions may show signs of systemic illness. These signs generally are mild and may include pyrexia, depression, and anorexia. Some cats may also have a slight, usually serous, coryza or a mild transient diarrhea.

I. More severe systemic signs and death are uncommon but may be associated with lower respiratory tract involvement or with extensive secondary bacterial infection, particularly of the primary lesion. Immunosuppressive conditions (e.g., feline leukemia virus [FeLV] infection or long-term corticosteroid treatment) may also exacerbate the disease.

J. Cheetahs and other cats in zoological collections often become severely ill and may die rapidly of pneumonia.

K. In most cases, however, the skin lesions gradually heal, the dried scabs separating within 4–6 weeks to reveal small, bald areas of healing epithelium. New hair growth soon follows, although extensive damage to hair follicles (e.g., at the site of the primary lesion) may result in small, permanently bald scars.

DIAGNOSIS

I. The key diagnostic features include a history of a single recent (primary) skin lesion on the head, neck, or forelimb and the development of widespread, well-circumscribed skin lesions that progress from small nodules to 1- or 2-cm scabbed ulcers. Given this typical history and a careful examination of the skin lesions, a fairly confident diagnosis of feline cowpox can often be made on clinical grounds alone.

II. Primary skin lesions should be differentiated from simple bite wounds, tumors, eosinophilic granuloma complex, and feline leprosy. Secondary skin lesions should be differentiated from parasitic conditions (especially flea infestation), miliary eczema, and secondary staphylococcal pyodermas. In addition, the possibility of other viral conditions, such as feline herpesvirus infection and feline calicivirus dermatitis, should not be ignored (see Ch. 13, Feline Respiratory Disease Complex).

III. Confirmation of the diagnosis requires laboratory testing. There are three main approaches to a laboratory diagnosis: virus detection [by electron microscopy (EM) and virus isolation in tissue culture], histopathology, and serology. Each approach, however, has its own inherent advantages and disadvantages with regard to sensitivity, accuracy, rapidity, and ability to confirm or deny differential diagnoses. It is therefore best to take samples suitable for several test approaches.

IV. For virus detection by EM and isolation, dry scab material can be sent by mail; no transport medium is necessary unless long postal delays are anticipated or other viruses are also sought. A rapid presumptive diagnosis can be made by EM in about 75% of cases, but isolation in tissue culture is a more sensitive technique and is required for specific identification of the virus.

V. Histologic examination of fixed biopsy material may enable a diagnosis to be made in most cases, although healing lesions or those with extensive bacterial infection may not exhibit characteristic pathology. The sensitivity and accuracy of diagnosis by histologic methods can be increased by the use of an immunoperoxidase technique.

VI. Various serologic tests are possible, including virus neutralization, hemagglutination inhibition, complement fixation, and enzyme-linked immunosorbent assay. For most tests either serum or plasma is suitable; however if doubt exists, the laboratory to which the samples will be sent should be consulted beforehand.

TREATMENT

I. Most cats recover uneventfully from poxvirus infection. There is no specific cure and therefore treatment is largely symptomatic. Secondary bacterial infection can usually be controlled with broad-spectrum antibiotics, and larger skin lesions can be bathed with antiseptics. Pruritus and scratching are rarely severe enough to warrant concern, but the effects of scratching may be controlled with an Elizabethan collar or by bandaging the paws.

II. Corticosteroids are contraindicated, because their use has been associated with worsening of the disease.

III. More severely ill cats may require rehydration and intensive nursing. However, the prognosis for cats with clinically evident pulmonary signs is poor. Underlying predisposing causes of severe poxvirus infection (e.g., FeLV infection or other debilitating or immunosuppressive conditions) should be investigated, and euthanasia might have to be considered.

IV. Generalized *orthopoxvirus* infections in humans have been treated with hyperimmune gammaglobulin. However, hyperimmune serum is in short supply, and its efficacy in cats is untested. It might, however, be considered for prophylactic use during outbreaks among big cats in zoological collections.

PREVENTION

There is no commercially available vaccine for use in cats. Vaccinia virus has been used to protect zoo elephants in Germany and might be considered for use in big cats believed to be at risk. However, the pathogenicity of vaccinia virus in felines has not been thoroughly investigated, although preliminary studies have suggested that the virus is probably of low virulence in domestic cats.

PUBLIC HEALTH CONSIDERATIONS

I. Although cowpox virus is infectious for humans and cat-to-human transmission can occur, most cases in cats have not resulted in disease in human contacts. However, human infection can result in quite a severe illness, particularly in people with a preexisting skin condition, and the owners of affected cats should take care to avoid becoming infected.

II. Gloves should be worn when handling affected cats. Cats should be kept apart from people at particular risk of infection (e.g., small children and people who have a preexisting skin complaint or who are immunocompromised for some reason). It is worth noting that even a recent smallpox vaccination may not provide complete protection against infection.

III. In both cases of cat-to-human transmission reported in Great Britain, human infection was the index case; cats were incriminated only retrospectively as the source of infection. The possibility of cat-to-human transmission should therefore be investigated whenever human cowpox is diagnosed.

SUGGESTED READINGS

Anonymous: What's new pussycat? Cowpox. Lancet 2:668, 1986

Baxby D: Identification and interrelationships of the variola/vaccinia subgroup of poxviruses. Prog Med Virol 19:215, 1975

Baxby D: Is cowpox misnamed? A review of 10 human cases. Br Med J 1:1379, 1977

Baxby D, Ashton DG, Jones DM, et al: An outbreak of cowpox in captive cheetahs: virological and epidemiological studies. J Hyg (Camb) 89:365, 1982

Baxby D, Gaskell RM, Gaskell CJ, et al: The ecology of orthopoxviruses and the use of recombinant vaccinia vaccines. Lancet 2:850, 1986

Baxby D, Shackleton WB, Wheeler J, et al: Comparison of cowpox-like viruses isolated from European zoos. Arch Virol 61:337, 1979

Bennett M, Baxby D, Gaskell RM, et al: The laboratory diagnosis of *Orthopoxvirus* infection in the domestic cat. J Small Anim Pract 26:653, 1985

Bennett M, Gaskell CJ, Gaskell RM, et al: Poxvirus infection in the domestic cat: some clinical and epidemiological observations. Vet Rec 118:387, 1986

Fenner F, Henderson DA, Arita I, et al: Smallpox and its eradication. World Health Organization, Geneva, 1987 (in press)

Gaskell RM, Gaskell CJ, Evans RJ, et al: Natural and experimental poxvirus infection in the domestic cat. Vet Rec 112:164, 1983

Hoare CM, Bennett M: Cowpox in the cat. Vet Annu 25:348, 1985

Marennikova SS, Shelukhina EM, Efremova EV: New outlook on the biology of cowpox virus. Acta Virol (Praha) 28:437, 1984

Martland MF, Poulton GJ, Done RA: Three cases of cowpox infection of domestic cats. Vet Rec 117:231, 1985

Thomsett LR, Baxby D, Denham EMH: Cowpox in the domestic cat. Vet Rec 103:567, 1978

Willemse A, Egberink HF: Transmission of cowpox virus infection from domestic cat to man. Lancet 1:1515, 1985

7

Rabies

John R. August

ETIOLOGY

I. Rabies is an infectious viral disease characterized by encephalitis. Rabies virus is a rhabdovirus containing negative-strand RNA and measures approximately 180 × 70 nm.

II. Rabies virus is a neurotropic virus, found primarily in nervous tissue and the salivary glands. It has been suggested that the receptor for rabies virus in mammalian tissues may be the acetylcholine receptor, which would explain the universal susceptibility of mammals to the virus and its predilection for nervous tissue. The virus is quite fragile in the environment and becomes inactivated in dried saliva.

III. Worldwide, the World Health Organization reports about 700 deaths per year from rabies. The number of deaths from rabies in the United States has fallen from about 40 per year in the 1940s, to an average of less than 2 per year since 1980.

IV. About 1 million persons in the United States are reported to have been bitten by animals each year, resulting in about 25,000 individuals receiving postexposure prophylaxis annually. Although most of the human deaths from rabies since 1960 have resulted from contact with rabid wild animals, the great majority of people now requiring postexposure prophylaxis have had contact with potentially rabid dogs or cats.

V. The present low incidence of rabies in human beings in the United States is due to the declining incidence of the disease in companion animals; the infrequent contact of most human beings with wildlife reservoirs of the disease; the relatively low susceptibility of human beings to infection with rabies virus; and the high efficacy of postexposure immunization and medical treatment.

VI. Before 1958 most cases of animal rabies were reported in domestic animals. Since that time the majority of cases have been reported in wild animals, and presently only 15% of reported cases occur in domestic species.

VII. Enzootic domestic animal rabies is now uncommon; most rabid domestic animals become infected through the bite of a rabid wild animal. In 1981 for the first time, the incidence of rabies in cats exceeded that reported in dogs.

VIII. The major wildlife species presently responsible for the maintenance of rabies in the United States are, in order of importance: skunks, raccoons, bats, and foxes. Terrestrial wildlife rabies tends to be localized to certain geographic regions of the country in accordance with the habitat and population density of these species. The exception is bat rabies, which is considered to be ubiquitous.

IX. Enzootic rabies, which is a density-dependent disease, is maintained in these feral populations by animals with primary infections and, most importantly, by latently infected carriers. In these latter animals stressful episodes may result in recrudescence of virus shedding. Nonfatal infections may result from low challenge doses of virus or infection with a strain of low virulence.

CLINICAL SIGNS

I. Pathogenesis

A. Dogs and cats usually become infected with rabies virus as a result of the deep bite of a wild animal that is shedding virus in its saliva. Less commonly, infection may result from a nonbite exposure, such as contamination of an open wound or scratch. Wild animals may become infected through ingestion of infected carrion, since the virus can remain viable in salivary glands and nervous tissue for 7 to 10 days after death. Transmammary and transplacental transmission may also occur in certain feral species. Aerosol infections of human beings have been reported following inhalation of virus in infected bat caves. Iatrogenic infections have occurred following the transplant of contaminated corneas.

B. In a deep bite wound rabies virus first replicates in local myocytes of striated muscle. Virus probably enters the peripheral nervous system through neuromuscular spindles and motor end plates. Passive transport of virus in perineural structures results in an ascending infection of the peripheral nerves. During this centripetal spread of virus, little stimulation is provided to the host's immune response, owing possibly to the small amount of initial inoculum or to sequestration of virus from the host's defense mechanisms. In spite of this poor response, only 15% of human beings who are bitten by proven rabid dogs and who do not receive postexposure prophylaxis will develop clinical disease.

C. Once virus reaches the spinal cord, spread of infection throughout the central nervous system (CNS) occurs within 48 to 120 hours. Early preferential infection of the limbic system results in signs of aggression, changes in character, and aberrant sexual behavior. Eventual widespread infection of the neocortex causes terminal depression and coma, with death usually resulting from respiratory arrest.

D. Centrifugal spread of virus from the brain to non-neural tissues occurs via the peripheral nerves. Virus appears in the salivary glands coincidental with or slightly before the appearance of clinical signs. In dogs virus has been isolated from the saliva up to 13 days prior to the onset of clinical disease. Effective transmission of virus is ensured because virus is present in the saliva during the furious stage of the disease.

E. Virus-neutralizing antibody and inflammatory cells are usually absent within the CNS at the time of appearance of encephalitic signs and only increase significantly at the time of death.

II. Clinical course

A. The incubation period of rabies virus infection varies from 9 days to more than 1 year. In most cases, however, clinical signs appear within 15–25 days of exposure.

B. Three classical phases of the disease have been described: the prodromal, furious, and paralytic phases. However, not all animals progress through each of these phases, and the furious and paralytic phases may occur concurrently.

1. Prodromal phase

This phase usually lasts 2–3 days. The animal may show subtle changes in temperament, mild pyrexia, slow palpebral and corneal reflexes, and self-mutilation at the bite site.

2. Furious phase

Affected animals become increasingly restless and irritable, with episodes of aggression and barking often being triggered by visual and auditory stimuli. Rabid dogs may roam long distances, attacking inanimate objects. Pica may be observed. Later in this phase muscular incoordination, disorientation, and generalized grand mal seizures may develop. Cats tend to show furious signs more consistently than dogs, and aggression is a common feature in this species.

3. Paralytic phase

Signs of paralysis usually appear within 2–4 days of the onset of clinical signs and persist for a similar length of time. Occasionally the signs ascend from the site of the bite wound until the entire CNS is affected. Often laryngeal and pharyngeal paralysis are the first signs of this phase, resulting in a change in character of the bark, drooling, dysphagia, and dyspnea. Death results from coma and respiratory paralysis.

C. In one study the average duration of clinical disease was 3.5 days, with the longest survival time being 7 days.

D. Of great concern is the observation that some dogs and wild animals may recover from clinical rabies and continue to shed virus for protracted periods of time in their saliva.

DIAGNOSIS

I. Prompt laboratory confirmation of rabies in a domestic or wild animal is important to facilitate early treatment of exposed human beings and to decrease spread of the disease in the environment.

II. The circumstances of human or animal exposure determine the steps that should be taken.

A. Healthy dogs and cats, vaccinated or unvaccinated for rabies, that bite a human being should be isolated for 10 days and observed for developing signs of rabies. During confinement contact with all other animals should be prohibited, and the animal in question should be kept in an escape-proof enclosure or building. Animals should be kept on a leash when outdoors under the control of an adult owner. However, if the offending animal is unwanted or is a stray, it should be destroyed immediately for laboratory examination.

B. Dogs and cats that have been exposed to rabies virus and that are currently vaccinated against rabies should be revaccinated immediately and observed under similar isolation conditions for 90 days. Domestic animals should be considered to have been exposed to rabies virus if they have been bitten by a known rabid animal or have been bitten or scratched by a wild carnivore or bat that is not available for testing. All animal exposures should be reported to local health authorities.

C. Unvaccinated dogs and cats that are exposed to rabies virus should be destroyed immediately and their tissues submitted for laboratory examination. If the owners are unwilling to agree to euthanasia, the animal must be placed in strict isolation for 6 months and vaccinated 1 month prior to release. Isolation should be in a veterinary hospital, a quarantine facility, or, less preferably, in a secure pen at home. No human or animal contact is allowed, and the animal should be carefully inspected from a distance each day.

D. Wild animals involved in unprovoked attacks on human beings, dogs, or cats should be destroyed if feasible and the head submitted for laboratory examination. All bats that have inflicted a bite should be examined for rabies.

III. Proper submission of specimens is essential because early diagnosis of rabies depends on the detection of viral antigen or viable virus in fresh tissues. Animals should be destroyed in a manner that will not damage the brain or salivary glands. The head should be placed on wet ice in a leakproof container and shipped by an express service, or preferably hand-delivered. Complete details should be enclosed, including the signalment of the offending animal, nature of the biting incident, and the names and addresses of all persons and animals exposed.

IV. Laboratory tests used to detect rabies virus infection include:

A. Histopathology

Rabies virus infection causes an acute nonsuppurative encephalomyelitis, characterized by cerebral edema, perivascular cuffing with mononuclear cells, neuronophagia, and the formation of intracytoplasmic inclusions (Negri bodies). In spite of widespread neuronal dysfunction and massive viral replication within affected cells, however, the histopathologic changes are often mild. Negri bodies, which are found most consistently in dogs in the pyramidal cells of the hippocampus, are present in only 75% of confirmed cases of rabies. If the dog is destroyed for examination early in the course of the clinical disease, Negri bodies may not have had sufficient time to form. Other intracytoplasmic inclusion bodies, such as those caused by canine distemper virus, must be distinguished from Negri bodies. Negri bodies are not commonly found in the neurons of rabid cats.

B. Direct immunofluorescent antibody (FA) test

This test is presently the method of choice for the rapid detection of rabies virus antigen in submitted tissues. The FA test is considered sensitive and reproducible as long as tissues have not been fixed in formalin, repeatedly frozen and thawed, or exposed to high environmental temperatures. The tissues of choice are the left and right horns of the hippocampus, the cerebellum, and the medulla oblongata. In human beings, the FA test has provided a means of confirming rabies virus infection antemortem, by detection of viral antigen in corneal smears, skin biopsies, and buccal cavity scrapings. The technique has similar applications for domestic and wild animals by utilizing frozen sections of the facial sensory papillae, which are surrounded by rich nerve plexuses. From the midpoint of clinical illness until death, correlation between results using skin and brain specimens approaches 100%.

C. Mouse inoculation test

Suspensions of brain material from animals reported positive on FA testing are inoculated intracerebrally into mice, which are then observed for 5 to 6 days. The brains from mice that die or show clinical signs suggestive of rabies are submitted for FA testing and examined for the presence of Negri bodies.

D. Tissue culture isolation test

Cultures of continuous baby hamster kidney cells or neuroblastoma cells are inoculated with suspensions of tissues positive on FA testing. The culture is examined after 24 to 72 hours by the FA test.

E. Monoclonal antibody techniques

These are used to differentiate street, fixed, and vaccinal strains of rabies virus isolated from human and animal patients.

TREATMENT

I. Because rabies is almost invariably fatal in domestic animals and because the threat of exposure to human beings and animals is so great, rabid animals should be humanely destroyed as soon as clinical signs appear. Attempts to prolong the life of the animal are inadvisable.

II. Management of companion animal species exposed to rabid animals has already been discussed in connection with diagnosis.

III. Choice of treatment for human beings potentially exposed to rabies virus depends on many factors, including:

A. Species of biting animal

  B. Geographic region of the country
  C. Circumstances of the biting incident
  D. Type of exposure (bite vs. nonbite)
  E. Availability of the biting animal for observation and laboratory examination
  F. Immunization status of the human being who has been bitten
IV. Factors contributing to the likelihood of significant exposure in human beings include:
  A. Location of bite on the body (bites on the head and neck carry a greater risk)
  B. Amount of clothing at the bite site
  C. Stage of disease of the biting animal
  D. Severity of the bite
  E. Amount of virus in the saliva of the biting animal
 V. Depending on the immunization status of the human patient, post-exposure therapy may include vigorous wound hygeine, induction of passive immunity, and induction of active immunity.
  A. Early wound cleansing helps to reduce the amount of virus remaining within the tissues. Wounds should be carefully debrided and flushed with copious amounts of water containing soap, detergent, or quaternary ammonium compounds because the lipoprotein envelope of the virus is susceptible to these cleansing agents. Also, 70% ethyl alcohol should be used, as it is rabicidal. Tetanus prophylaxis and antimicrobial therapy should be initiated as indicated.
  B. Unimmunized persons are those who are not currently immunized with human diploid cell vaccine (HDCV) or who have a serum antibody titer of less than 0.5 IU/ml. In addition to the wound hygeine measures described above, these patients should receive rabies immune globulin (RIG) at the beginning of postexposure treatment. A total dosage of 20 IU per kilogram body weight is administered, of which half is infiltrated at the bite site, while the remainder is given by intramuscular injection.
  C. Five 1-ml doses of HDCV are administered intramuscularly. The first dose is given on the same day as the RIG (day 0), with subsequent doses on days 3, 7, 14, and 28.
  D. Patients who are currently immunized with HDCV should not receive RIG because the latter may interfere with an anamnestic response to the vaccine. In addition to wound hygeine, these patients should receive two 1-ml doses of HDCV intramuscularly on days 0 and 3.

PREVENTION AND PUBLIC HEALTH
CONSIDERATIONS

I. Because the control of rabies in wildlife species is presently not feasible, protection of human beings currently depends on the following measures:
   A. Creation of an immune barrier of dogs and cats between wildlife reservoirs and human beings
   B. Reduction of contact between companion animals and wildlife through stringent enforcement of leash laws
   C. Preexposure immunization of individuals at high risk of exposure to rabies virus, including veterinarians, veterinary hospital employees, animal control officers, and wildlife control officers. They should receive 0.1 ml of HDCV by intradermal injection on days 0, 7, and 21 and single booster vaccinations every 2 years thereafter.
II. Principles of rabies immunization for companion animals:
   A. Presently only 40% of owned dogs and 4% of owned cats are immunized against rabies. Concerted efforts must be made to vaccinate many more cats because this species now outnumbers the dog in reported cases of rabies.
   B. Because 3-year rabies vaccines appear to be as effective as 1-year vaccines, the use of 3-year products is to be encouraged in order to maximize the number of animals that are immunized.
   C. Manufacturers' recommendations should be followed carefully in order to prevent vaccine failures through improper handling and administration.
   D. Dogs and cats that bite human beings and are currently immunized against rabies should *not* be presumed free of the disease.
III. In order to decrease the risk of rabies virus exposure to themselves, their employees, clients, and patients, veterinarians should take the following precautions:
   A. Familiarize themselves with the Compendium of Animal Rabies Vaccines, published annually by the National Association of State Public Health Veterinarians, Inc.
   B. Vaccinate all dogs and cats against rabies, keeping their patients' immunization status current
   C. Promote rabies vaccination of pets in the community
   D. Deter clients from keeping wild animals as pets and avoid vaccinating any wild animal against rabies

    E. Report all human and animal exposures to the local health department

    F. Report all cases of rabies in currently vaccinated animals to the vaccine manufacturer, in addition to the local health authority

    G. Advise against contact with any unusually friendly wild animals

    H. Ensure that all hospital employees receive proper preexposure prophylaxis with HDCV and that proper medical treatment is sought after all potential exposures to rabies virus

SUGGESTED READINGS

Diesch SL, Hendricks SL, Currier RW: The role of cats in human rabies exposures. J Am Vet Med Assoc 181:1510, 1982

Dreesen DW, Sumner JW, Brown J, et al: Intradermal use of human diploid cell vaccine for preexposure rabies immunizations. J Am Vet Med Assoc 181:1519, 1982

Johnson KP, Swoveland PT: Rabies. Neurol Clin 2:255, 1984

Martin ML, Sedmak PA: Rabies. Part I. Epidemiology, pathogenesis, and diagnosis. Compend Contin Ed Pract Vet 5:521, 1983

Sedmak PA, Martin ML: Rabies. Part II. Prophylaxis and control. Compend Contin Ed Pract Vet 6:49, 1984

Veterinary Learning Systems: Report on Rabies. Fromm Laboratories, Grafton, Wis., 1983

8

Canine Distemper

Max J. G. Appel

ETIOLOGY

I. Canine distemper (CD) has been recognized as an important and often fatal disease of dogs for at least two centuries. The disease occurs worldwide not only in dogs but also in many other species in the order Carnivora. The mortality rate varies greatly among species.

II. The causative agent was shown by Carré (1905) to be a filterable virus. Detailed studies on the transmission, pathogenesis, and prevention of the disease in dogs and ferrets were made in England in the late 1920s by Dunkin and Laidlaw. Together with Puntoni, they developed an inactivated virus vaccine that was used for several decades with limited success. Live-attenuated-virus vaccines became available in the late 1950s after Cabasso and Haig attenuated the virus to chick embryos and Rockborn to canine tissue culture. These modified-live virus vaccines still dominate the market today and have been instrumental in controlling the disease in dogs. Distemper is still fairly common among a variety of wildlife species, however, and its eradication, as has been proposed for measles, the related disease of humans, is presently impossible.

III. Canine distemper virus (CDV), together with measles virus, rinderpest virus, and peste des petits ruminants virus, belongs to the genus *Morbillivirus* in the Paramyxoviridae family. The virus has a spherical or sometimes filamentous structure and may be highly pleomorphic, with a diameter ranging from 100 to 700 nm.

IV. The genetic information of CDV, a single-stranded, negative-sense RNA, is located in the center of the virus in a filamentous form, together with three of six structural proteins (NP, P, and L). This nucleocapsid is surrounded by a lipoprotein envelope with a membrane (M) protein on the inside and two glycoproteins (H and F) in spike form on the outside of the envelope.

V. The virus replicates in the cytoplasm of infected cells and matures by budding from the plasma membrane.

VI. Only one CDV serotype is recognized although a variety of CDV "biotypes" exist, which vary greatly in pathogenicity and tissue tropism within the central nervous system (CNS) (see below). The commercial vaccines presently available protect against all CDV strains that have been tested. By the use of monoclonal antibody, minor differences between CDV strains have been detected.

VII. Like most enveloped viruses, CDV is not very stable outside the host. Heat, radiation, and drying destroy CDV rapidly. Above 50°C the virus is destroyed within minutes, above 20°C within hours, and at 4°C within days. The virus can survive in a frozen state for years, and lyophilized CDV is stable for at least 3 years at 4°C.

VIII. Lipid solvents such as ether and chloroform destroy the virus rapidly. Hypochlorite solution, oxidizing agents, phenol (0.75%), and quaternary ammonium disinfectants inactivate CDV within minutes. The pH stability range is pH 4.5–9.0, with an optimal range of pH 7.2–8.0.

IX. Transmission of CDV occurs mostly by aerosol, directly from animal to animal. The virus does not survive outside the host under moderate environmental conditions. Acutely infected dogs shed virus in all body secretions regardless whether they show clinical signs or not. Virus shedding begins approximately 7 days postexposure. Dogs with subacute distemper encephalitis and persistent virus infection of the CNS may still transmit the virus to susceptible contact dogs for up to 2–3 months. By contrast, virus shedding ceases much earlier in dogs that recover.

X. Susceptible dogs of any age may succumb to CDV infection. In a vaccinated dog population, pups are protected by maternal antibody until approximately 6–12 weeks of age. They are then susceptible to virulent virus infection until they are protected by vaccination. Vaccination with modified-live virus induces long-lasting immunity in some dogs, while others lose their immunity; reports of distemper in dogs with a history of vaccination several years earlier are not uncommon. The denser the population of susceptible animals, the greater the risk of infection.

XI. Transplacental infection of fetuses has been reported. Cesarean-derived pups that were raised under gnotobiotic conditions developed clinical distemper when they were several weeks old. The importance of this route of viral spread, in the field, is probably limited because most bitches are immune to CDV.

XII. Infected dogs are not the only source of CDV. Most of the terrestrial carnivores are susceptible to natural CDV infection. All species in the Canidae family (e.g., dog, dingo, fox, coyote, wolf, jackal), the Mustelidae family (e.g., weasel, ferret, mink, skunk, badger, stoat, marten, otter), and the Procyonidae family (e.g., kinkajou, coati, bassarisk, raccoon, panda) may succumb to distemper or at least develop clinical signs of disease. Epizootics in raccoons, skunks, or foxes are not uncommon. They all shed virus during the acute infection and remain a constant source of virus for infection of dogs. Because of wildlife infection and the worldwide distribution of CDV, eradication in dogs is not feasible.

CLINICAL SIGNS

I. Pathogenesis

    A. Early events in the pathogenesis of CD appear to be quite similar in all susceptible dogs, regardless of virus strain or individual host response. Aerosolized virus is inhaled and infects macrophages in the respiratory tract. Infected macrophages carry the virus to lymphoid tissues, where it spreads rapidly. Within 1 week cells (T and B lymphocytes and macrophages) in virtually all lymphoid tissues become infected and virus can be found in blood lymphocytes. During this period of viral growth in lymphoid cells the first elevation of body temperature can be seen, usually 3 or 4 days postinfection (PI). At the same time interferon appears in serum.

    B. After the first week of infection an enormous variation in disease development may be seen that depends both on the virus strain and on the immune response of individual animals. It is still unknown today why 100% of ferrets and 30%–50% of dogs succumb to CDV infection while some dogs and other species experience only subclinical infection. A vigorous cellular and humoral immune response can be found 2 weeks PI in animals that fail to show clinical signs or that recover early, while only a very limited response is found in dying animals. These differences can be observed in pups within the same litter, and it is assumed that genetic variations are responsible. Variations in breed susceptibility appear to exist but have not been tested under controlled conditions. Long-nosed breeds of dog (German shepherds, greyhounds, pointers, setters, etc.) are believed to be more susceptible to CD than others.

    C. Different virus strains induce strikingly different but predictable diseases. This is perhaps not surprising because certain other mutants (e.g., modified-live vaccine virus) induce only an immune response but no disease. Most of the virulent CDV strains that have been tested induce either an acute encephalitis with predominant destruction of cells in the gray matter (including neurons) or a subacute encephalitis with predominantly white-matter lesions (demyelination). Hard-pad disease in the 1940s and 1950s was considered at that time to be a different disease; however, the disease was caused by a mutant strain of CDV that produced subacute to chronic infection.

    D. In dogs that develop clinical disease and encephalomyelitis, virus continues to spread after the first week of infection. Infected lymphocytes and macrophages carry the virus to the surface epithelium of the respiratory, alimentary, and urogenital tracts, to endocrine and exocrine glands, and to the CNS. In acute disease virus can be found in all these tissues. In more subacute or chronic forms, late cellular and humoral immune responses clear the virus from lymphoid and peripheral tissues; virus tends to persist in the CNS, however, and sometimes in the eyes and footpads (depending upon the virus strain).

II. Clinical course

    A. The first sign of disease is always pyrexia 3–6 days PI, when interferon appears in the blood. This sign probably passes unnoticed in most cases, however. Several days later the second fever (103°–105°F) evolves and is present intermittently thereafter, often in association with anorexia and depression. At that time serous nasal and ocular discharges may be present, which can become mucopurulent later on. Respiratory and gastrointestinal signs may follow, and they are often enhanced by secondary bacterial infections, owing to the immunosuppressive nature of the distemper infection. Coughing, dyspnea, and sometimes frank pneumonia may be seen. Vomiting and diarrhea, often watery or mucoid, may appear at the same time. Fluid losses may result in severe dehydration and emaciation. Skin pustules can be seen in some cases, predominantly on the ventral part of the abdomen.

    B. The acute multisystemic disease usually lasts for 2–4 weeks; it may be fatal or it may be followed by recovery or by CNS signs. In some dogs the acute disease is so mild that it passes unnoticed and it is the subsequent CNS signs that appear to mark the onset of the disease. A great variation in duration and severity of disease has been found experimentally in dogs infected with different strains of virulent CDV. In addition, age and individual host resistance greatly influence the outcome of the disease. A range from virtually no disease to severe disease with 50% mortality, therefore, can be expected. The mortality rate may increase to 100% in pups less than 6 weeks of age if they are not protected by maternal antibody.

C. The CNS signs may be concomitant with or follow upon recovery from systemic disease or may result from a subclinical systemic infection. Depending upon the virus strain, the signs may be referable to infection of primarily gray matter or white matter. Gray-matter disease, where many neurons are infected, is more often seen in the acute stage. Animals are depressed, recumbent, with convulsive seizures and champing or frothing from the mouth. Myoclonus, meningeal signs of hyperesthesia, and cervical rigidity are sometimes seen at this stage. White-matter disease tends to follow a more subacute or chronic form, incoordination, ataxia, paresis, paralysis, muscle tremors, and torticollis being the more common clinical signs. Overlapping symptoms of both forms, however, are often seen. Of the CNS signs, myoclonus is the only symptom that is not seen in other diseases. Optic nerve signs, retinal lesions, and sometimes blindness are not uncommon in distemper. Neurologic deficits at two or more levels of the brain and spinal cord can often be demonstrated.

D. Dogs with nervous signs often die, sometimes after weeks of progressive disease. Some dogs recover. Residual signs, such as myoclonus, may persist indefinitely. Persistent virus may induce hyperkeratosis of the foot pads and nose ("hard-pad disease").

E. Another form of distemper is "old dog encephalitis" (ODE), a disease of middle-aged or older dogs, which is quite rare today. Progressive motor and mental deterioration are the predominant clinical signs, with a fatal outcome in all cases. Clinically it may be difficult to differentiate between typical distemper in older dogs and ODE, but the neuropathology of the two forms of CDV infection is quite distinct.

F. Enamel hypoplasia of the teeth in growing dogs subsequent to CDV infection is a common lesion. The resulting enamel loss can be seen for several weeks after recovery.

III. Immune responses

A. During the first 2 or 3 weeks of CDV infection, dogs are always lymphopenic and immunosuppressed. Depletion of lymphocytes and necrosis of lymphoid tissues appear to be direct effects of CDV infection. Dogs that recover early respond to the infection with vigorous humoral and cellular immune reactions. Depending upon the virus strain, neutralizing antibody appears between 10 and 20 days PI and reaches maximal levels soon afterwards. Cell-mediated immune responses, as indicated by circulating virus-specific cytotoxic T cells, appear by 10–14 days PI and are maximal by 14–21 days PI. While the humoral immune response in recovered dogs persists for several years (and perhaps for a lifetime), measurable cell-mediated immune responses are of short duration. Recovered dogs surviving virulent CDV infection are probably immune for life. Experimentally such dogs have resisted virulent challenge-exposure following 7 years in isolation.

B. Dogs that succumb to acute CD 2–4 weeks PI have little or no virus-neutralizing antibody in serum, and cell-mediated immune responses are either absent or delayed. Great variability in the immune responses is seen in dogs that succumb to subacute or chronic CD and in dogs that recover from persistent infection of the CNS. Chronically infected dogs usually show delayed humoral (production of virus-neutralizing antibody) and cellular immune responses, and the response to other antigens is suppressed.

C. Cerebrospinal fluid (CSF) from dogs that recover early from the infection is free of viral antibody and interferon. Virus-neutralizing antibody may be found in some, but not all, dogs with persistent CDV infection.

DIAGNOSIS

I. Classical acute distemper in 3- to 6-month-old dogs, with coughing, diarrhea, dehydration, catarrhal discharge from the eyes or nose, and nervous manifestations with a duration of several weeks, is not common today. Attenuated-virus vaccines and antibiotics have kept this type of disease under control. Seen today are the less acute cases, frequently in dogs with a subacute encephalomyelitis in which pathognomonic CNS symptoms are absent (unless the dog has myoclonus). Demonstration of multifocal lesions in the CNS by neurologic examination may be helpful. Persistently infected dogs often have injected scleral blood vessels, a consequence of uveitis.

II. In exceptional cases postvaccinal encephalitis may be seen in pups 7–14 days postvaccination with modified-live CDV. Acute encephalitis, often with convulsions and a short and fatal disease course, is typical for such postvaccinal CD encephalitis.

III. Hematology in dogs with CD is fairly non-specific. In acute cases lymphopenia and thrombocytopenia may be marked owing to atrophy and necrosis of lymphoid tissue. The number of monocytes may be increased. Erythrocyte counts, hemoglobin concentration, and packed cell volume (PCV) may be on the low side of the normal range. The total plasma protein level usually is normal, but may be considerably increased with severe dehydration. Decreased albumin and increased globulin concentrations have been reported. The total IgG and IgA levels may be reduced while IgM levels remain in the normal range. In more subacute and chronic forms of encephalitis, the lymphoid tissues recover and most of the changes listed above would return to normal levels.

IV. Abnormalities of the CSF may be useful in diagnosis of CD. Cell counts and protein levels are usually elevated. Interferon in the CSF appears to be a reliable indicator of virus persistence. If CDV-specific antibody is found in the CSF, the diagnosis of CD encephalitis is confirmed. Negative test results, however, do not rule out the diagnosis.

V. Demonstration of viral antigen or inclusion bodies in conjunctival or vaginal imprints, in cells from tracheal washings, or in buffy-coat cells confirms the diagnosis. Immunofluorescence (IF) in acetone-fixed imprints, immunoperoxidase staining, or staining for inclusion bodies in formalin-fixed imprints is commonly used. Unfortunately, in subacute and chronic forms of CD viral antigen has disappeared from the buffy coat and surface epithelium, and so negative test results do not rule out a diagnosis of CD.

VI. Serologic demonstration of levels of neutralizing, precipitating, or cytotoxic antibody does not suffice for a diagnosis of CD. Titers are often high at the onset of clinical disease and may not increase thereafter. Furthermore, antibody may be induced by vaccination. The only specific serologic test would be demonstration of virus-specific IgM in dogs that have not been vaccinated within the 3 weeks prior to sampling. Dogs vaccinated for CD have virus-specific IgM in serum for up to 3 weeks, while dogs exposed to virulent CDV may have virus-specific IgM for 3 months. Detection of CDV antibody in the CSF is pathognomonic, unless the blood-brain barrier has been damaged by other means. Changes in the cellular immune response in dogs with distemper are difficult to test for and are fairly nonspecific and therefore unreliable for diagnostic purposes.

VII. Attempts at virus isolation from dogs with distemper are not practical unless fresh postmortem tissues are available. Virus can be isolated from buffy-coat cells at 7–14 days PI, when clinical signs begin to occur. Bronchial washings and ocular or nasal discharge may also contain virus. However, CDV is very fragile and may not survive transportation to a diagnostic laboratory, and many laboratories do not have indicator cells available for CDV isolation. An expensive and time-consuming but quite reliable test would be the inoculation of isolated, CD-susceptible ferrets with suspect material. When distemper in dogs progresses to the more subacute and chronic forms, the only known method to retrieve CDV from the living animal appears to be by direct transmission to CD-susceptible dogs.

VIII. With fresh postmortem tissues the diagnosis of CD is easier to achieve. Evidence that is usually sufficient to confirm the diagnosis is provided by imprints from lymph nodes, urinary bladder epithelium, and cerebellum that have been dried, fixed on glass slides in acetone, and stained with CDV-specific fluorescent antibody or by immunocytochemical methods. In acute cases all three tissues are usually positive. In subacute or chronic cases, in which serum antibody levels are high, CDV antigen cannot be demonstrated in lymphoid tissues but often is still present in bladder epithelium and cerebellum. Demonstration of histopathologic changes by conventional methods—especially inclusion bodies in brain cells, lung, and bladder epithelium—is more time-consuming but still reliable. Demonstration of viral antigen in formalin-fixed tissues can be made by IF or immunocytochemical techniques under light or electron microscopy.

IX. If virus isolation is desired, cells from minced lungs and brain, from scraped urinary bladder epithelium, and from trypsinized kidneys or testes can be cultured providing that the animal has died or been euthanized within a few hours of the postmortem. In acute cases lung macrophages show syncytium formation within 12 to 24 hours; unfortunately, lung cells from postmortem cases often are contaminated with bacteria or fungi. In urinary bladder epithelium cultures CDV antigen can be demonstrated by IF as soon as the cells are attached. In kidney, testes, and brain cells virus may not be demonstrable until 1 or 2 weeks in culture.

X. Virus isolation from lymph nodes, spleen, and thymus cells is usually positive from acute cases. Best results may be obtained by mitogenic stimulation and culture of these cells for 3–5 days, with infection confirmed by IF. These cells also can be overlaid on dog or ferret kidney or testicle cells or cocultivated with canine or ferret macrophages for virus isolation.

XI. Attempts at virus isolation from ground fresh or frozen tissues from subacute or chronic CD cases usually are less successful than attempts at isolation from live cells because antibody present in the tissues neutralizes the virus.

XII. If postvaccinal CD encephalitis is suspected, inoculation of susceptible ferrets with brain suspension appears to be the safest method to confirm this diagnosis: if, indeed, attenuated virus is involved, ferrets seroconvert without developing clinical signs. If virulent virus is present, ferrets die 10–30 days PI, depending on the virus strain. In subacute and chronic distemper cases ferret inoculation usually does not yield positive results because virus in brain (or other tissue) suspension is neutralized by antibody. Virus still can be isolated by direct growth of brain or kidney cells. However, the isolated virus rapidly becomes attenuated in these cells and thus is no longer suitable for testing by ferret inoculation.

TREATMENT

I. A specific antiviral drug having an effect on CDV in dogs is not presently available. Treatment of CD, therefore, is nonspecific.

II. Antibiotic therapy is indicated because of the common occurrence of secondary bacterial infections of the conjunctiva and respiratory and alimentary tracts. Antibiotic sensitivity testing should be considered, if possible. The route of administration may be important: for example, respiratory infection with *Bordetella bronchiseptica* is common in dogs with CD, but oral or parenteral administration of common antibiotics has little effect. Best results are obtained instead by aerosol treatment with polymyxin B, gentamicin, or kanamycin.

III. Symptomatic and supportive therapies are indicated when respiratory and/or gastrointestinal signs occur. Care should be taken to eliminate parasitic and protozoal infections, which may be more severe than in normal dogs because of the immunosuppressive nature of CDV. Because dogs with CD and diarrhea are often dehydrated, fluid and electrolyte support may be the most important therapy for CD.

IV. Treatment of neurologic forms of CD is usually not very rewarding. Sedatives and anticonvulsants may ameliorate clinical signs, but they do not have a healing effect. If CNS signs are progressive and dogs become recumbent, euthanasia would be indicated. Some dogs with CNS symptoms, however, recover quite well, and residual signs such as myoclonus or optic neuritis can improve with time.

V. Favorable results have been obtained by some investigators with short-duration (1- to 3-day) corticosteroid therapy. Prolonged treatment would be contraindicated because of the immunosuppressive effect.

VI. A variety of questionable "remedies" have been reported for the treatment of CD, such as high doses of ascorbic acid or ether inhalations. None of these has been tested under controlled conditions, and there is no evidence that they are effective.

VII. Intravenous administration of modified-live vaccine virus in dogs with CD has been common practice. Unfortunately, this treatment is only effective if given *before* clinical signs appear. It thus would be indicated for a dog with unknown immune status that has been in contact with a dog with CD.

PREVENTION

I. Immunization by controlled vaccination is the only effective approach to CD prophylaxis at the present time. Active immunization with modified-live virus vaccines induces long-lasting immunity and has kept the disease in dogs under control during the last 20 years. With a few exceptions the modified-live CDV vaccines available today are derived from either egg and avian cell or canine cell culture adaptations. Both methods of adaptation produce vaccines that are very effective in inducing an immunity that lasts for at least 1 year and probably for several years in most dogs. There are minor disadvantages to both products: Canine cell–adapted strains immunize virtually 100% of susceptible dogs but may induce sporadic postvaccinal encephalitis. They also are virulent for gray foxes. The avian cell-adapted strains are safer for dogs and avirulent for gray foxes, but the onset of the immune response in dogs may be 2 or 3 days later than with the canine cell–adapted vaccines, and not all susceptible dogs may become immunized.

II. Maternal antibody interferes with immunization, and the persistence of maternal antibody in young pups greatly influences the proper time of vaccination. Transplacental uptake of maternal antibody may range from 3% to 20% of the bitch's serum level. The predominant portion (approximately 80%) is absorbed in the intestine from colostral antibody, mainly during the first day of life. The half-life of maternally derived antibody is about 9 days. Pups with detectable serum antibody titers to CDV, with few exceptions resist imunization with CDV and do not seroconvert after vaccination. In order to determine the proper time for vaccination, a nomograph has been devised to predict the earliest age at which pups become susceptible to vaccination based upon the serum antibody titer of the bitch. Unfortunately, the level of maternal antibody varies in pups within the same litter and the nomograph, although quite useful for predicting the approximate age of vaccination, does not preclude repeated vaccination of litters for safe immunization.

III. Heterotypic (measles) virus vaccination has been one approach to overcome maternal antibody interference with immunization. Measles virus (MV) is not neutralized by CDV antibody. As with inactivated CDV vaccines, MV induces a limited immunity that can protect dogs against CDV disease but not against CDV infection. The use of MV vaccines was originally recommended for pups 2–4 weeks of age. It was not successful under natural conditions, although safety and efficacy were tested in 2- to 4-week-old pups that were free of maternal antibody. An explanation for this discrepancy was later found: although low titers of CDV maternal antibody in 6- to 10-week-old pups were tolerated, CDV antibody titers of 1 : 300 in 2- to 4-week-old pups did interfere with MV vaccination. While the use of MV vaccine in 2- to 4-week-old pups has been discontinued, a combination of attenuated MV and CDV is still commonly used in 6–10-week-old pups. It offers the advantage of complete protection in the absence of, and partial protection in the presence of, maternal antibody. In addition, MV antibody titers induced by vaccination usually are below a level that would interfere with MV vaccination in the next generation when used in 6–10-week-old pups.

IV. Reports are becoming more numerous about postvaccinal encephalitis, especially when combined modified-live CDV and parvovirus are administered. In most cases it is unknown whether the dogs were infected with virulent virus before or at the time of vaccination. The problem can be avoided by heterotypic vaccination with MV or combined MV-CDV in pups 6–8 weeks of age, followed by parvovirus vaccination 7–10 days later. Combined products can be used thereafter.

V. Thus, a vaccination schedule for pups against CD should include a combined modified-live MV-CDV vaccination at 6–8 weeks of age, with a second CDV vaccination at 14–16 weeks. If MV is not included in the first vaccination, two additional CDV vaccinations at 3- to 4-week intervals should be given. Annual booster inoculations are recommended because some dogs lose antibody titers in that time period. Colostrum-deprived pups should not be vaccinated with modified-live CDV before they are 3 or 4 weeks of age. Modified-live CDV can be fatal in unprotected younger pups, as it can be in some wild or zoo animals, e.g., lesser pandas, black-footed ferrets, and gray foxes.

VI. Passive immunization against CDV was used extensively before attenuated CDV vaccines became available. Because passive immunization enhances the effect of maternal antibody in interfering with active immunization, its use has been almost entirely discontinued. Only a few situations—for example, colostrum-deprived pups or susceptible dogs known to have been exposed to virulent CDV—warrant passive immunization.

VII. Besides immunization, strict isolation of dogs with CD appears to be the most important step in controlling the disease. Virus is shed in all body excretions during the acute systemic disease and direct dog-to-dog contact appears to be the main route of viral spread. Dogs with subacute CD encephalitis still may infect susceptible contact dogs. Disinfection of CDV in the environment can be accomplished with commonly used products because the enveloped virus is rapidly destroyed outside the host.

PUBLIC HEALTH CONSIDERATIONS

I. There was speculation several years ago that CDV might cause multiple sclerosis (MS) in humans. The speculation was based on epidemiologic observations involving prior exposure of MS patients to dogs and even to dogs with CD. This proposition has not been substantiated in many subsequent reports published over the past 5 years.

II. Another point of concern has been the possible shedding of modified-live MV from vaccinated dogs. The concern was that dogs may excrete a mutant virus that is virulent for humans. This concern is not justified because MV replicates only to a very limited extent in dogs and only in lymphoid tissues; dogs vaccinated with modified-live MV, like those vaccinated with modified-live CDV, do not shed vaccine virus.

SUGGESTED READINGS

Appel M, Gillespie JH: Canine distemper virus. p. 1. In Gard S, Hallauer C, Meyer KF (eds): Virology Monographs. 11. Springer-Verlag, New York, 1972

Appel M (ed): Virus diseases of carnivores. In Horzinek M (ed): Virus Diseases of Vertebrates. Elsevier Science Publishers, Amsterdam (in press)

Cornwell HJC, Campbell RSF, Vantsis JT, Penny W: Studies in experimental canine distemper. I. Clinico-pathological findings. J Comp Pathol 75:3, 1965

DeLahunta A: Veterinary Neuroanatomy and Clinical Neurology. 2nd ed. WB Saunders, Philadelphia, 1983

Fisher CA, Jones GT: Optic neuritis in dogs. J Am Vet Med Assoc 160:68, 1972

Gorham JR: The epizootiology of distemper. J Am Vet Med Assoc 149:610, 1966

Greene CE: Canine distemper. p. 386. In Greene CE (ed): Clinical Microbiology and Infectious Diseases of the Dog and Cat. WB Saunders, Philadelphia, 1984

Hartley WJ: A post-vaccinal inclusion body encephalitis in dogs. Vet Pathol 11:301, 1974

Krakowka S, Confer A, Koestner A: Evidence for transplacental transmission of canine distemper virus: two case reports. Am J Vet Res 35:1251, 1974

Krakowka S, Higgins RJ, Koestner A: Canine distemper virus: review of structural and functional modulations in lymphoid tissues. Am J Vet Res 41:284, 1980

Schalm OW, Gribble DH: Viral inclusions in blood cells and hemograms in canine distemper. Calif Vet 28(12):23, 1974

Vandevelde M, Zurbriggen A, Higgins, RJ, Palmer D: Spread and distribution of viral antigen in nervous canine distemper. Acta Neuropathol 67:211, 1985

9

Feline Infectious Peritonitis

Jeffrey E. Barlough
Fredric W. Scott

ETIOLOGY

I. Feline infectious peritonitis (FIP) is an important and complex disease of domestic and exotic cats. The causative agent is a virus belonging to the family Coronaviridae, a large and widely distributed group of enveloped, single-stranded RNA viruses that infect several species of birds and mammals. Feline infectious peritonitis virus (FIPV), canine coronavirus (CCV), transmissible gastroenteritis virus (TGEV) of swine, and human respiratory coronaviruses of the 229E group together comprise a cluster of antigenically related viruses within the Coronaviridae. In fact, the major structural polypeptides of FIPV, CCV, and TGEV are so closely similar that some regard these three viruses as host-range mutants rather than as individual viral species.

II. Cats are susceptible to natural infection not only with FIPV but also with certain enteric coronaviruses, which may or may not be variants of FIPV (or vice versa). These feline enteric coronaviruses (FECVs) can produce a range of effects, from asymptomatic infection of the gastrointestinal tract to mild to severe enteritis, the latter primarily in kittens. The nature of the relationship between FIPV and FECVs is perhaps illuminated by the observation that certain FIPV strains are capable of producing either FIP or enteritis, or both. It has been suggested that these agents represent pathogenetic (rather than host-range) mutants of a single coronavirus type—mutants possessing, however, a relatively broad spectrum of virulence from asymptomatic infection to enteritis to lethal, disseminated FIP.

III. Recent reports have shown that at least two other coronaviruses in the FIPV antigenic cluster can infect cats under experimental conditions: TGEV, which produces an asymptomatic infection and is excreted in feces for as long as 3 weeks postexposure, and CCV, which also produces an asymptomatic infection and is excreted from the oropharynx for at least 1 week. At present the frequency of infection of cats in nature with these two coronaviruses is completely unknown.

IV. In nature FIPV infections appear to be restricted to members of the cat family, including domestic breeds as well as certain exotic species—sand cats, caracals, lynx, cougars, cheetahs, jaguars, leopards, and lions. An outbreak of FIP in captive cheetahs can be particularly devastating to an incipient or established colony. Additionally, there has been a single report of an FIP-like illness in Asian short-clawed otters, but to date no conclusive association of this disease with FIPV has been demonstrated.

V. The major route(s) by which FIPV is transmitted in nature is/are still unknown. However, it is most likely that initial infection results from ingestion and/or inhalation of the virus. Virus is probably excreted into the environment in a number of ways: in oral and respiratory secretions, in feces, and possibly in urine as well. Close contact between cats is probably required for the most effective transmission to occur, although the possibility of transmission by indirect methods (on fomites) also exists. The potential for transmission by hematophagous arthropod vectors is unknown. Transmission of FIPV across the placenta to the developing fetus, as suggested by several reports, has not yet been conclusively proved to occur.

VI. On the basis of serosurvey data it has been proposed that most FIPV infections in nature result only in seroconversion without progression to inevitably fatal disease. This is because serum coronavirus antibody can be found not only in cats with lethal, disseminated FIP but also in many healthy cats and in many cats with diseases other than FIP, which indicates that exposure of cats to coronavirus(es) is much more widespread than was once believed.

A. In the general healthy feline population—*excluding* cats in catteries and multiple-cat households—approximately 10–40 percent of cats will have positive coronavirus antibody titers (*Note*: "Positive" refers only to the presence of antibody and not to the presence of the FIP disease process).

B. A special situation is encountered when cats are clustered together in catteries or multiple-cat households, in which case positive titers are either completely absent (i.e., there has been no exposure to virus), or are present in 80–90% of the cats within a household (reflecting efficient spread of virus once it has been introduced).

C. The presence of coronavirus antibody in a cattery does not necessarily correlate with its FIP history (i.e., antibody has been detected in healthy cats in catteries that have experienced death losses to FIP as well as in catteries that have never lost a cat to FIP).

D. Most cats with histopathologically confirmed FIP have serum coronavirus antibody, often of high titer. Because many cats with undiagnosed illnesses can also have elevated titers (indicating previous coronavirus exposure *but not confirming an active infection*), interpretation of such titers can be challenging. Further complexity has been contributed by the recent reports of other coronaviruses (FECVs, TGEV, CCV) that are capable of infecting cats and stimulating production of coronavirus antibody. Because these viruses are all serologically cross-reactive to varying degrees with each other and with FIPV and because several of them can be used relatively interchangeably in commercially available coronavirus antibody tests, the nonspecificity of these tests should be readily apparent. The serodiagnostic potential of these tests (i.e., their ability to identify cats with FIP and/or possible virus carriers and/or excreters) has thus been diminished, not only by the widespread occurrence of serum coronavirus antibody in the general feline population but also by the possibility that non-FIPV coronaviruses may be responsible for some of the seroconversions that they detect. The actual distribution of antibodies in the general feline population to each of these coronaviruses is unknown and will remain unknown until highly specific tests, capable of distinguishing antibody to one coronavirus (e.g., FIPV) from antibody to another (e.g., CCV), are developed.

VII. Reports indicate that FIP has been observed since the early 1950s. In the United States FIP has been reported in California since at least 1954, in the New York City area since 1956, and in the Midwest since at least 1962. The disease is worldwide in occurrence.

VIII. The FIPV is heat-labile, ether-sensitive, and inactivated by most commonly used household detergents and disinfectants. Maintenance of the virus at room temperature results in complete loss of infectivity within 24 to 48 hours. Household bleach (sodium hypochlorite), diluted 1 : 32 in water or in combination with the quaternary ammonium compound A-33 (Airkem) to give a final concentration of 1 : 32 bleach and 1 : 64 A-33, has been recommended for disinfection of FIPV-contaminated premises.

CLINICAL SIGNS

I. Following infection of large mononuclear cells in regional lymphoreticular tissue at or near the site of initial FIPV penetration, a primary viremia involving virus and/or virus-infected cells occurs within 1 week after exposure. In this way virus is transported to other regions of the body, especially to organs such as the liver, spleen, and lymph nodes—organs containing sizable populations of macrophages, which appear to be the primary target cells for FIPV infection. Hematogenous dissemination of virus also results in infection of circulating mononuclear cells (primarily monocytes) and, importantly, in localization of virus and virus-infected cells on or within the walls of small blood vessels, especially venules and small veins. A secondary cell-associated viremia may occur after initial infection of target tissues and result in further spread of virus throughout the body. Deposition of virus, virus-infected mononuclear cells, and immune complexes on or within blood vessel walls produces an intense perivascular inflammatory response that is Arthus-like (type III hypersensitivity) in nature. The response is pyogranulomatous and complement-dependent and results in vessel damage, with escape of fibrin-rich serum components into intercellular spaces and the eventual accumulation of characteristic "FIP fluid" within body cavities.

II. Studies have shown that some cats with serum coronavirus antibody experience a more rapid, fulminating disease course after FIPV exposure than do coronavirus antibody–negative cats receiving a similar exposure. Moreover, intravenous administration of anti-FIPV hyperimmune serum to antibody-negative cats results in the more fulminating form of the disease following FIPV challenge. A potential state of antibody-mediated hypersensitivity thus exists in FIP, wherein coronavirus antibody may act by accelerating the uptake of FIPV (in the form of virus antibody–immune complexes) into receptive monocytes and macrophages, where production of additional infectious virus is enhanced, and also by mediating the widespread destructive inflammatory reactions in blood vessel walls and tissues. It is thus the immune response itself that helps to fuel the escalating FIP disease process, a process that reflects an inability to control FIPV replication and thereby reaches its inexorable conclusion only upon death of the host.

III. Hypersensitization by coronavirus antibody is dependent upon the identity of the coronavirus(es) that generated the antibody response. Thus, antibody resulting from exposure to FIPV or FECVs usually hypersensitizes, while antibody produced by TGEV, CCV, or human coronavirus 229E usually does not. It should be emphasized at this point that the mere presence of coronavirus antibody in an animal's serum does not mean that FIP will ever develop in that animal, even after repeated FIPV exposure. In actuality FIP is a relatively *uncommon* disease in nature, even in crowded catteries (i.e., the vast majority of coronavirus antibody–positive cats never develop lethal, disseminated FIP).

IV. There is some evidence to indicate that in a certain percentage of cats initial exposure to FIPV results in a localized upper respiratory disease, which is usually mild and is characterized by conjunctivitis and/or rhinitis. Although most cats undergoing this primary form of FIP recover, some of them probably become healthy but chronically infected virus carriers. Only a very small number of exposed cats will proceed to develop the lethal, disseminated (secondary) form of the disease weeks, months, or years later.

V. Most cases of FIP occur in young cats less than 3 or 4 years of age. The onset of clinical signs may be sudden (especially in kittens), or it may be slow and insidious, with the severity of signs gradually increasing over a period of weeks. Some of these signs can be quite nonspecific: intermittent or complete anorexia, depression, dehydration, weight loss, fever. In many cases affected cats continue to eat and remain alert and responsive for a considerable period of time. Fever, however, is a consistent finding and usually persists until the last few hours of life.

VI. Three major forms of disseminated FIP are recognized: effusive ("wet") FIP, noneffusive or parenchymatous ("dry") FIP, and combinations of the two.

A. Accumulation of fibrin-rich fluid within the peritoneal cavity with progressive, usually painless enlargement of the abdomen is probably the most common clinical manifestation of effusive FIP (Fig. 9-1). Respiratory distress may develop when abdominal fluid accumulation becomes excessive or, more commonly, when accumulation of fluid occurs within the thorax, resulting in compression of the lungs and exudation of fluid into the airways. As

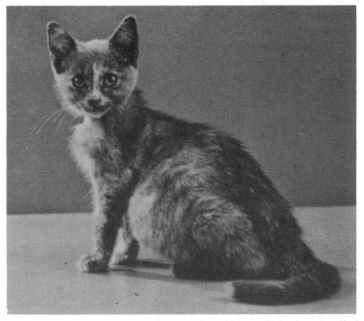

Fig. 9-1. Distention of the abdomen in a 6-week-old kitten suffering from the effusive form of FIP. (Courtesy of R.G. Sherding, Ohio State University.) (Sherding RG: Feline infectious peritonitis. Compend Contin Ed Sm Anim Pract 1:95, 1979.)

outlined earlier, this fluid apparently is the end product of the disseminated, immunologically mediated vasculitis that is characteristic of the disease. Other signs that may be seen include icterus and nonregenerative anemia. Rarely, the inflammatory process in the abdomen damages the pancreas, so that clinical pancreatitis, pancreatic enzyme deficiency, or even diabetes mellitus develops. The course of effusive FIP is quite variable, but the usual survival time after onset of clinical signs is about 2 or 3 months. Some young kittens may survive for no longer than a few days, while some adults may live for 6–8 months with active clinical disease.

B. The onset of noneffusive FIP is often insidious, with clinical signs reflective of pyogranulomatous involvement of specific organ systems in the FIP inflammatory process. Weight loss, depression, anemia, and fever are almost always present, but fluid accumulation is usually minimal. Clinical signs of renal and/or hepatic

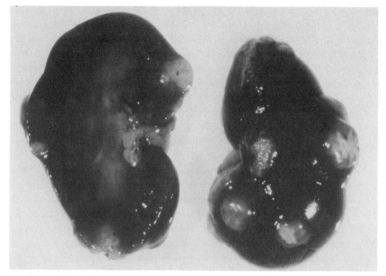

Fig. 9-2. Disseminated pyogranulomas in the kidney of a cat with experimentally induced FIP. Note the subcapsular distribution of the lesions and their superficial resemblance to renal lymphoma. (Courtesy R.C. Weiss, Auburn University.)

insufficiency, pancreatic disease, or ocular/central nervous system disease may be observed in cats with severe organ impairment (Fig. 9-2). Ocular lesions that may be seen include iritis, hyphema, keratic precipitates, retinal hemorrhage or detachment, chorioretinitis, and panophthalmitis. Neurologic signs can include posterior paresis, ataxia, nystagmus, behavioral changes, increased muscle rigidity, paralysis, and seizures. The disease course is usually more chronic than in effusive FIP. Some cats, especially those with primary ocular involvement, may survive for as long as 1 year or more.

C. It has also been proposed that FIPV is a possible cause of reproductive problems in breeding queens—infertility, fetal resorptions, abortions, stillbirths, birth of weak or "fading" kittens, congenital malformations, and neonatal heart disease (acute congestive cardiomyopathy). As of this writing there is still no conclusive evidence that FIPV plays a role in any of these disease processes. However, much additional research in this area will be required before the possibility of FIPV involvement in feline reproductive disorders can be entirely excluded.

DIAGNOSIS

I. The clinical diagnosis of FIP is made by evaluation of history and presenting signs and the results of supportive laboratory tests. Clinicopathologic and serologic procedures useful in diagnosis include analysis of thoracic or abdominal fluid, hemogram, serum protein electrophoresis, clinical chemistry profiles, biopsy (when possible), and serum coronavirus antibody titers.

   A. The volume of fluid present in cases of effusive FIP is variable but generally a reflection of disease chronicity. In the more chronic cases as much as 1 L or more of fluid may accumulate within the abdomen. Typically, this fluid is clear to slightly opaque, straw-colored to bright yellow, and viscid; contains fibrin strands or flakes; and often clots upon exposure to air. The fluid is an exudate of high specific gravity (1.017–1.047) and protein content (5–10 g/dl) and of variable cellularity (1,600–25,000 cells or more per microliter). In very acute cases the differential leukocyte count consists primarily of neutrophils, with smaller numbers of mononuclear cells. In chronic cases mononuclear and mesothelial cells predominate. In contrast to septic peritonitis, the majority of the leukocytes are intact, and bacterial, fungal, mycoplasmal, and chlamydial isolations are usually negative.

   B. Alterations in the hemogram are variable and not specific for FIP. Commonly observed changes include leukocytosis due to an absolute neutrophilia (which may be accompanied by either a regenerative or degenerative left shift), moderate monocytosis, eosinopenia, and lymphopenia. Occasionally leukopenia may develop, especially in more fulminating or in terminal cases. Many cats with FIP also develop a mild to moderate, normocytic normochromic anemia, which may be exacerbated by coinfection with feline leukemia virus (FeLV) and/or *Haemobartonella felis*. An increase in the icterus index may occur when there is extensive liver involvement. In some cases total plasma proteins may be as high as 10 g/dl or more. The hyperproteinemia of FIP is usually the result of a polyclonal hypergammaglobulinemia (elevations in IgG_1 and IgG_2 isotypes), with variable elevations of α_2- and β- globulins (Fig. 9-3). However, FIP may occasionally be associated with a monoclonal gammopathy. Although these changes are suggestive of FIP, *they are not diagnostic*; hypergammaglobulinemia may also occur in other chronic inflammatory conditions associated with persistent antigenic stimulation of antibody-producing cells.

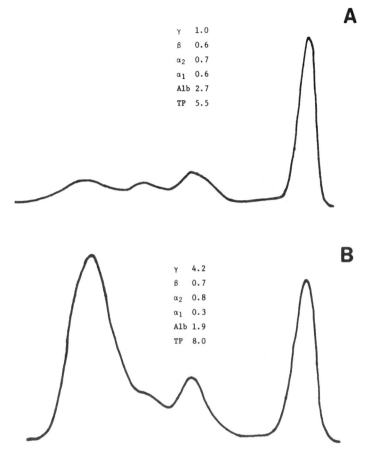

Fig. 9-3. Polyclonal hypergammaglobulinemia characteristic of FIP. Cellulose acetate zone electrophoresis of **(A)** normal cat serum and **(B)** serum from a case of FIP.

1. Experimentally, disseminated intravascular coagulation (DIC) has been observed in cats with FIP. Multiple in vitro clotting abnormalities, including prolonged prothrombin and partial thromboplastin times, depression of coagulation factors VII, VIII, IX, X, and XII, elevation of fibrinogen and fibrin-fibrinogen degradation products, and thrombocytopenia, have been documented in these cases.

2. Single or multiple acidophilic intracytoplasmic inclusion bodies, morphologically resembling canine and equine *Ehrlichia* structures, have been observed within small numbers of circulating neutrophils in both spontaneous and experimentally induced FIP cases. Their occurrence is rare; less than 1% of cells examined in one report were found to contain them. While the exact significance of these inclusions is not appreciated, it has been suggested that they may represent phagocytized immune complexes rather than aggregates of nascent virus.

C. In general, abnormalities in clinical chemistry profiles reflect the extent of involvement of different organ systems in the FIP disease process. Extensive liver involvement may produce hyperbilirubinemia, mild to moderate elevations in hepatic enzymes, and urobilinogenuria. A proteinuria with or without increased blood urea nitrogen and serum creatinine and electrolyte disturbances may be seen in cases with renal involvement. Analysis of cerebrospinal fluid from cats with extensive meningeal lesions may reveal a nonseptic fluid high in protein (90 to 2,000 mg/dl or more) and leukocytes (90–9,000 cells per microliter), the latter predominantly neutrophils. Similar changes may occur in aqueous humor from cats with anterior chamber involvement.

D. It is important to remember that biopsy is the only test procedure that can provide a *definitive* diagnosis of FIP in the living animal. Exploratory laparotomy with organ punch biopsy of affected tissues (especially liver, spleen, omentum, and mesenteric lymph nodes) is the preferred method of obtaining FIP biopsy specimens. Percutaneous needle biopsy cannot be recommended owing to the friability of diseased organs and the potential for serious hemorrhage. Similarly, a complete postmortem examination with histologic evaluation of suitable tissues will provide a definitive diagnosis after death. *Any FIP diagnosis made in the absence of histologic examination either on biopsy or on necropsy must be considered presumptive*; hence the vast majority of clinical FIP diagnoses will not be definitive in nature. This is so because of the large number of "FIP look-alike" diseases that can affect cats, such as lymphoma and other neoplasms (especially those involving the liver, biliary tract, kidneys, lungs, and brain), cardiomyopathy, nephrotic syndrome, septic peritonitis, diaphragmatic hernia, pyothorax, chylothorax, internal abscessation, pansteatitis, toxoplasmosis, cryptococcosis, and tuberculosis. Thus, in individual cases clinicopathologic and serologic test procedures will assist in ruling out possible diagnoses, but only biopsy or necropsy examination will definitively identify the FIP disease process. It therefore follows that, as indicated below, the diagnosis of FIP must *never* be made solely on the basis of a coronavirus antibody titer determination.

E. The presence of serum coronavirus antibody in any cat, whether healthy or diseased, is indicative *only* of prior exposure to a coronavirus in the FIPV antigenic group, and does not necessarily diagnose an active infection. A positive coronavirus antibody titer, while *consistent with* a clinical diagnosis of FIP (*recall*: This type of FIP diagnosis is always presumptive), does not indicate that a cat actually has FIP, because many healthy cats and many cats with diseases other than FIP will also be coronavirus antibody–positive. Neither, however, does a positive titer indicate that a cat is protected from developing FIP, because most cats with FIP are coronavirus antibody–positive. Considering that FIP occurs only sporadically in the general feline population and that most cats in FIP-problem households are coronavirus antibody–positive and yet do not contract FIP, it would appear that many (if not most) cats with coronavirus antibody are protected against developing the disease. The question remains: Is it coronavirus antibody that confers this protection, or are other, cellular immune mechanisms involved? It must also be kept in mind that present-day coronavirus antibody tests have absolutely no predictive value (i.e., a positive titer in no way indicates that a cat is doomed to develop FIP at some time in the future).

F. Recent research has shown that antibody directed against *bovine* serum components can be found in the serum of certain cats—antibody capable of reacting with antigenically similar bovine serum components present in cell cultures used to propagate target viruses for many coronavirus antibody tests. Because these components adhere tightly to both cells and virus, reactivity against them can be mistaken for a coronavirus antibody response unless the appropriate internal test controls are provided. One possible explanation for the presence of this antibovine reactivity is routine vaccination. Cell culture vaccines prepared for use in cats (as well as vaccines for many other species) frequently contain bovine serum components that could conceivably be the source of this noncoronavirus activity. Studies have shown further that this reactivity dissipates with time and that the probability of encountering it (and hence of producing a false positive result) can be minimized if serum samples for elective serotesting are drawn no sooner than 3–4 months after the most recent vaccination. A low positive antibody test thus should be viewed with some degree of skepticism when it occurs within 3–4 months after vaccination with any of the commercially available feline vaccines.

G. Some testing laboratories have stated that the only reliable means of diagnosing FIP in the laboratory is by detection of a rising coronavirus antibody titer over a period of a few days to a few weeks. In our experience some cases may indeed show a markedly rising titer, but more often the rise is moderate or nonexistent and sometimes the titer even declines, especially in the terminal stages of the disease. This latter phenomenon may be related to immune complexing and an apparent disappearance of antibody from the circulation during antigen excess. Thus the only definitive method for diagnosis of FIP still is histologic examination of biopsy or necropsy tissues.

H. General recommendations regarding the use of coronavirus antibody tests include the following:

1. Determination of antibody titers can be used for screening purposes, to detect the presence or absence of antibody in a previously untested household, and to detect *potential* (but not proven) virus carriers when introducing new cats into coronavirus antibody–negative households. Based on our current understanding of feline coronaviral serology, screening would appear to be the major use for coronavirus antibody testing today. Screening of cats in a household experiencing undiagnosed disease problems may be especially useful. Only about 10–20% of the cats (a minimum of three) in such a household need to be tested, because antibody will either be completely absent or will be present in 80–90% of the animals. While the discovery of coronavirus antibody–positive cats in such households will not diagnose the problem, knowledge that coronavirus antibody is absent will be helpful in ruling out an FIPV-group coronavirus as the culprit.

2. Determination of antibody titers can also be used as an aid (and nothing more) in the clinical diagnosis of a diseased cat with signs suggestive of FIP. A coronavirus antibody titer should be given no more weight than any of the other routine procedures (hemogram, clinical chemistry profiles, fluid cytology and analysis, radiography, etc.) used in arriving at a clinical diagnosis. If a conflict occurs between the clinical or clinicopathologic picture and the antibody titer determination, *the antibody titer should be ignored* and the diagnosis based on the other relevant data. In many cases fluid cytology and analysis will be especially

helpful because the characteristic alterations (high specific gravity, elevated protein level and fibrin content, variable cellularity, etc.) seen in effusive FIP will be present even when serum coronavirus antibody titers are low.

TREATMENT

I. Although mild cases of FIP, wherein clinical signs are minimal and spontaneously resolve, may occasionally occur, the vast majority of cats that develop disseminated FIP will die, usually within a few weeks or months of onset.

II. Present-day treatment of cats with FIP is purely palliative because no curative therapy yet exists. There are no effective antiviral compounds or prophylactic vaccines for FIP, and there is no way to eliminate the virus from infected animals. However, some treatment regimens may induce temporary, short-term (usually weeks) remissions in a small percentage of carefully chosen patients. The best candidates for palliative therapy are cats that are still in good physical condition preferably are still eating, do not show severe anemia, neurologic signs, or other significant organ dysfunction, and are not coinfected with FeLV. The FeLV status of *all* suspect FIP cases should be determined prior to commencing treatment, because the prognosis for cats infected with both viruses is extremely poor.

III. The basic aim of palliative therapy in FIP is to alleviate the disseminated inflammatory response, which represents the immune system's unsuccessful efforts at eliminating the virus from the patient's body. The most effective treatment protocols combine high levels of corticosteroids (prednisolone 2–4 mg/kg PO sid in the evening), cytotoxic drugs (either cyclophosphamide [Cytoxan, Bristol-Myers Oncology] 2 mg/kg PO sid for four consecutive days of each week, or melphalan [Alkeran, Wellcome] 1 mg PO every third day), and broad-spectrum antibiotics (ampicillin 20 mg/kg PO tid), together with maintenance of nutrient intake and fluid and electrolyte balance. Cats receiving cytotoxic drugs should be routinely monitored for evidence of bone marrow suppression or kidney dysfunction. If the patient shows a positive response to therapy over the first few weeks, treatment should be continued for at least 3 months. If the patient is in complete remission at this time (unfortunately, an infrequent occurrence), corticosteroids and cytotoxic drugs should be slowly withdrawn. Treatment should be reinstated, however, if signs of FIP reappear. Progressive physical deterioration in the face of treatment is a poor prognostic sign.

IV. There has been some indication that the use of certain immunomodulators affecting primarily T-cell and macrophage activities may have some beneficial effect early in the course of the FIP disease process. To date, however, no controlled studies of these products have been published.

V. Interferon treatment of FIP has not been reported as of this writing.

VI. Currently there is no documented scientific evidence that supplemental multivitamin therapy (including the use of vitamin C in megadoses) is of any benefit in treating FIP.

PREVENTION

I. A safe and efficacious FIP vaccine is still unavailable. Studies have been underway for several years to develop such a vaccine, but because of the hypersensitization without protection that is produced by the antibody response to FIPV and FECVs, all attempts to date to develop an effective vaccine have been unsuccessful. Neither has the use of nonsensitizing, cross-reactive coronaviruses (such as TGEV and CCV) produced any encouraging results. Thus, until an effective vaccine is produced, control of FIPV infections must be based on accurate identification and isolation of diseased animals and suspected chronic virus carriers.

II. A test-and-removal program for coronavirus antibody–positive cats, similar to that utilized for FeLV infection, cannot be recommended on the basis of current scientific information. Because there is no available serodiagnostic test that can specifically identify virus carriers, there is no logical medical reason for destroying healthy coronavirus antibody–positive cats. It is readily apparent, however, that such a test is urgently needed so that rational FIPV control measures may be devised. Until such a test is available, control must depend on isolation of cats suspected of having FIP and on maintenance of coronavirus antibody–negative catteries and households, when possible. Destruction of coronavirus antibody–positive cats to achieve this latter purpose, however, *cannot be justified*. Control must be exerted at the level of admission, and all cats tested negative must be quarantined for 4–6 weeks and then retested negative before entry into antibody–negative households. In FIP-problem households cats may be segregated into antibody–positive and antibody–negative groups to minimize further exposure of antibody–negative cats to potential FIPV carriers, and litters should be raised in isolation with individual queens. In coronavirus antibody–positive households without an FIP history, however, control measures cannot be recommended because there is no way of ascertaining to which coronavirus (FIPV, FECV, CCV, or TGEV) the cats were exposed.

SUGGESTED READINGS

Barlough JE: Cats, coronaviruses and coronavirus antibody tests. J Small Anim Pract 26:353, 1985

Barlough JE, Jacobson RH, Pepper CE, et al: Role of recent vaccination in production of false-positive coronavirus antibody titers in cats. J Clin Microbiol 19:442, 1984

Barlough JE, Jacobson RH, Scott FW, et al: Effect of recent vaccination on feline coronavirus antibody test results. Feline Pract 15(5):17, 1985

Barlough JE, Stoddart CA: Feline infectious peritonitis. p. 93. In Scott FW (ed): Contemporary Issues in Small Animal Practice. Vol. 3. Infectious Diseases. Churchill Livingstone, New York, 1986

Barlough JE, Weiss RC: Feline infectious peritonitis. p. 1186. In Kirk RW (ed): Current Veterinary Therapy. Vol. 8. WB Saunders, Philadelphia, 1983

Evermann JF, Roelke ME, Briggs MB: Feline coronavirus infections of cheetahs. Feline Pract 16(3):21, 1986

Hayashi T, Watabe Y, Nakayama H, et al: Enteritis due to feline infectious peritonitis virus. Jpn J Vet Sci 44:97, 1982

Horzinek MC, Lutz H, Pedersen NC: Antigenic relationships among homologous structural polypeptides of porcine, feline, and canine coronaviruses. Infect Immun 37:1148, 1982

Horzinek MC, Osterhaus ADME: The virology and pathogenesis of feline infectious peritonitis. Arch Virol 59:1, 1979

Hoshino Y, Scott FW: Replication of feline infectious peritonitis virus in organ cultures of feline tissue. Cornell Vet 68:411, 1978

Lutz H, Hauser B, Horzinek MC: Feline infectious peritonitis (FIP)—the present state of knowledge. J Small Anim Pract 27:108, 1986

Ott RL: Feline infectious peritonitis. p. 116. In Pratt PW (ed): Feline Medicine. 1st Ed. American Veterinary Publications, Santa Barbara, 1983

Pedersen NC: Feline infectious peritonitis and feline enteric coronavirus infections. Feline Pract 13(4):13–19; 13(5):5–20, 1983

Pedersen NC: Feline coronavirus infections. p. 514. In Greene CE (ed): Clinical Microbiology and Infectious Diseases of the Dog and Cat. WB Saunders, Philadelphia, 1984

Pedersen NC: Coronavirus diseases (coronavirus enteritis, feline infectious peritonitis). p. 193. In Holzworth J (ed): Diseases of the Cat. Vol. 1. WB Saunders, Philadelphia, 1987

Pedersen NC, Boyle JF: Immunologic phenomena in the effusive form of feline infectious peritonitis. Am J Vet Res 41:868, 1980

Pedersen NC, Evermann JF, McKeirnan AJ, et al: Pathogenicity studies of feline coronavirus isolates 79-1146 and 79-1683. Am J Vet Res 45:2580, 1984

Pedersen NC, Floyd K: Experimental studies with three new strains of feline infectious peritonitis virus: FIPV-UCD2, FIPV-UCD3, and FIPV-UCD4. Compend Contin Ed Pract Vet 7:1001, 1985

Scott FW: Feline infectious peritonitis and other feline coronaviruses. p. 1059. In Kirk RW (ed): Current Veterinary Therapy. Vol. 9. WB Saunders, Philadelphia, 1986

Stoddart CA, Barlough JE, Scott FW: Experimental studies of a coronavirus and coronavirus-like agent in a barrier-maintained feline breeding colony. Arch Virol 79:85, 1984

Stoddart M: Feline infectious peritonitis. Vet Annu 26:324, 1986

Weiss RC, Dodds WJ, Scott FW: Disseminated intravascular coagulation in experimentally induced feline infectious peritonitis. Am J Vet Res 41:663, 1980

Weiss RC, Scott FW: Laboratory diagnosis of feline infectious peritonitis. Feline Pract 10(2):16, 1980

Weiss RC, Scott FW: Pathogenesis of feline infectious peritonitis: nature and development of viremia. Am J Vet Res 42:382, 1981

Weiss RC, Scott FW: Pathogenesis of feline infectious peritonitis: pathologic changes and immunofluorescence. Am J Vet Res 42:2036, 1981

Weiss RC, Scott FW: Antibody-mediated enhancement of disease in feline infectious peritonitis: comparisons with dengue hemorrhagic fever. J Comp Immunol Microbiol Infect Dis 4:175, 1981

10

Feline Leukemia Virus

Dennis W. Macy

ETIOLOGY

I. The virus
   A. The feline leukemia virus (FeLV) is an RNA virus belonging to the subfamily Oncovirinae of the family Retroviridae (retroviruses). It contains a single strand of RNA, the enzyme reverse transcriptase, and core protein and is enclosed by a lipoprotein envelope.
   1. The envelope protein is a glycosylated polypeptide of 70,000 mol wt known as *gp70*. Antigenic variation in this polypeptide serves to subdivide FeLV strains into three subgroups, A, B, and C. Most field isolates consist of one or more subgroups, most commonly subgroup A. The combination of subgroups present may dictate the clinical manifestations of FeLV observed in a particular infected cat.
      a) Antibodies to gp70 have been shown to be protective against the development of persistent viremia. These antibodies do not in themselves protect against proliferative diseases such as lymphosarcoma resulting from FeLV-induced malignant transformation of cells, but in the presence of complement they may produce lysis of infected cells (cytotoxic antibody).
      b) The presence of antibodies to gp70 in cats indicates previous exposure to FeLV.
      c) Persistently viremic cats have low or nondetectable levels of gp70 antibody.
   2. The envelope also contains a 15,000 mol wt polypeptide, *p15E*, which is believed to be responsible, at least in part, for the marked immunosuppression often associated with persistent viremia.

    3. The major core protein is composed of a 27,000 mol wt polypeptide, *p27*. This protein is present in infected leukocytes and platelets and can also be found in soluble form in the blood of infected cats. It is the marker protein used for the identification of FeLV by the commercially available antigen detection tests.

    4. The enzyme, reverse transcriptase, is an RNA-dependent DNA polymerase, which allows the virus to produce DNA copies of its RNA genome. The DNA versions of the viral genome are then capable of integrating into host-cell chromosomal DNA.

    5. The virus is capable of replicating within many tissues, including the bone marrow, salivary glands, and respiratory epithelium. The virus is noncytopathic and escapes from infected cells by budding from the plasma membrane.

    6. The feline oncornavirus–associated cell membrane antigen (FOCMA) is a tumor-specific antigen found on the surface of FeLV-infected cells that have undergone malignant transformation. The presence of this antigen thus is used as a marker for identification of tumors induced by FeLV. Antibody to FOCMA in the presence of complement can produce lysis of FeLV-transformed cells.

II. Transmission

    A. All persistently viremic cats are excreters of infectious FeLV and probably remain so for the remainder of their lives.

       1. Excretion of FeLV in persistently infected cats occurs primarily by way of salivary secretions. Saliva may contain high concentrations of virus (10^6 virions per milliliter). Respiratory secretions, blood, milk, colostrum, feces, and urine also contain variable quantities of virus.

       2. Fighting and grooming are believed to be primary routes of transmission of FeLV. Blood transfusions, milk from infected queens, litter pans, and food and water bowls also may be potential sources of virus.

       3. Cats living in multiple-cat households are considered to be at higher risk of contracting FeLV infections.

III. Epizootiology

    A. In nature FeLV infections are limited to members of the cat family.

       1. The incidence of persistent FeLV infection in cats is reported to be in the 1–9% range and to be higher for males than for females. The frequency of viremia in cats with known previous exposure to FeLV may be as high as 33%.

2. The number of cats that have had contact with FeLV (based on the presence of antibodies to gp70 and/or FOCMA) depends on the population sampled but is reported to be in the 17–50% range.

3. Among the feline population FeLV and its associated diseases are the most important infectious cause of morbidity and mortality today.

    a) As many as 85% of persistently infected cats may be expected to die within 3 years of the initial diagnosis. As many as 30% may be expected to die within the first year.

    b) As many as 20% of FeLV-infected cats may be expected to die of neoplastic disease. The remainder may be expected to succumb to associated diseases, such as anemias and secondary infections. The incidence of secondary infections is fivefold greater in persistently viremic cats as compared with nonviremic cats.

CLINICAL SIGNS

I. Pathogenesis

  A. The virus usually enters the body through the mucous membranes or through the skin following a bite. Initial infection and replication occur in the lymphoid tissues surrounding the site of virus penetration.

    1. The virus attaches to receptors on the plasma membrane and is taken into the cell.

    2. Through the action of reverse transcriptase, a DNA copy of the viral RNA is made and is integrated into host cellular DNA. The integrated viral information is known as a *provirus* or *proviral DNA*. It divides whenever the host cell divides and thus is transmitted to all daughter cells produced by the infected cell and can serve as a template for the intracellular production of new virus particles.

    3. Following this localized infection, a low-grade mononuclear cell viremia occurs, which allows the virus to be transported to other areas of the body. Areas of greatest importance include systemic lymphoid tissue, intestinal tissue, and the bone marrow—areas containing populations of rapidly proliferating cells wherein FeLV replication can be enhanced.

    4. Infection of leukocyte and platelet precursors in the bone marrow and the subsequent release of infected cells into the circulation can produce a second, more profound viremia. Cats that resist widespread infection apparently contain the virus during the early lymphoid stage of infection. In those destined to become persistently viremic, however, widespread infection of the bone marrow, pharynx, esophagus, stomach, bladder, respiratory tract, and salivary glands occurs.

B. There are several possible outcomes to FeLV exposure. In determining these use is made of the two major antigen detection tests available, namely, immunofluorescence assay (IFA) and enzyme-linked immunosorbent assay (ELISA), and of serologic testing for antibodies to gp70 and to FOCMA.

    1. *Persistent viremia* develops in as many as 33% of exposed cats, usually within 2 months of infection. Cats become first ELISA-positive and then IFA-positive 1–2 weeks later. Cats remain viremic for life. Antibodies to gp70 and FOCMA are low.

    2. *Transient viremia* of 1–8 weeks' duration can develop following exposure. Cats first become ELISA-positive, then both IFA- and ELISA-positive, then ELISA-positive and IFA-negative, and finally negative on both tests. Cats develop elevated antibody titers to gp70 and FOCMA on recovery.

    3. *Immune cats* are those that never become ELISA- or IFA-positive following exposure but develop significant antibody titers to gp70 and FOCMA.

    4. *Discordant cats* are those that never become IFA-positive but remain ELISA-positive. Although not viremic, these cats harbor the virus in isolated tissues such as salivary glands, mammary tissue, or local lymph nodes. Of these cats, 50% will become negative on both ELISA and IFA tests within 2 years, while 5–10% will become viremic during the same time period. Some cats develop high gp70 and FOCMA antibody titers.

    5. *Latent infections.* Of cats exposed to FeLV, 30–80% will develop latent infections, which may be transient or persistent. The virus latency is believed to be a transient (for most cats), previously unrecognized phase of recovery in transiently viremic and immune cats, which lasts for several weeks to several months. Latency is difficult to detect because latently infected cats remain both IFA- and ELISA-negative. Isolation of the virus from bone marrow is required to identify these cats.

    C. Several factors influence the consequences of FeLV exposure and can alter FeLV pathogenesis. These include the following:
      1. Amount of virus
      2. Strain of virus
      3. Age at time of exposure. Of kittens under 6 weeks of age, 80% become viremic, while only 14% of cats over 1 year of age become viremic.
      4. Colostral antibody titers
      5. Drug therapy. Cats receiving corticosteroids have a sevenfold greater chance of developing persistent viremia.
    D. Susceptibility to disinfectants
      1. The FeLV is unstable outside the host and may easily be inactivated by dessication and by the lysing action of most household detergents and disinfectants on the viral envelope. Food bowls, litter pans, and other utensils may be disinfected by routine soap-and-water washing.
      2. The virus probably does not persist in the household environment for more than a few hours in most situations. However, under moist conditions it has been known to survive for several days.
      3. It is recommended that approximately 1 week be allowed to elapse prior to repopulating a house that has been occupied by an FeLV-positive cat. All food bowls, litter pans, and other utensils used by the previous cat should be thoroughly washed or replaced. The same should apply to towels or bedding utilized by the FeLV-positive cat.

II. Clinical course
    A. Proliferative disease
      1. *Lymphoproliferative* disease includes lymphosarcoma (LSA) and lymphoid leukemia, the clinical forms varying with geographic location. Mediastinal, alimentary, leukemic, and miscellaneous forms are recognized. Histologic categories include lymphocytic and histiocytic types.
        a) The *mediastinal* form is the most common and is seen more often in younger cats (median age 3 years). Tumor masses arise from lymphoid tissues in the anterior mediastinum and produce compression of the trachea and esophagus, resulting in clinical signs of dysphagia and dyspnea. Pleural effusion is a frequent sequela. The effusion fluid contains many malignant lymphocytes and can be used for making the diagnosis.

b) The *alimentary* form is a relatively uncommon presentation and occurs more often in older cats (median age 8 years). The tumor tissue arises in mesenteric lymph nodes or in parenchymatous organs within the abdomen and may be either focal or diffuse in distribution. Clinical signs frequently are vague: weight loss, fever, protein-losing enteropathy, vomiting. Complete obstruction of the gastrointestinal tract may occur. The ileocecal valve is a frequent site of focal lesions.

c) The *leukemic* or *lymphoblastic* form is a relatively common presentation, especially in the eastern United States. The origin of the proliferating lymphoid mass in this form is the bone marrow, and variable numbers of abnormal lymphocytes are found in the peripheral circulation. Tumor tissue may be found in other locations as well. Clinical signs associated with this form of the disease are vague and include anemia, which may be quite severe (packed cell volume (PVC) less than 15%), as well as lethargy and anorexia.

d) The *miscellaneous* form category includes other clinical presentations involving, for example, the skin, nasal cavity, eye, liver, or central nervous system. Tumors in these sites may also be seen in combination with other forms of the disease.

2. The *myeloproliferative* disorders are characterized clinically by severe anemia, secondary infections, and hepatosplenomegaly owing to extramedullary hematopoiesis. Histologically, myeloproliferative disease may be classified as myelogenous (granulocytic), erythroid, megakaryocytic, or combinations of these forms.

a) *Erythroid myelosis* is the most common myeloproliferative disease form, resulting in proliferation of erythroid precursor cells in the bone marrow. There is evidence of asynchrony in maturation of the nucleus and cytoplasm in many affected rubricytes. The peripheral blood picture is characterized by low PCVs, nucleated red cells, and anisocytosis without polychromasia or reticulocytosis characteristic of regeneration.

b) *Erythroid leukemia* may involve both myeloid and erythroid lines. In addition, switches between pure red cell leukemia and leukemia involving the granulocytic series may be seen during the course of the disease. Clinically and therapeutically, however, erythroid leukemia should be considered essentially the same as erythroid myelosis.

    c) *Myelogenous* (*granulocytic*) *leukemia* affects granulocytic precursor cells in the bone marrow and is characterized by proliferation of promyeloblasts. Myelomonocytic leukemia associated with FeLV is rare. Eosinophilic leukemia and hypereosinophilic syndromes are not believed to be associated with FeLV.

B. Nonneoplastic disease

  1. Aplastic anemia

    a) Nonregenerative anemia is a common sequela to FeLV infection. The mechanism of the anemia is unknown.

    b) The bone marrow is hypocellular and contrasts with that seen in erythroid myelosis, wherein the marrow is cellular with megablastic changes.

  2. Leukopenia

    a) A profound leukopenia (less than 1,000 cells per microliter) may be seen alone or in combination with aplastic anemia. Leukopenia may involve one or all cell lines (in the latter case it is termed *panleukopenia*).

    b) Leukopenia may be cyclic and may respond temporarily to corticosteroids (not recommended).

    c) Leukopenia associated with FeLV is considered to be a preleukemic condition and may progress to frank leukemia in 1–33 months.

    d) Leukopenia may be associated with diarrhea, in which case the disease can be confused with feline parvovirus-induced panleukopenia. The leukopenia and diarrhea associated with FeLV are chronic in nature, however, which contrasts with the parvoviral disease.

  3. Lymphadenopathy

    a) A nonneoplastic enlargement of peripheral lymph nodes, with or without associated systemic signs, has been reported in young FeLV-positive cats.

    b) Histopathologically, the lymph nodes in these animals are hyperplastic rather than neoplastic. A minority of these cases may progress to lymphoma, however.

  4. Secondary infections

    a) Immunosuppression may be seen with or without associated anemia or leukopenia. The suppression appears to reflect a T cell deficit. In vitro lymphocyyte blastogenesis may be depressed up to 90% in affected cats.

    b) Patients usually are leukopenic and may have thymic atrophy.

    c) Defects in neutrophil, macrophage, and lymphocyte functions have been described.

    d) The humoral response is altered, as exemplified by depressed class switching from IgM to IgG.

    e) Many of the alterations have been attributed to the viral envelope protein p15E.

    f) It has been suggested that FeLV may interrupt transmission of lymphokine signals through T cells and/or the T-cell response to lymphokines, acting more as an "immunologic anesthetic" than as an immunotoxin because the suppression may be generally reversible.

    g) Immunosuppression is associated with a fivefold increase in secondary infections, such as bacterial stomatitis, abscesses, pyothorax, upper respiratory infections, feline infectious peritonitis, toxoplasmosis, haemobartonellosis, cryptococcosis, and dermatophytosis. Any cat presented with a history of chronic infection should be evaluated for FeLV infection.

5. Reproductive failures

    a) Queens infected with FeLV may experience one or more reproductive disorders, including fetal resorption, abortion, infertility, endometritis, and birth of "fading kittens." Abortions characteristically occur late in gestation.

    b) It has been reported that nearly 75% of FeLV-infected queens may experience abortions and/or fetal resorptions.

6. Osteochondromas

    a) These involve a multicentric proliferation of cartilage and bone (flat bones, axial skeleton).

    b) Histologically, they are considered benign.

    c) They may pose limitations in limb movement.

7. Glomerulonephropathy

    a) Up to 80% of glomerulonephropathies in cats have been associated with chronic FeLV infection.

    b) It is believed that immune complexes involving especially the FeLV p27 protein are deposited in the glomeruli.

    c) Most affected cats develop only a mild proteinuria. A small number may develop more severe lesions and the nephrotic syndrome.

8. Ocular disease

    a) Feline leukemia virus has been associated with a variety of ocular changes, including bilateral or unilateral anterior

uveitis, and wtih retinal hemorrhages associated with tumor involvement.
  b) Pupillary abnormalities include anisocoria, bilateral mydriasis, and miosis in the absence of ocular inflammation.
9. Urinary incontinence
  a) Urinary incontinence has been associated with persistent FeLV infection and may or may not be associated with anisocoria.
  b) The urinary incontinence associated with FeLV must be differentiated from that associated with the Key-Gaskell syndrome (feline dysautonomia), which does not appear to be FeLV-related.

DIAGNOSIS

I. Virus and viremia
  A. There are a number of basic laboratory procedures available to assist the veterinarian in determining the FeLV and FeLV-immune status of an animal. The procedure selected depends upon the requirements of the individual case (i.e., whether test results are to be used for diagnosis, prognosis, colony disease control, prevaccination screening, etc.)
    1. Tests for FeLV detection include those for viremia/antigenemia (ELISA, IFA, concentration immunoassay technology (CITE), virus isolation), bone marrow culture, antibody to gp70 and FOCMA, and mixed FeLV antibody.
    2. The ELISA procedure detects soluble p27 viral antigen in body fluids and is considered approximately 100 times more sensitive than IFA. The most frequently evaluated sample is blood, but serum, tears, or other body fluids may also be used. The advantage of the test is that it may detect infections up to 5 weeks sooner than the IFA; in addition, it is an in-house laboratory procedure. Its principal disadvantage is its subjectivity: colorimetric changes may not be clear-cut, and interpretation relies upon personnel training, the presence of hemolysis in the sample, etc. The results may not always correlate with actual viremia: 5–30% of ELISA-positive cats may not be viremic but instead may have a local infection in regional lymph nodes or mammary tissue that may shed enough p27 antigen to produce a positive reaction.

3. The CITE procedure is a variant of the microwell ELISA technique. The principal advantages are speed, simplicity, and the presence of an internal control. The technology has been only recently developed, and comparisons with standard microwell ELISA procedures have not yet been reported.

4. The IFA is the oldest test for FeLV detection and identifies p27 in circulating infected white cells and platelets. The required sample is a thin blood film or buffy coat smear. The principal advantage of the IFA is the correlation with viremia and virus shedding. Its disadvantages include the fact that the test must be read in a commercial laboratory and there is thus a delay in the availability of results. False positives may occur as a result of thick smears, platelet clumping, or eosinophilia; false negatives may occur because of leukopenia and thrombocytopenia. The IFA may also be negative in aviremic cats that nevertheless harbor FeLV.

5. The determination of specific antibody levels has been used to classify immunity and the probability of developing an FeLV-related disease. Categories are based on specific levels of virus-neutralizing antibody and antibody to FOCMA. Virus-neutralizing (anti-gp70) antibodies protect against viremia, while high levels of antibody to FOCMA protect against tumor development. Unfortunately these specific tests are not usually available commercially, and what is available is thus a mixed antibody level. Because virus-neutralizing and FOCMA antibodies are not always equivalent in the magnitude of response, the ability to provide a long-term prognostic determination based on a mixed antibody response (which may include nonprotective antibodies, such as those directed against p27) is questionable. In addition, antibody levels (and thus protection) tend to decrease with time unless restimulation occurs. Because of the lack of specificity and durability, the use of antibody levels as long-term or short-term prognostic indicators is of limited clinical value.

6. Virus isolation is the most accurate means of evaluating virus shedding. However, because this procedure is confined to research laboratories and is limited by the fragility of the virus, it is not a practical alternative for practitioners. The results correlate well with IFA results.

7. Another research tool is bone marrow culture, involving collection of bone marrow cells and their propagation in in vitro culture. Under such conditions virus can be found in 30–60% of ELISA- and IFA-negative cats following exposure to FeLV. It is the most sensitive test for the detection of virus in tissues

and is the only test available for the detection of latent infections.

B. Testing patterns

1. Persistently viremic: ELISA- and IFA-positive
2. Transiently viremic: ELISA- and IFA-positive for 1–8 weeks. The ELISA-positive state precedes IFA-positivity by 1–2 weeks and may persist for 1–2 weeks after the IFA becomes negative.
3. Transiently discordant: ELISA-positive and IFA-negative, eventually becoming IFA- and ELISA-negative after months to years
4. Persistently discordant: ELISA-positive and IFA-negative, persisting for months to years
5. Negative on both tests: Either there has been no exposure to an infective dose, or the animal is immune and possibly harbors the virus (latent infection).

C. Test selection

1. Diagnosis

Use of an FeLV test for diagnosis should be made only if the patient's condition might be associated with FeLV infection. The most sensitive test available is ELISA.

2. Prognosis

The prognosis will vary depending upon the testing pattern. A persistent viremia is usually determined by two consecutive IFA-positive tests 4–6 weeks apart. Persistent viremia is associated with an 83% chance of death within 3 years of the date of the first positive test. A persistently discordant cat (ELISA-positive, IFA-negative) has approximately a 50% chance of death within the same time period. Latently infected cats whose bone marrow still contains the virus have perhaps a 10% chance of developing disease. Mixed antibody titers are of little value in determining the long-term prognosis.

3. Control

Test-and-removal is an established method by which losses associated with FeLV infection can be reduced. Infection rates in multiple-cat households have been reduced from 20 to 0.5% by testing cats every 3 months and isolating and removing those that are positive. For individual situations or one- or two-cat households, the IFA correlates best with the potential risk to housemates. In breeding colonies a potentially different situation exists, wherein aviremic discordant cats may pose a risk. These animals are not classic shedders except under special situations (e.g., pregnancy or lactation, during which the queen may pass the virus by transplacental or transmammary transmission to offspring). Under these circumstances the most sensitive tests available for FeLV should be used; thus the ELISA would be recommended.

II. Proliferative disease

A positive ELISA or IFA for p27 viral antigen is not a diagnosis of leukemia, lymphoma, or myeloproliferative disease. A positive test confirms the presence of FeLV but does not necessarily indicate that neoplastic transformation has occurred. Conversely, a negative IFA or ELISA does not exclude a diagnosis of viral lymphoma, leukemia, or myeloproliferative disease. Up to 30% of cats with these conditions will test negative for the virus despite the fact that the disease was caused by FeLV and that FOCMA is present. The definitive diagnosis of a proliferative disorder in the cat is the same as it is in other species—a morphologic diagnosis made by cytologic or histologic means.

A. Lymphoid neoplasia

1. Mediastinal form

Cytologic evaluation of fluid from the chest cavity or cells aspirated from the anterior mediastinal mass is usually diagnostic, revealing large numbers of abnormal lymphocytes or lymphoblasts. This form of the disease is usually (75%) associated with persistent viremia. Virus-negative animals must be differentiated from those with nonlymphoid tumors such as thymoma, which are predominantly epithelial.

2. Abdominal form

This is probably the most difficult form to diagnose, and more than 50% of the cases are ELISA-negative. The diagnosis is usually made by intestinal, hepatic, or mesenteric lymph node biopsy. This may be accomplished by fine-needle percutaneous aspiration or by exploratory celiotomy.

3. Leukemic form

This form is usually diagnosed by identification of lymphoblasts in a peripheral blood smear or bone marrow aspirate. Cats with aleukemic leukemia will have abnormal cells in the marrow but not in the blood. Some cats may also experience a preleukemic phase for months or years prior to development of frank leukemia. In these cases, patients may shed abnormal cells into the peripheral blood but may not have neoplastic disease at the time. Other cats will have a preleukemic leukopenia. All patients should undergo bone marrow examination in order to confirm the presence of neoplastic cells in the marrow.

B. Myeloproliferative disease

   1. Erythroid leukemia

     a) Diagnosis is based on a complete blood count and bone marrow evaluation. Cases are characterized by an anemia that is often severe (PCV below 15%), presence of nucleated red cells, and anisocytosis without evidence of regeneration, polychromasia, or reticulocytosis.

     b) Although 70% of anemic cats are FeLV-positive, only 10% of these will have a regenerative anemia. In these cats FeLV must be differentiated from haemobartonellosis and immune-mediated causes of anemia.

     c) There appears to be a maturation defect characterized by megaloblastic changes in the erythrocytes. These changes result in asynchronous development of the nucleus and cytoplasm in rubricytes. The bone marrow is infiltrated by large numbers of erythroid precursor cells. Nonanemic cats with mean corpuscular volumes (MCVs) greater than 50 are likely to be FeLV-positive.

   2. Acute myelogenous leukemia

     a) The diagnosis is based on identification of abnormal myelocytes in the bone marrow and peripheral blood.

     b) Differentiation between cells of the lymphoid and myelogenous series may be difficult. The myelogenous cells contain more cytoplasm and multiple, more prominent nucleoli.

III. Nonneoplastic disease

A. The diagnosis of FeLV-associated nonneoplastic disease is usually made by the detection of p27 and a process of elimination.

   1. Aplastic anemia

     A severe nonregenerative anemia, with a PCV often less than 10%, is most often seen in young cats (less than 3 years of age). Bone marrow is hypocellular, and MCV is normal. The ELISA is positive in 70% of cases.

   2. Leukopenia

     Cyclic (10–14 days) or persistent leukopenia may be accompanied by both lymphopenia and neutropenia. This must be differentiated from feline parvoviral disease, which is noncyclic and transient (1–5 days). The ELISA is positive in 70% of cases.

3. Lymphadenopathy

Histologic evidence of hyperplasia is obtained on biopsy; test for FeLV is positive.

4. Secondary infections

Many chronic infections, including bacterial (nonhealing abscesses, chronic rhinitis), fungal (resistant dermatophytosis, cryptococcal rhinitis) viral (feline infectious peritonitis) and protozoal (toxoplasmosis) have been associated with FeLV. Virtually all cats with chronic infections should be tested for FeLV.

5. Reproductive disorders

All breeding colonies experiencing abortions, stillbirths, infertility, and neonatal losses should be tested for FeLV.

6. Osteochondroma

Multicentric bone tumors are rare. Biopsy and ELISA determination are necessary for the diagnosis.

7. Glomerulonephropathy

Up to 80% of cases are associated with FeLV. Clinical diagnosis is based on a positive ELISA test and proteinuria in the absence of active urine sediment. Cats may also be hypoproteinemic and have elevated serum cholesterol levels.

8. Ocular disease

Ocular symptoms must be differentiated from those due to feline infectious peritonitis, toxoplasmosis, etc. Aspiration of material from the anterior chamber may be helpful. Pupillary abnormalities, especially in the absence of an anatomic cause, are an indication for FeLV testing.

9. Urinary incontinence

This is uncommon in cats. An ELISA should be performed on all incontinent cats.

TREATMENT

I. Proliferative disease
   A. Lymphoid neoplasia
      1. Untreated lymphomas usually are fatal within 1–2 months.
      2. Although lymphoma is not generally considered curable, complete remissions may be obtained in up to 80% of cases, with a median remission time of 5 months. Over 25% of these cats can be expected to remain in remission for at least 1 year.

3. The prognosis is adversely affected by the degree of debilitation and severity of hematologic abnormalities (leukopenia, anemia, thrombocytopenia) and major organ dysfunction.

4. The FeLV status and the histologic classification of the tumor do not significantly alter the prognosis.

5. Response to therapy often is dramatic; objective improvement is usually seen in 24–48 hours.

6. Combination therapy is superior to single-drug therapy. The combination most frequently used includes cyclophosphamide (Cytoxan, Bristol-Myers Oncology), vincristine (Oncovin, Lilly), and prednisolone (COP regimen). Cyclophosphamide and prednisolone are given PO, while vincristine is given IV.

7. Cyclophosphamide is supplied as 25- and 50-mg tablets and is administered at a dose of 2.2 mg/kg for 4 consecutive days each week. The principal toxicity is myelosuppression, which usually peaks in 7–10 days. Cystitis, although common in dogs, is rarely seen in cats.

8. Prednisolone or prednisone is given daily at a dose of 1 mg/kg. Cats are much more resistant to the adverse effects of glucocorticoids than are dogs and tolerate high doses for prolonged periods very well.

9. Vincristine is supplied in 1-mg vials and is given IV (0.75 mg/m^2) once weekly for 2–3 consecutive treatments and is then reduced to once every 3–4 weeks. This drug is a vesicant and will cause sloughing if deposited outside the vein. Neurotoxicity has not been described in cats, and the drug is considered nonmyelosuppressive. All drug therapies are continued until relapses are seen.

10. Up to 50% of cats demonstrating resistance to the COP regimen may undergo a second remission with doxorubicin (Adriamycin, Adria), given at 15 mg/m^2 IV once every 3 weeks. Doxorubicin is associated with cumulative cardiotoxicity when doses greater than 250 mg/m^2 are achieved in dogs and with a potential for renal toxicity in cats when cumulative doses greater than 100 mg/m^2 are given.

11. Thymic lymphomas respond better to treatment than do intestinal or cutaneous forms of the disease (Table 10-1). Resistant solitary intestinal masses producing obstruction may be managed by surgical resection.

TABLE 10-1.   TREATMENT RESULTS OF FELINE LYMPHOMA BY
CYTODISEASE FORM

Disease Form	Frequency of Complete Remission (%)	Median Duration of Remission (months)
Mediastinal	92	6
Alimentary	86	4.5
Multicentric	100	5
Leukemic	27	7
Miscellaneous	50	10

12. Lymphoid leukemia carries a much poorer prognosis than the solid lymphoid tumors. This may be due in part to the fact that affected cats frequently are quite anemic and perhaps even pancytopenic. Despite the severity of the condition, however, a complete remission can be expected in up to 40% of patients by use of the COP regimen described for lymphoma. Blood transfusions should be given to severely anemic cats (PCV below 10%) until regenerative cell mass can be established. Blood transfusions may have to be repeated. Cyclophosphamide should be withheld if neutrophil counts drop below 1,000 per microliter.

B. Myeloproliferative disease
1. Erythroid and myeloid myelosis are the most difficult of the FeLV-associated proliferative diseases to treat. An effective chemotherapeutic regimen for these forms has not been reported.
2. Palliative therapy includes appetite stimulants—diazepam (Valium, Roche Products) 1 mg IV daily or oxazepam (Serax, Wyeth) 2.5 mg PO—along with B vitamins and blood transfusions. The therapeutic value of transfusion may be associated with the supply of FOCMA or virus-neutralizing antibodies, complement, or other constituents in addition to red cells. The first transfusion usually lasts for approximately 2 weeks; subsequent transfusions usually must be repeated weekly.

II. Nonneoplastic disease
A. A variety of nonneoplastic conditions associated with myelosuppression occur and must be treated aggressively. Most of these

are secondary and infectious in nature; thus antibacterial, antifungal, and antiparasitic therapies are frequently used. These therapies should be initiated promptly and must be continued for a longer time in cats with FeLV infection than in those that are FeLV-negative.

B. Although corticosteroids may alter the cyclic neutropenia observed in some cats with FeLV, it is doubtful whether they benefit cats long-term; they may in fact result in a more profound immunosuppression.

C. A small percentage (6%) of cats with aplastic anemia will respond long-term (6 years) following whole blood transfusions. However, the majority of responses are short-term in nature (less than 2 weeks), and the patients usually succumb to their disease.

D. Of cats with panleukopenia-like syndromes (diarrhea, leukopenia), 50% may be expected to survive the initial crisis with aggressive supportive therapy (transfusion, antibiotics, fluids).

PREVENTION

I. Vaccination

A. A USDA-approved, commercially available vaccine against FeLV was introduced early in 1985 (Leukocell, Norden). Although the effectiveness of this vaccine has been challenged by some, it remains the only available product for FeLV immunoprophylaxis.

B. The vaccine is made from soluble antigens naturally released from lymphoid tumor cells grown in serum-deprived medium in vitro. Preservatives and adjuvants are then added.

C. Cats have been demonstrated to develop antibodies to gp70, p15E, p27, and FOCMA following immunization with this product. It has been shown by its developers to protect against viremia (80%) and tumor development (92%). A higher percentage of young cats (2–6 months of age) seroconvert with higher titers than older cats completing the vaccine series. Cats with evidence of previous FeLV exposure demonstrate titer rises.

D. The vaccine may be administered either IM or SC, the first dose being given no earlier than 9 weeks of age. This is followed by a second dose 2–4 weeks later and a third dose 2–4 months later. Annual boosters are recommended.

    E. The vaccine reaction rate is relatively high (17%). Most of the reactions (84%) are local or of a mild generalized type. Recent alterations in adjuvant, preservatives, and route of administration have claimed to reduce this rate.

    F. Given the fact that cats are most susceptible to FeLV when under 1 year of age and the evidence of increased exposure with age, vaccine programs should be targeted at but not limited to kittens and young cats.

    G. Prevaccination testing is of questionable value in most situations because only 1–9 percent of the population will be positive, and it will not prevent vaccination of latently infected cats testing negative on ELISA and IFA. Testing in multiple-cat households in conjunction with vaccination and test-and-removal, however, appears to be cost-effective.

II. Test-and-removal program

Test-and-removal has been demonstrated to be an effective means of controlling FeLV infection in over 50 multiple-cat households and has reduced the rate of viremia from a preprogram incidence of 22% to less than 0.5%. The program involves quarantine of all household cats until the procedure is completed. *All* cats are tested for FeLV (ELISA), and positive cats are removed or isolated. Food bowls and litter pans are cleaned or replaced. The remaining cats are retested 3 months after the first test. Positive cats are again removed or isolated. This procedure is repeated until two negative test results 3 months apart are obtained for all cats. New cats that are to be introduced into the household or colony are allowed entry only following quarantine and three negative test results 3 months apart.

III. Management of FeLV-positive cats in single-cat households

Persistently viremic cats warrant special management considerations. Because many of these cats may be immunosuppressed, they should not receive modified-live virus vaccines. These cats should not be subjected to the stress of boarding and should be kept confined in order to prevent spread of the virus to other cats. Probably the biggest risk to these cats is contraction of infectious diseases other than FeLV; thus confinement benefits both the FeLV-positive cat and the healthy FeLV-negative cats to which it will not be exposed.

PUBLIC HEALTH CONSIDERATIONS

I. Controversy still exists regarding the public health aspects of FeLV infections.

A. Basis for concern
   1. In vitro replication of FeLV in human cell lines has been observed.
   2. The feline sarcoma virus (FeSV, a replication-defective mutant of FeLV) produces tumors experimentally when inoculated into nonhuman primate species.
   3. So far as is known, FeLV is the only oncogenic animal virus to which humans are exposed on a regular basis.
   4. These facts should be tempered by the realization that natural transmission of FeSV is unlikely to occur and that FeLV is rapidly inactivated by human complement.
B. Epidemiologic studies involving veterinarians and the general human population have over the years produced conflicting or equivocal results.
   1. For example, veterinarians have been shown to be at increased risk for the development of Hodgkin's and non-Hodgkin's lymphoma when compared with the general population. However, this increased risk also exists for their physician counterparts, who do not have regular contact with cats.
   2. The most recent and most complex study searched for the presence of FeLV p27, FOCMA, and antibodies to p27 and FOCMA in 239 human cancer patients; all results were negative. This finding is significant in that both FeLV-positive and FeLV-negative lymphomas in cats carry FOCMA on tumor cell membranes.
   3. Despite these facts, retroviruses have crossed species lines in the past (FeLV from rat to cat, approximately 5 million years ago), and a theoretical possibility for future trans-species transmission remains.

SUGGESTED READINGS

Beck ER, Harris CK, Macy DW: Feline leukemia virus: infection and treatment. Compend Contin Ed Pract Vet 8:567, 1986

Cotter SM: Anemia associated with feline leukemia virus infection. J Am Vet Med Assoc 175:1191, 1979

Cotter SM: Treatment of infectious tumors in dogs and cats. p. 129. In Scott FW (ed): Contemporary Issues in Small Animal Practice. Vol. 3. Infectious Diseases. Churchill Livingstone, New York, 1986

Gerstman BB: The epizootiology of feline leukemia virus infection and its associated diseases. Compend Contin Ed Pract Vet 7:766, 1985

Hardy WD: The feline leukemia virus. J Am Anim Hosp Assoc 17:951, 1981

Hardy WD: Oncogenic viruses of cats: the feline leukemia and sarcoma viruses. p. 246. In Holzworth J (ed): Diseases of the Cat. Vol. 1. WB Saunders, Philadelphia, 1987

Hardy WD, Essex M, McClelland AJ (eds): Feline Leukemia Virus. Elsevier, New York, 1980

Hardy WD, Hess PW, Essex M, et al: Horizontal transmission of feline leukaemia virus. Nature 244:266, 1973

Hardy WD, Hirshaut Y, Hess P: Detection of the feline leukemia virus and other mammalian oncornaviruses by immunofluorescence. Bibl Haematol 39:778, 1973

Hawkins EC, Johnson L, Pedersen NC, et al: Use of tears for diagnosis of feline leukemia virus infection. J Am Vet Med Assoc 188:1031, 1986

Jarrett O, Golder MC, Weijer K: A comparison of three methods of feline leukaemia virus diagnosis. Vet Rec 110:325, 1982

Kiehl AR, Macy DW: Feline leukemia virus: testing and prophylaxis. Compend Contin Ed Pract Vet 7:1038, 1985

Lewis MG, Mathes LE, Olsen RG: Protection against feline leukemia by vaccination with a subunit vaccine. Infect Immun 34:888, 1981

Lutz H, Pedersen NC: Immunodiagnosis of feline leukemia virus infection. p. 448. In Kirk RW (ed): Current Veterinary Therapy. Vol. 9. WB Saunders, Philadelphia, 1986

Madewell BR, Jarrett O: Recovery of feline leukaemia virus from non-viraemic cats. Vet Rec 112:339, 1983

McMichael JC, Stiers S, Coffin S: Prevalence of feline leukemia virus infection among adult cats at an animal control center: association of viremia with phenotype and season. Am J Vet Res 47:765, 1986

Orosz CG, Zinn NE, Olsen RG, et al: Retrovirus-mediated immunosuppression. I. FeLV-UV and specific FeLV proteins alter T lymphocyte behavior by inducing hyporesponsiveness to lymphokines. J Immunol 134:3396, 1985

Orosz CG, Zinn NE, Olsen RG, et al: Retrovirus-mediated immunosuppression. II. FeLV-UV alters in vitro murine T lymphocyte behavior by reversibly impairing lymphokine secretion. J Immunol 135:583, 1985

Osterhaus A, Weijer K, Uytdehaag F, et al: Induction of protective immune response in cats by vaccination with feline leukemia virus iscom. J Immunol 135:591, 1985

Ott RL: Feline leukemia virus infection. p. 123. In Pratt PW (ed): Feline Medicine. 1st ed. American Veterinary Publications, Santa Barbara, 1983

Pacitti AM, Jarrett O, Hay D: Transmission of feline leukaemia virus in the milk of a non-viraemic cat. Vet Rec 118:381, 1986

Pedersen NC, Meric SM, Ho E, et al: The clinical significance of latent feline leukemia virus infection in cats. Feline Pract 14(2):32, 1984

Pedersen NC, Theilen GH, Werner LL: Safety and efficacy studies of live- and killed-feline leukemia virus vaccines. Am J Vet Res 40:1120, 1979

Reimann KA, Bull RW, Crow SE, et al: Immunologic profiles of cats with persistent, naturally acquired feline leukemia virus infection. Am J Vet Res 47:1935, 1986

Rojko JL, Hoover EA, Mathes LE, et al: Pathogenesis of experimental feline leukemia virus infection. JNCI 63:759, 1979

Rojko JL, Hoover EA, Quackenbush SL, et al: Reactivation of latent feline leukaemia virus infection. Nature 298:385, 1982

11

Canine Viral Enteritis

Roy V. H. Pollock
Leland E. Carmichael

ETIOLOGY

I. Several different viruses can cause viral enteritis in dogs. By far the most important of these is canine parvovirus. Canine coronavirus is probably the second most important cause of virus-induced vomiting and diarrhea, while canine rotavirus and other viruses appear to be very infrequent agents of disease.

II. Canine parvovirus is a "new" canine pathogen.
   A. Retrospective studies suggest that the virus first appeared in the dog population in 1976–1977.
   B. The virus is closely related to feline panleukopenia virus. The two viruses cross-react extensively in serologic tests and cross-immunize against one another.
   C. The predominant form of transmission is believed to be fecal-oral. Canine parvovirus is shed in large quantities in the feces of acutely infected dogs and can survive in the environment for at least several weeks.
   D. Canine parvovirus is resistant to many common disinfectants; based on studies of panleukopenia virus, chlorine bleach has been recommended as an effective virucidal agent.
   E. The virus is panzootic, and serologic surveys reveal that it is prevalent in both wild and domestic canids.

III. Canine coronavirus is also widely distributed.
   A. Serologic surveys in several countries indicate that most adult dogs have already been exposed to the virus despite the relatively low incidence of clinical disease.
   B. The primary route of infection is likely to be fecal-oral.
   C. Canine coronavirus can apparently be shed intermittently for long periods from otherwise healthy dogs.
   D. The virus is relatively labile in the environment and is readily inactivated by most common germicidal agents.

IV. Although the principal clinical manifestation is enteritis, canine parvovirus infection is a systemic disease.
   A. Viremia precedes intestinal viral replication and shedding.
   B. Viral replication occurs in many organs. Parvoviruses replicate only in dividing cells; hence virus-induced lesions are most evident in tissues with rapid cell proliferation.
   C. Lymphocytolysis is observed in most lymphoid organs; it is especially prominent in the mesenteric lymph nodes and thymus. In young dogs thymic atrophy may be evident on gross examination.
   D. Enteritis results from destruction of the germinal epithelium of the intestinal glands (crypts). This results in shortening and collapse of villi, malabsorption, and maldigestion.
V. Canine coronavirus is believed to be primarily an infection of the intestinal epithelium.
   A. Mature epitheliocytes of the distal half of the intestinal villi are the primary target cells.
   B. In enteric coronavirus infections of other species, intraluminal antibody is essential for resistance; serum antibody is not protective. The same situation is believed to apply to canine coronavirus.

CLINICAL SIGNS

I. The principal clinical signs of viral enteritis are diarrhea and/or vomiting, but the range of clinical manifestations is extremely broad (from subclinical to rapidly fatal). It is usually impossible to differentiate viral enteritis from other causes of gastrointestinal disease on the basis of clinical signs alone.
II. The simultaneous or rapidly progressive appearance of disease among a group of dogs with a common exposure strongly suggests a viral etiology.
III. Serologic evidence suggests that the majority of infections with either canine parvovirus or coronavirus are nonfatal and frequently nonclinical.
IV. It is believed that signs of canine coronaviral enteritis are most often relatively mild and confined to the gastrointestinal tract.
   A. A mucoid, fetid, orange-colored stool has been described as classic, but it is doubtful that a clinical diagnosis of coronaviral enteritis can be made with any certainty in an individual case.

B. Other clinical signs are nonspecific (lethargy, low-grade fever, etc.) and extremely variable.

V. Parvoviral enteritis is more likely to be accompanied by severe systemic signs, especially in young dogs.

    A. Fever is common and frequently marked.

    B. Hematologic abnormalities, including a relative or absolute lymphopenia, leukopenia, or the presence of abnormal "reactive" lymphocytes in the peripheral blood occur in the majority of dogs with parvoviral enteritis. These changes are transient, and repeated hemograms may be necessary to detect them.

    C. In general, the severity of the leukopenia is a useful prognostic indicator. Dogs with very low white blood cell counts are less likely to survive.

    D. Puppies develop clinical disease more frequently than older dogs; infections in dogs more than 1 year of age are usually subclinical. Certain breeds, especially Doberman pinschers, rottweilers, and English springer spaniels appear to be at higher risk of developing clinical disease.

    E. Concurrent illnesses and parasitisms are believed to exacerbate the severity of parvoviral enteritis.

DIAGNOSIS

I. Definitive diagnosis requires laboratory confirmation.

II. Leukopenia or lymphopenia occurring together with enteritis constitutes very strong presumptive evidence of a parvoviral etiology. The absence of leukopenia, however, is not sufficient to rule out the diagnosis.

III. Because of the prevalence of preexisting antibody, serologic diagnosis requires evidence of seroconversion (paired samples) or of recent infection (predominant class of antiviral antibody is IgM).

IV. Demonstration of virus in fecal specimens is unambiguous evidence of active infection.

    A. Both viruses are shed in large numbers during the period of acute illness.

    B. Electron microscopy, where available, is a relatively rapid and inexpensive diagnostic method for either virus.

    C. Because canine coronavirus is labile, false negatives are likely if there are lengthy shipping or processing delays.

D. Several other methods for detecting virus in feces have been developed for canine parvovirus. These include the stool hemagglutination test and an enzyme-linked immunosorbent assay (ELISA) technique.
V. In cases of parvoviral infection the histopathologic changes in the intestine and lymphoid organs are usually sufficiently specific to allow a definitive postmortem diagnosis. Gross lesions are variable and nonspecific.
VI. The postmortem lesions of canine coronaviral enteritis are more subtle, less specific, and easily obliterated by autolysis. Hence, a definitive histopathologic diagnosis is seldom possible.

TREATMENT

I. Treatment of viral enteritis is purely supportive and independent of the specific diagnosis.
II. The goals of therapy are to rest the gut, maintain fluid and electrolyte balance, and prevent secondary complications.
III. Food should be withheld for a minimum of 12–24 hours. If vomiting is severe or if drinking induces vomiting, water should also be withheld.
   A. At the end of this time or when gastrointestinal signs subside, a small amount of a bland diet purée should be offered.
   B. If this is tolerated, small amounts should be given frequently and the normal diet gradually reintroduced over several days. If feeding results in an exacerbation of clinical signs, food should be withheld for an additional 12–18 hours.
IV. Most animals with vomiting and diarrhea become dehydrated and require fluid therapy. This is especially important in puppies.
   A. If the animals can retain oral liquids without vomiting, it may be possible to maintain hydration with oral electrolyte solutions (e.g., Resorb, Gatorade).
   B. Subcutaneous administration of a balanced electrolyte solution may be sufficient in mildly dehydrated animals.
   C. Intravenous fluid therapy is indicated for animals with profuse or uncontrollable vomiting and diarrhea or for those that have already become severely dehydrated.
   D. Ideally, fluids should be selected on the basis of electrolyte and acid-base evaluations. If these are unavailable, lactated Ringer's solution supplemented with 10–20 mEq/L potassium chloride and 1–4 mEq/kg sodium bicarbonate should be used.

    E. Fluids should be given to effect.

  V. Locally acting gastrointestinal medications (e.g., kaolin-pectin preparations) have limited efficacy. Pepto-Bismol (1–2 mg/kg) may be of some benefit, probably as a result primarily of its subsalicylate moiety.

  VI. Motility modifiers, particularly anticholinergic compounds, have fallen into disfavor among most gastroenterologists.

 VII. Antiemetics may be of some value in cases of severe vomiting. Metoclopramide (Reglan, Robins) (0.2–0.4 mg/kg SC) has proved useful for viral enteritis. It can be given continuously as an intravenous drip (1–2 mg/kg per 24 hours) in exceptional cases.

VIII. Antibiotic therapy is no longer considered warranted in the routine management of diarrhea. Signs indicative of severe intestinal damage (e.g., hematochezia, melena) or the presence of leukopenia, however, justify prophylactic antimicrobial therapy in order to reduce the likelihood of secondary bacterial infections.

    A. Oral antibiotics should be avoided. Absorption is uncertain and enteric pathogens may be favored by disruption of the normal flora.

    B. Therapy should be selected to provide broad-spectrum protection against both gram-negative and gram-positive aerobes and anaerobes.

    C. A suggested combination is ampicillin (5–10 mg/kg) together with gentamicin (2.2 mg/kg) tid or qid.

    D. If aminoglycosides are used, hydration must be maintained and the urine sediment should be monitored for granular casts, which herald the development of tubular nephrosis.

PREVENTION

    I. Commercial vaccines are available for the prevention of both canine parvovirus and canine coronavirus infection.

   II. While there are ample field and experimental data on the efficacy of parvovirus vaccines, data are limited and contradictory for canine coronavirus vaccines.

    A. Both modified-live and inactivated parvovirus vaccines appear to be capable of immunizing *fully susceptible* dogs for periods of 1 year or more.

    B. In most instances there is good correlation between antibody titer and resistance to infection with canine parvovirus.

    C. There does *not* appear to be good correlation between serum antibody and resistance to enteric coronavirus infection.

    D. The duration of protection afforded by canine coronaviral vaccines remains to be rigorously demonstrated.

III. The principal impediment to control of parvoviral enteritis appears to be maternal antibody interference with immunization.

    A. High levels of maternal antibody protect against infection.

    B. High levels of maternal antibody also inhibit an immune response to vaccination.

    C. In some pups the interference with immunization may persist for as long as 18 weeks.

    D. Vaccines may differ in the amount of maternal antibody required to suppress an immune response. There are insufficient data to categorically rank vaccines in this regard.

    E. There is no readily available means to predict when an individual pup will respond to vaccination.

    F. As a result puppies should be vaccinated periodically from the time of first presentation until they are 16–18 weeks of age.

    G. The number and timing of inoculations depend upon professional assessment of the risk, the value of the animal(s), and the expense involved for the owner.

IV. In large breeding colonies an enzootic cycle of infection may become established.

    A. Heavily exposed pups can be infected while their maternal antibody levels are high enough to inhibit immunization by vaccination.

    B. *Thus, it has proved nearly impossible to break these enzootic infection cycles by means of vaccination.*

    C. While it has not proved possible to eliminate *infection* in such kennels, improving the overall health of pups has often reduced mortality to acceptable levels.

  V. No vaccine is a guarantee of freedom from disease.

PUBLIC HEALTH CONSIDERATIONS

  I. There is good evidence that canine parvovirus does *not* infect humans.

 II. Coronaviruses may be less host-specific. Canine coronavirus is not believed to be a human pathogen; however, definitive data are lacking.

SUGGESTED READINGS

Carmichael LE, Binn LN: New enteric viruses in the dog. Adv Vet Sci Comp Med 25:1, 1981

Greene CE: Canine viral enteritis. p 437. In Greene CE (ed): Clinical Microbiology and Infectious Diseases of the Dog and Cat. WB Saunders, Philadelphia 1984

Hammond MM, Timoney PJ: An electron microscopic study of viruses associated with canine gastroenteritis. Cornell Vet 73:82, 1983

Helfer-Baker C, Evermann JF, McKeirnan AJ, et al: Serologic studies on the incidence of canine enteritis viruses. Canine Pract 7(3):37, 1980

Macartney L, McCandlish IAP, Thompson H, Cornwall HJC: Canine parvovirus enteritis 2. Pathogenesis. Vet Rec 115:453, 1984

Moreau PM: Canine viral enteritis. Compend Contin Ed Pract Vet 2:540, 1980

Pollock RVH, Carmichael LE: Canine viral enteritis. Vet Clin North Am [Small Anim Pract] 13:551, 1983

Pollock RVH: The parvoviruses. Part 2. Canine parvovirus. Compend Contin Ed Pract Vet 6:653, 1984

Zimmer JF: Clinical management of acute gastroenteritis including virus-induced enteritis. p 1171. In Kirk RW (ed): Current Veterinary Therapy. Vol. 8. WB Saunders, Philadelphia, 1983

12

Canine Respiratory Disease Complex

Cheryl R. Dhein

ETIOLOGY

I. Numerous infectious agents may produce respiratory disease in the dog, including viruses, bacteria, mycoplasmas, fungi, and parasites. This chapter will address the commonly diagnosed and highly contagious respiratory disease of dogs known as *infectious tracheobronchitis* or *kennel cough*. Infectious tracheobronchitis is a clinical syndrome generally characterized by the acute onset of a dry, hacking, paroxysmal cough, which lasts from several days to several weeks.

II. The following agents, either alone or in combination, may cause infectious tracheobronchitis:

A. *Bordetella bronchiseptica*

1. This gram-negative organism is the most frequent bacterial isolate from dogs with upper respiratory tract disease, but it can also be isolated from normal dogs.

2. *Bordetella bronchiseptica* can also be isolated from rabbits, cats, guinea pigs, horses, and humans. Although no occurrences have been documented, the possibility for cross-species transmission exists.

3. The organisms attach to the cilia of the upper airways and slow their motion. This may lead to an impaired clearance of foreign debris from the airways by the mucociliary transport system.

4. *Bordetella bronchiseptica* may persist in the respiratory tract for as long as 14 weeks. Apparently healthy dogs may shed the organism, providing a source of infection for susceptible dogs.

B. Canine parainfluenza virus (CPIV)

1. This virus is frequently isolated from dogs with infectious tracheobronchitis. The virus spreads rapidly from dog to dog by aerosol exposure.

    2. Pure CPIV infections are mild. Mixed infections with other viruses, bacteria, or mycoplasmas can result in more severe clinical signs.

    3. In young dogs CPIV has also been associated with encephalomyelitis.

C. Canine adenovirus (CAV)

    1. Two adenoviruses can cause respiratory disease in the dog: CAV-1, which causes canine infectious hepatitis and is infrequently isolated from dogs with infectious tracheobronchitis, and CAV-2, which is commonly isolated from dogs with infectious tracheobronchitis.

    2. Alone, CAV-2 produces mild clinical signs, whereas in combination with other agents the signs are often more severe.

    3. Experimental production of disease with CAV-1 produces mild to severe clinical signs, depending on the route of exposure.

    4. CAV-2 invades both the respiratory and intestinal epithelia and can be shed from both sites. Shedding of the virus and subsequent dog-to-dog transmission occur for approximately 8 days postexposure.

D. Canine herpesvirus (CHV)

    1. This virus causes a fatal, generalized, hemorrhagic, necrotizing disease of neonatal puppies.

    2. Puppies over 3 weeks of age and adult dogs may develop signs of mild upper respiratory disease following infection with CHV.

    3. The virus may also be isolated from the respiratory tract of apparently healthy dogs.

    4. Canine herpesvirus may exist in a latent state and be associated with respiratory disease during times of stress. It is not readily transmitted between dogs, however, and is only sporadically isolated in cases of infectious tracheobronchitis.

    5. Infection with CHV is probably lifelong, with intermittent shedding of the virus from the respiratory and intestinal tracts.

E. Reovirus

    1. Three types of canine reovirus have infrequently been isolated from dogs with infectious tracheobronchitis.

    2. There is serologic evidence that the frequency of infection with reoviruses is higher than virus isolation results would suggest.

F. Mycoplasmas

    1. Mycoplasmas are part of the normal flora of the oral and nasal cavities and pharynx of the dog.

2. Mycoplasmas generally act as opportunists, exacerbating the disease produced by viruses or bacteria.

G. Canine distemper virus may infect a dog concurrently with other agents of infectious tracheobronchitis, but the disease process is then canine distemper rather than infectious tracheobronchitis.

III. Epizootiology

A. Infectious tracheobronchitis is a highly contagious disease complex.

B. The condition occurs most commonly where groups of dogs of different ages and susceptibilities are congregated (e.g., pet shops, humane shelters, veterinary clinics, research facilities). Morbidity in affected groups of dogs may be in the 10–50% range.

C. There may be a history of recent exposure to a group of unfamiliar dogs at a dog show, field trial, or similar event.

D. The etiologic agents of infectious tracheobronchitis are present in high concentration in the respiratory tract secretions of infected dogs and may be spread by coughing and sneezing. In the cases of CAV-2 and CHV intestinal shedding may also occur.

E. The infectious agents may also be carried on the hands and clothing of animal handlers and on food and water dishes.

F. The agents enter susceptible dogs through the nasopharynx.

G. Disinfectants effective against the agents of infectious tracheobronchitis include sodium hypochlorite (bleach), chlorhexidine (Nolvasan, Fort Dodge; Virasan, Bio-Ceutic), and benzalkonium chloride (Roccal-D, Winthrop).

CLINICAL SIGNS

I. The clinical signs of infectious tracheobronchitis are generally mild and self-limiting. A severe form of the disease may occur when a patient is concurrently infected with several agents or is immunocompromised. Occasionally the mild form of the disease may progress.

II. The most consistent clinical sign is a dry, hacking, and often paroxysmal cough. The coughing episode may terminate in expectoration of mucus or gagging. Coughing is most frequent following exercise, excitement, or changes in temperature or humidity of inspired air.

III. A mild serous and/or ocular discharge may infrequently be present.

IV. A dog with the mild form of infectious tracheobronchitis is generally healthy in other respects.

V. The severe form of infectious tracheobronchitis is difficult to distinguish from canine distemper. Animals with this form are usually less than 6 months of age. Clinical signs may include a moist productive cough, serous to mucopurulent nasal and/or ocular discharge, anorexia, and fever. Of dogs with this form, 10–20% may die.

VI. Infrequently an acute episode of infectious tracheobronchitis can result in a chronic cough by inducing chronic bronchitis or tracheal collapse in predisposed individuals.

DIAGNOSIS

I. History

A diagnosis of infectious tracheobronchitis can be made on the basis of circumstantial evidence alone in the case of an otherwise healthy dog with sudden onset of a dry, hacking cough within 5–10 days of exposure to unfamiliar dogs in a kennel or at a dog show.

II. Physical examination

A. A cough can often be elicited with gentle tracheal palpation.

B. A mild serous nasal and/or ocular discharge may infrequently be present. With the severe form the discharge may be purulent.

C. Occasionally the tonsils may be hyperemic and protrude from the crypts.

D. Thoracic auscultation reveals no abnormalities in mild cases but may reveal abnormal lung sounds in the severe form of the disease.

E. Fever may be present in animals with the severe form of infectious tracheobronchitis.

III. Clinicopathologic evaluation

A. Hemograms from dogs with mild disease are usually normal or may demonstrate a stress response characterized by mild mature neutrophilia, lymphopenia, and eosinopenia. Neutrophilia with or without a left shift may be present in animals with the severe form of the disease.

B. Cytological evaluation of samples obtained by transtracheal aspiration may reveal increased numbers of neutrophils and bacteria in both forms of the disease.

IV. Radiographic examination

A. Thoracic radiographs are normal in animals with mild disease.

B. Thoracic radiographs of patients with severe disease may demonstrate an interstitial pattern if viral agents predominate, but more often a bronchopneumonia consistent with bacterial infection is present.

V. Other diagnostic tests

A. Bacterial or mycoplasmal isolations can be made from samples obtained by nasal or pharyngeal swabs or by transtracheal aspiration. Transtracheal aspirations generally yield more specific results by bypassing the normal oropharyngeal flora. Nasal swabs are better than pharyngeal swabs for isolation of *Bordetella bronchiseptica*.

B. Virus isolation in appropriate cell cultures can be attempted with material obtained by any of the methods used to obtain material for bacterial culture.

C. Serologic evaluation of paired serum samples obtained 2–3 weeks apart may be performed in order to identify a rise in the level of virus-specific antibodies.

TREATMENT

I. Because infectious tracheobronchitis is often self-limiting in 7–14 days, dogs with mild clinical signs require no specific therapy.

II. Enforced rest and avoidance of stress- and cough-precipitating situations, such as leash-walking, exercise, excitement, and draft and temperature extremes, may reduce the frequency of cough as the disease runs its course.

III. Cough suppressants may be utilized if the frequency of the cough interferes with the dog's or the owner's rest.

TABLE 12-1. BRONCHODILATOR ANTITUSSIVES

Generic Name	Trade Name	Dosage for Dogs
Aminophylline	Available as generic	11 mg/kg q 6–8 hr PO, IM
Ephedrine sulfate	Available as generic	2 mg/kg q 8 hr PO
Oxtriphylline	Choledyl	10–15 mg/kg q 6–8 hr PO
Terbutaline	Bricanyl, Brethine	1.25–5 mg q 8–12 hr PO
Theophylline	Bronkodyl, Slo-Phyllin and others	5–7 mg/kg q 6–8 hr PO

(Compiled by Christine Schultz, R.Ph.)

TABLE 12-2.   NARCOTIC AND NON-NARCOTIC CENTRALLY ACTING
ANTITUSSIVES

Generic Name	Trade Name	Dosage for Dogs
Butophanol	Torbutrol, Torbugesic Stadol	0.05–0.1 mg/kg q 6–12 hr PO or SC
Codeine	Available as generic	1–2 mg/kg q 4–8 hr PO
Dextromethorphan	Benylin DM, Pertussin and others	1–2 mg/kg q 6–8 hr PO
Hydrocodone	Hycodan (with homatropine hydrobromine)	0.22 mg/kg q 6–24 hr PO
Morphine	Available as generic	0.1 mg/kg q 6–12 hr SC

(Compiled by Christine Schultz, R.Ph.)

A. Cough suppressants should only be used if the cough is nonproductive.

B. Mucosal irritation may lead to bronchoconstriction, which in turn stimulates cough. Bronchodilators may therefore act as cough suppressants. Dosages for several commonly used bronchodilator antitussives are listed in Table 12-1.

C. Centrally acting cough suppressants act on the cough center in the medulla to depress its sensitivity to stimuli.

   1. Narcotic antitussives may result in analgesia and sedation in addition to cough control.

   2. Dextromethorphan (non-narcotic) and butorphanol (narcotic) are both very effective in controlling the cough associated with infectious tracheobronchitis.

   3. Dosages for several centrally acting antitussives are listed in Table 12-2.

IV. Specific antibiotic therapy is indicated when the dog manifests systemic signs of illness, when the course of the disease is prolonged, or when specific bacteria are isolated.

A. The selection of an antibiotic is made on the basis of culture and subsequent susceptibility testing.

   1. Because *Bordetella bronchiseptica* is the most common bacterial isolate from dogs with infectious tracheobronchitis, antibiotics with known efficacy against *Bordetella* should be administered pending the results of bacterial culture.

    2. Isolates of *Bordetella bronchiseptica* from 27 dogs with infectious tracheobronchitis were all susceptible to chloramphenicol, gentamicin, kanamycin, and tetracycline. Most isolates were resistant to cephaloridine, nitrofurantoin, streptomycin, and trimethoprim-sulfadiazine, and 58% of the isolates were resistant to ampicillin.

  B. If the infection is confined to the upper airways (which is true of most cases of infectious tracheobronchitis), the aerosol administration of antibiotic solutions (gentamicin, kanamycin, or polymyxin B) via a face mask may prove beneficial in reducing clinical signs.

  C. The intratracheal injection of antibiotics is of questionable value.

V. Glucocorticoids are occasionally administered to patients with infectious tracheobronchitis. Care should always be exercised in the administration of systemic glucocorticoids to patients with respiratory tract disease because their immunosuppressive effects may potentiate bacterial and fungal infections.

VI. Patients with radiographic evidence of a bacterial pneumonia may require intensive treatment.

  A. The mainstay of therapy for animals with bacterial pneumonia is antibiotics. Rational antibiotic therapy should be based on culture and susceptibility results on material obtained by transtracheal aspiration, bronchial lavage, bronchial brushing, or fine-needle lung aspiration. Antibiotics should be continued for a minimum of 10 days after resolution of clinical signs.

  B. Maintenance of adequate hydration is an essential component of therapy for pneumonia. As the water content of tracheobronchial secretions decreases, the secretions increase in viscosity, making them difficult to remove by the mucociliary system or by expectoration. Hydration may be maintained by either the oral or parenteral routes.

  C. Aerosol therapy may be used to loosen tracheobronchial secretions.

    1. Aerosol therapy is accomplished by nebulization, which is the process of suspending particles of a liquid in a gas.

    2. The dog should be nebulized with a face mask or in a closed cage nebulizer for 30–45 minutes, three to four times daily, for 3–5 days.

    3. Pretreatment with bronchodilators is indicated to reduce bronchospasm caused by the procedure.

4. In the treatment of pneumonia the nebulization of antibiotics or mucolytic agents has no benefit over saline nebulization. Mucolytic agents administered by aerosol may be detrimental to the patient.

5. Humidification is the conversion of a liquid to a gas. Humidification achieved by a humidifier or by placing the dog in a steamy bathroom may deliver small amounts of water to the lower airways but is not as effective as nebulization in loosening airway secretions.

6. Physiotherapy, in the form of mild exercise or chest wall coupage, should follow each episode of aerosol therapy to facilitate the removal of secretions.

D. Cough suppressants are contraindicated in dogs with pneumonia.

PREVENTION

I. Numerous vaccines are available to immunize dogs against the principal viral and bacterial agents causing infectious tracheobronchitis. A partial list of available vaccines is presented in Table 12-3.

II. Some of the vaccines contain single agents while others are polyvalent.

III. Some of the vaccines are for parenteral use and others for intranasal instillation. The rationale of intranasal vaccination is to stimulate the production of local secretory IgA antibodies, which play a major role in protection of the upper respiratory tract against pathogens.

IV. The decision to employ these vaccines should be determined by the potential exposure of the individual animal. It appears that some degree of natural immunity develops to the infectious agents involved.

V. Specific vaccine constituents and vaccination techniques have given the following results:

A. More consistent protection against *Bordetella bronchiseptica* is afforded by intranasal vaccination. A field test of one intranasal vaccine containing *Bordetella bronchiseptica* and CPIV in a kennel of 5,000 dogs reduced the incidence of clinical disease from 40 to 8%. No adverse effects were observed. Vaccination every 10–12 months is recommended.

B. Administration of a parenteral CPIV vaccine will protect against disease but not infection and thus does not limit the spread of this virus among dogs. Administration of an intranasal CPIV vaccine protects against both infection and disease and is effective in the face of maternal immunity. Annual revaccination with the intranasal product is recommended.

TABLE 12-3. VACCINES FOR THE PREVENTION OF INFECTIOUS TRACHEOBRONCHITIS

Company	Name	Route	Etiologic Agent(s)[a]
Beecham	Sentryvac DHP	Parenteral	3
	Sentryvac DHP/L	Parenteral	3
	Sentrypar DHP	Parenteral	3
	Sentrypar DHP/L	Parenteral	3
Bio-Ceutic	Naramune 2	Intranasal	1, 3
	D-VAC 7	Parenteral	3
Coopers	EPIvaxine DA$_2$P	Parenteral	2, 3
	EPIvaxine DA$_2$PL	Parenteral	2, 3
	EPIvaxine DA$_2$PPv	Parenteral	2, 3
	EPIvaxine DA$_2$PPvL	Parenteral	2, 3
Fort Dodge	Duramune DA$_2$P + PV	Parenteral	2, 3
	Duramune DA$_2$LP + PV	Parenteral	2, 3
Norden	Vanguard DMP	Parenteral	3
	Vanguard DA$_2$	Parenteral	2
	Vanguard DA$_2$L	Parenteral	2
	Vanguard DA$_2$P	Parenteral	2, 3
	Vanguard DA$_2$MP	Parenteral	2, 3
	Vanguard DA$_2$PL	Parenteral	2, 3
	Vanguard 5	Parenteral	2, 3
	Vanguard 5L	Parenteral	2, 3
	Vanguard 5B	Parenteral	1, 2, 3
	Coughguard B	Parenteral	1
	Coughguard BP	Parenteral	1, 3
Pitman-Moore	Tissuvax 5	Parenteral	3
	Tissuvax 6	Parenteral	3
	Quantum 4	Parenteral	3
	Quantum 6	Parenteral	3
Schering	Intra-Trac-II	Intranasal	1, 3
Solvay	Galaxy DA$_2$L	Parenteral	2
	Galaxy DA$_2$PL	Parenteral	2, 3
	Galaxy 6-MPL	Parenteral	2, 3
	Galaxy 6-MHP	Parenteral	2, 3
	Galaxy 6-MHPL	Parenteral	2, 3
TechAmerica	Adenomune 7	Parenteral	2, 3
	Adenomune 7-L	Parenteral	2, 3
	Adenomune 5-L	Parenteral	2, 3
	Bronchicine	Parenteral	1

[a] Etiologic Agents: 1. Bordetella bronchiseptica 2. Canine adenovirus type 2 3. Parainfluenza virus

(Compiled by Christine Schultz R.Ph. and Jeff Ronngren R.Ph.)

C. Protection against the clinical signs of CAV-2 infection may be induced by the parenteral administration of vaccines containing either CAV-1 or CAV-2. Experimental use of an intranasal CAV-2 vaccine has proved effective in the face of maternal immunity, but a commercial product is not yet available.

SUGGESTED READINGS

Appel MJG: Canine infectious tracheobronchitis (kennel cough): a status report. Compend Contin Educ Pract Vet 3:70, 1981

Bemis DA, Appel MJG: Aerosol, parenteral, and oral antibiotic treatment of *Bordetella bronchiseptica* infections in dogs. J Am Vet Med Assoc 170:1082, 1977

Dhein CR, Gorham JR: Canine respiratory infections. p. 177. In Scott FW (ed): Contemporary Issues in Small Animal Practive. Vol. 3. Infectious Diseases. Churchill Livingstone, New York, 1986

Ott RL, Miller JB, Barrett RE: The respiratory system. p. 1035. In Catcott EJ (ed): Canine Medicine. 4th Ed. Vol 2. American Veterinary Publications Inc. Santa Barbara, 1979

Roudebush P, Fales W: Antibacterial susceptibility of *Bordetella bronchiseptica* isolates from small companion animals with respiratory disease. J Am Anim Hosp Assoc 17:793, 1981

Roudebush P: Antitussive therapy in small companion animals. J Am Vet Med Assoc 180:1105, 1982

Thayer GW: Canine infectious tracheobronchitis. p. 430. In Greene CE (ed): Clinical Microbiology and Infectious Diseases of the Dog and Cat. WB Saunders, Philadelphia, 1984

Thayer GW: Infections of the respiratory system. p. 238. In Greene CE (ed): Clinical Microbiology and Infectious Diseases of the Dog and Cat. WB Saunders, Philadelphia, 1984

13

Feline Respiratory Disease Complex

Rosalind M. Gaskell

This chapter covers those infectious diseases that predominantly affect the respiratory tract of cats, although they also commonly have ocular and oral components.

ETIOLOGY

I. The two major causes of respiratory disease in cats are two viruses: feline viral rhinotracheitis (FVR) virus, or felid herpesvirus-1 (FHV-1), and feline calicivirus (FCV). Both viruses are widespread throughout the world and are probably of equal importance in causing the disease. Together they probably account for at least 80% of cases.

II. The feline strain of *Chlamydia psittaci* (previously known as the feline pneumonitis agent) can also cause mild respiratory signs, but in general the major feature of *C. psittaci* infection is a marked persistent conjunctivitis.

III. Feline reovirus has been shown to produce a mild, predominantly conjunctival disease experimentally, but it is probably not a very significant cause of respiratory disease in the field.

IV. Bacteria, such as staphylococci, β hemolytic streptococci, *Pasteurella* spp. and coliforms, are probably important mainly as secondary invaders. The role of *Bordetella bronchiseptica,* which has been detected in some laboratory colonies, has yet to be determined.

V. *Mycoplasma* spp. are also probably important mainly as secondary invaders, although a more primary role, particularly for *Mycoplasma felis* in conjunctivitis, has been suggested by some. The significance of mycoplasmas is difficult to assess because of the frequency with which they are also isolated from apparently normal cats.

FHV-1 AND FCV INFECTIONS

Epizootiology

I. Both FHV-1 and FCV are highly successful pathogens of the cat: most animals tested prior to vaccination were shown to have neutralizing antibodies to both viruses.

II. Infection is generally less common in isolated household pets when compared with colony animals. Thus the disease occurs mainly in boarding colonies, breeding colonies, stray cat homes, or other situations in which a large number of cats have been brought together.

III. The feline respiratory viruses persist in such populations in three main ways:

   A. By passing directly from acutely infected to susceptible animals. This depends on the presence of a sufficient number of animals in the population and on sufficient opportunities for contact among them.

   B. By persisting in the environment. Although both viruses survive outside the cat for relatively short periods of time, it is nevertheless long enough for indirect transmission to occur, particularly within the close confines of a cattery.

   C. By persisting in the recovered cat by means of a carrier state. Such carriers are widespread in the population and are of considerable importance as a source of virus.

IV. There are no known reservoir or alternative hosts for the viruses, and vertical transmission does not generally seem to occur.

V. Because the carrier state probably is responsible in large part for the success of the feline respiratory viruses as pathogens, the features of each virus carrier state will be described more fully.

   A. Features of the FHV-1 carrier state (Fig. 13-1)

   1. This state is characterized by a latent phase, with only intermittent episodes of virus shedding in oronasal and conjunctival secretions.

   2. At least 80 percent of FHV-1 recovered cats remain as virus carriers. Approximately half of these cats are likely to be of epizootiologic importance (i.e., they will shed virus under natural conditions).

   3. Shedding may occur spontaneously but is most likely following stress (e.g., corticosteroid treatment; a change of housing, as upon entering a boarding cattery, or on going to a cat show, or to stud; or during lactation).

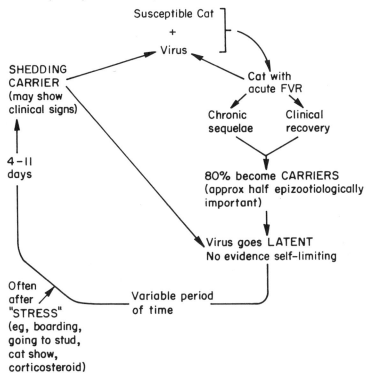

Fig. 13-1. Felid herpesvirus 1 (feline viral rhinotracheitis virus) carrier state: epizootiology. (Modified from Gaskell C, Gaskell R: Respiratory diseases of cats. Practice 2(6):5, 1980.)

4. Shedding does not occur immediately after the stress; there is a lag period of about 1 week, followed by a shedding episode lasting for up to 2 weeks. Therefore a carrier animal is likely to be infectious for about 3 weeks following stress.
5. Carriers may show mild clinical signs during the shedding episode.
6. There is no indication that the carrier state is self-limiting, although there is some evidence that animals are less likely to shed in the immediate few months after an episode.
7. The site of latency is probably the trigeminal ganglia, although other sites cannot be ruled out.
B. Features of the FCV carrier state (Fig. 13-2)

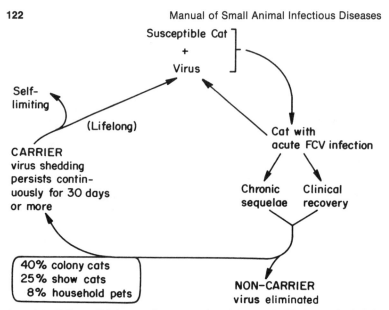

Fig. 13-2. Feline calicivirus carrier state: epizootiology. (Modified from Gaskell C, Gaskell R: Respiratory diseases of cats. Practice 2(6):5, 1980.)

1. Unlike FHV-1 carriers, FCV carriers shed virus more or less continuously.
2. A carrier has been defined as a cat that excretes FCV for at least 30 days after the acute infection.
3. Although in most cases, the FCV carrier state appears to be self-limiting at some point, in others it may be lifelong. In one group of cats studied, 50% of the animals were still shedding virus 75 days after infection. The decline was exponential, however, with some cats still shedding virus after 150 days.
4. Each carrier sheds a fairly constant amount of virus, which fluctuates around a mean for that individual. Carriers may be arbitrarily divided into high, medium, and low-level excreters. High-level shedders are highly infectious and easily detected upon swabbing. Low-level shedders are less infectious, and a series of swabs may be necessary to identify them.
5. Carriers of FCV are very widespread: a survey of 1,500 clinically healthy cats in the United Kingdom before vaccination showed that 40% of colony cats, 25% of cats at cat shows, and 8% of single household pets were shedding FCV.

      6. Virus persists in tonsil and other oropharyngeal tissues; unfortunately tonsillectomy does not terminate the carrier state.

VI. Thus, in breeding or boarding catteries respiratory virus infection often is introduced by the clinically normal carrier. Once enzootic, the disease is generally seen in the acute form in young kittens at the stage during which passive immunity is lost. In older cats the presence of FCV may be noted by the existence of chronically affected cats with persistent or recurrent rhinitis, sinusitis, or conjunctivitis.

VII. Transmission

    A. Transmission occurs mainly by direct cat-to-cat contact via infectious discharges. Both viruses are shed primarily in ocular, nasal, and oral secretions. Feline calicivirus may also be shed in urine and feces, but this is probably not of great epizootiologic significance.

    B. Indirect transmission via contaminated secretions on cages, feedbowls, cleaning utensils, personnel, etc. may also occur. However, the environment is not usually a long-term source of virus because both agents are relatively fragile outside the cat (FHV-1 survives for 1–2 days at most, FCV for 8–10 days).

    C. Aerosol transmission is not thought to be of major significance, although sneezing may propel macrodroplets a distance of several feet.

    D. Transmission is reduced where measures are taken to minimize external virus survival (e.g., optimal environmental temperature, low relative humidity, and adequate ventilation as by 15–20 air changes per hour). Disinfection is best achieved with hypochlorite and/or quaternary ammonium compounds.

    E. Transmission efficacy depends on the amount of virus shed by the infecting animal and the duration and intimacy of contact. Transmission is more easily achieved by animals in the acute phase of the disease, although carriers are also undoubtedly of importance, particularly in view of the close contact that occurs in colonies.

Clinical Signs

The natural route of infection of the feline respiratory viruses is intranasal, oral, or conjunctival; experimentally, other routes have also been investigated. The incubation period is typically 2–6 days, although it may be longer. A higher infecting dose can lead to a shorter incubation period and more severe clinical signs.

I. Feline viral rhinotracheitis
   A. There is only one serotype of FHV-1 known. Although different biotypes may exist, most naturally occurring strains are of generally uniform pathogenicity.
   B. Characteristic features of the disease include:
      1. Early signs of depression, sneezing, inappetance, pyrexia, and sometimes hypersalivation.
      2. Subsequent development of ocular and nasal discharges, often conjunctivitis, and sometimes dyspnea and coughing.
      3. Usually, leukocytosis with a left shift.
      4. More rarely, ulcerative or interstitial keratitis.
      5. Occasionally, lingual ulcers (much more common with FCV infection).
      6. Rarely, other signs, including skin ulcers, primary viral pneumonia, and neurologic signs.
      7. Occasionally, generalized disease in young or immunosuppressed animals.
      8. Abortion, but only as a result of severe debilitating disease and not as a direct effect of the virus itself.
   C. The mortality rate usually is not high, except occasionally in young kittens. Fatalities are usually due to dehydration and secondary bacterial infection.
   D. Resolution usually requires 2–3 weeks, although severe necrosis of the mucous membranes may lead to chronic rhinitis and sinusitis.
   E. Persistent or recurrent signs may also follow recurrent virus shedding in carriers.
II. Feline calicivirus infection.
   A. A number of different strains of FCV exist, which differ in virulence and pathogenicity. However, most are sufficiently closely related antigenically to be considered as a single serotype.
   B. Feline calicivirus infection is typically milder than FVR; however, the large number of strains can cause a spectrum of disease ranging from a more severe syndrome similar to that seen in FVR to subclinical infection.
   C. Certain features may be helpful in differentiating FCV infection from FVR (Table 13-1):
      1. Typically the disease is milder, with little general malaise.
      2. Only mild sneezing and conjunctivitis usually are present.
      3. Ocular and nasal discharges are less prominent.

TABLE 13-1.   A COMPARISON OF THE ESSENTIAL FEATURES OF RESPIRATORY INFECTIONS IN CATS

	Feline Viral Rhinotracheitis	Feline Calicivirus Infection	Feline *Chlamydia psittaci* Infection
General malaise	+ + +	+	+
Sneezing	+ + +	+	+
Conjunctivitis	+ +	+	+ + +*
Hypersalivation	+ +	–	–
Ocular discharge	+ + +	+ +	+ + +
Nasal discharge	+ + +	+ +	+
Oral ulceration	+	+ + +	–
Keratitis	+	–	+

* Often persistent.

4. No hypersalivation or keratitis occurs.
5. Oral ulceration is a frequent and characteristic feature and may be the only clinical sign.
6. Ulcers usually occur on the tongue and hard palate, but erosions may also be seen on the lips and nose. Occasionally lesions may occur elsewhere on the skin (e.g., the paws).
7. Some strains can produce an interstitial pneumonia.
8. Some strains can cause pyrexia, muscle pain, and limping that is unassociated with respiratory signs.

Diagnosis

I. To a large extent FCV infection and FVR may be distinguished on presenting clinical signs. Table 13-1 summarizes the essential features of each condition and includes feline chlamydial infection as a differential. The latter should always be suspected where there is persistent or recurrent conjunctivitis.

II. Diagnosis may be confirmed by isolation of the agent in feline cell cultures. Oropharyngeal swabs should be sent to the laboratory in specialized viral transport media. Samples should be taken ideally within 1 week of the onset of clinical signs.

Treatment

I. No antiviral drugs for these conditions are in widespread use. However, idoxuridine (Stoxil, Smith Kline & French; Herplex, Allergan; others) has been used for ulcerative keratitis in FVR, and it is possible that other antiherpesvirus drugs such as acyclovir (Zovirax, Wellcome), which has been used successfully in other species, may find application in FVR.

II. Use of a broad-spectrum antibiotic is indicated for at least 1 week to control secondary bacterial infection. Pediatric syrups may be helpful. Reexamination after 1 week is indicated; bacterial culture and sensitivity testing should be performed if purulent discharges are still present.

III. Multivitamin supportive therapy may be helpful in aiding mucosal regeneration.

IV. Corticosteroids are contraindicated because they retard the healing process and may potentiate the virus infection.

V. Nebulizers and steam inhalation to clear airways are better tolerated by cats than are nasal decongestants.

VI. Subcutaneous or IV fluid therapy may be indicated for dehydration. In severe or prolonged cases of anorexia and dehydration, a pharyngostomy tube may be useful.

VII. Aromatic and strongly flavored foods should be offered because affected cats may lose their sense of smell. Baby food or liquidized food may be helpful when oral ulceration makes eating painful. The food may also be diluted with water if there is dehydration.

VIII. Good nursing care is essential and is best given by the owner. Hospital intensive care requires scrupulous attention to hygiene to prevent cross-infection.

Prevention

I. The prevention and control of feline respiratory disease should be approached through a combination of vaccination and management.

II. A number of vaccines (modified-live and inactivated parenteral and modified-live intranasal) are available for protection of cats against the feline respiratory viruses.

III. In general these vaccines are relatively successful in preventing viral respiratory disease in the majority of healthy, previously unexposed cats. Ideally, vaccination of the entire cat population should be the aim.

IV. Nevertheless, because of the epizootiology of the disease vaccine reactions and breakdowns may occur from time to time (see below); thus management procedures are still necessary in many cases to aid in controlling the disease.

V. Different individual circumstances may require different approaches to prevention and control, as outlined below.

A. Household pet
   1. Pets are most likely to be exposed after entering a boarding cattery or veterinary hospital.
   2. Stress and social contact should be avoided (i.e., pet is best cared for at home when the owner is on vacation).
   3. Pets should be vaccinated routinely and with an extra booster if a boarding situation is unavoidable.

B. Boarding cattery
   1. All cats should be vaccinated. However, cattery owners should not rely on this alone because virus will often be present in the cattery both in cats incubating the disease and in carriers.
   2. Measures should therefore still be taken to prevent cross-infection within the cattery, as outlined in Table 13-2.

C. Stray cat homes
   1. The same guidelines given for boarding catteries apply, but often it is difficult to separate animals to the same extent. However, animals should be segregated or batched and quarantined as far as possible and those with clinical signs kept apart.
   2. Unless animals can be isolated on arrival for 3–4 weeks, parenteral vaccines may not have sufficient time to become effective. In these circumstances the intranasal route may be preferable because protection has been shown to develop within 4 days following such vaccination.

D. Breeding colonies (disease-free)
   1. All cats should be vaccinated routinely if there is any contact, direct or indirect, with other cats.
   2. Inactivated vaccines are preferable although, with care, modified-live products should be satisfactory.
   3. Care should be taken to avoid entry of carriers (i.e., *any* cat with a history of association with respiratory disease).
   4. All incoming cats should be quarantined for 3 weeks and, ideally, screened virologically and if not previously vaccinated, also serologically.

E. Breeding colonies (disease enzootic)

TABLE 13-2. RECOMMENDATIONS TO PREVENT THE SPREAD OF RESPIRATORY VIRUSES IN A BOARDING CATTERY

1. Be sure all incoming cats are fully vaccinated.

2. Cats should be housed individually unless they are from the same household.

3. The cattery should be constructed with solid partitions between pens. Ensure that frontages are at least 1.5 m apart and that the surface of the pens is easily washable.

4. Arrange pens so that food bowls and litter pans can be routinely removed without entering each pen (i.e., avoid handling cats more than is necessary).

5. Either hands should be washed in a bucket of disinfectant solution between visits to each pen, or individual pairs of rubber gloves kept on a peg beside each pen should be worn and used only for that particular pen. Gloves should be thoroughly disinfected before use with a new boarder.

6. Rubber boots should be worn and, if it is necessary to enter the pen, a disinfectant bath should be provided.

7. Either use disposable food bowls or have two sets of bowls for use on alternate days. In the latter case, the used set should be soaked in a 1:32 bleach/detergent solution for several hours, then thoroughly rinsed and dried before reuse 24 hours later.

8. Food should be prepared in a central area.

9. Badly soiled litter pans should be replaced by pans previously disinfected and prefilled in a central area (i.e., a similar system to that for food bowls should be employed).

10. After a boarder has gone home, the cage should be thoroughly disinfected, allowed to dry, and preferably left empty for 2 days before reuse.

11. Any cats with signs of previous respiratory infection (e.g., ocular discharge, chronic rhinitis), cats known to have had respiratory disease, and cats suspected from past experience of being carriers should be placed in one separate section or at the end of the cattery and fed last.

12. Cats should be fed in the same order every day. Each pen should be attended to completely before moving on to the next.

13. The concentration of virus in the environment should be reduced by adequate ventilation, low relative humidity, and optimal ambient temperature.

(Modified from Gaskell RM, Wardley RC: Feline viral respiratory disease: a review with particular reference to its epizootiology and control. J Small Anim Pract 19:1, 1978.)

1. In some circumstances it may be feasible to eliminate the virus by hand rearing kittens in isolation and, with a barrier system, to maintain a virus-free colony. The feline respiratory viruses are very widespread, however, and with most domestic situations reinfection is quite possible despite vaccination.
2. Thus in most situations it is best to try and control the disease by the following measures:
   a) Regular vaccination programs
   b) Booster-vaccinating queens either prior to mating, or during pregnancy (inactivated vaccine only)
   c) Maintaining cats in as stress-free an environment as possible
   d) Avoiding the use of particular queens with a history of respiratory disease in their kittens
   e) Moving queens into isolation at least 3 weeks before term so that kittens are not exposed to carriers in the colony and any shedding episode from the queen resulting from the move will be over before kittening
   f) Weaning kittens early (e.g., at 4–5 weeks) into isolation away from their mother if it is likely that she herself is a carrier
   g) Vaccinating all kittens as soon as maternal antibodies are at a noninterfering level (normally 9–10 weeks) and certainly before exposure to any other cats
   h) Earlier vaccination schedules (e.g., starting at 6 weeks with parenteral vaccines or possibly by using the intranasal route in very young kittens in whom maternal antibody is still present)

VI. Vaccine reactions and breakdowns

There are a number of possible reasons for these, the major points being listed below.

A. Vaccine reactions

1. The most likely cause is that the animal is already incubating the disease; vaccination programs are, of course, generally implemented in kittens just when their maternal antibody has waned.
2. The cat may already be a field virus carrier, and although the effect of vaccinating carriers is not clear, they are undoubtedly still of importance both to themselves and to other cats as sources of infectious virus. It is also possible that for FVR, the mild "stress" of vaccination and the attendant disruption of routine may initiate an episode of virus shedding.

3. Ideally, vaccine virus should be attenuated so that it does not itself cause disease. Nevertheless, there may be one or two individuals in whom this is not so. This may be due to individual idiosyncrasy, to intercurrent disease (e.g., with feline leukemia virus or panleukopenia virus), or perhaps to variations in microbial flora.

4. However, it does also seem that, even in apparently normal cats, modified-live vaccines given by the intranasal route may produce mild signs of disease.

5. In contrast, live parenteral vaccines should be safe if administered properly, but there have been suggestions that if they are inadvertently given by an incorrect route (e.g., by making an aerosol with a syringe, or by the cat's licking the injection site), signs of respiratory disease might develop.

B. Vaccine breakdowns

1. First, it should be emphasized that although the feline upper respiratory disease vaccines generally are effective in the majority of cases, even under ideal conditions protection is not necessarily complete in all animals.

2. Factors that may adversely affect an individual's immune response include: intercurrent disease; overwhelming challenge dose of virus; maternal antibody interference with the initial vaccination program. Infection with other respiratory pathogens (e.g., chlamydiae) or a variant strain of calicivirus may also occur.

3. In colonies with enzootic disease, breakdowns may occur relatively commonly. There are two main reasons for this. The first is the variable and sometimes short duration of passive immunity (particularly with FHV-1), which often leads to outbreaks of disease in young kittens. The second is that carriers are widespread in such colonies and represent a continual source of virus.

4. It is important to note also that although vaccinated animals generally are free from disease, they are not necessarily free from infection; such cats may already have been carriers before vaccination or may have become infected subclinically afterwards. Clearly, carriers may be of considerable epizootiologic importance, particularly in colonies wherein close contact encourages transmission.

FELINE *CHLAMYDIA PSITTACI* INFECTION

Epizootiology

I. Although at one time, feline *Chlamydia psittaci* infection was thought to be confined to North America, there is now evidence of this infection from Europe and Australia.

II. Although many species of animals and birds are susceptible to *C. psittaci* infection, there are a variety of strains of the organism with different tropisms, pathogenicity, and host specificity.

III. Thus, the feline strain, for example, is generally species-specific, and although there are isolated reports of its possible involvement in cases of human conjunctivitis, this would not normally appear to be a problem. The only animal species from which isolates of *C. psittaci* appear to have a clearly established zoonotic potential are birds and sheep.

IV. Chlamydiae, like the feline respiratory viruses, are relatively unstable outside their host, being inactivated by a number of lipid solvents and detergents.

V. Like the feline respiratory viruses, chlamydial infection is probably transmitted primarily by direct or fomite contact with infectious discharges, and possibly over short distances by aerosol.

VI. The organism is shed predominantly in ocular secretions. Following experimental infection, however, chlamydiae have also been detected for several months in vaginal and rectal swabs. The clinical and epizootiologic significance of this is not known.

VII. Once the infection is enzootic in a colony, clinical signs may persist in some individuals for weeks, and recurrent episodes are common. It has been suggested that some of these recurrent episodes may be induced by stress.

VIII. Thus, natural immunity to the disease appears to be relatively inefficient and incomplete, and infection appears to be perpetuated in a colony situation for some months, if not for years.

Clinical Signs

I. The original term *feline pneumonitis* for feline *C. psittaci* infection is really a misnomer because the predominant clinical sign is a persistent conjunctivitis.

  II. In the acute stages there are blepharospasm and marked serous and mucopurulent discharges; the conjunctivae are reddened and swollen.

  III. Initially only one eye may be affected, but usually both eyes eventually become involved.

  IV. Mild nasal discharge, sneezing, and coughing may also occur.

  V. Mild pulmonary lesions may be detected occasionally at necropsy, but pneumonitis is not usually apparent clinically.

  VI. In more severe cases follicular hyperplasia of the conjunctival lymphoid tissue has been reported, and corneal ulceration and keratitis have been described; however, the possibility that other agents may be involved in such cases should be considered.

  VII. The conjunctivitis may persist for up to 6 weeks or so; although most animals eventually recover, recurrent episodes may occur.

  VIII. Experimentally, there is some evidence that chlamydiae may infect the genital tract of cats, but the relevance of this to the field situation is not known.

Diagnosis

  I. Chlamydial infection may be diagnosed to a large extent on the characteristic clinical signs, specifically a persistent conjunctivitis (Table 13-1).

  II. Another aid in differentiation between chlamydial and viral infection of the respiratory tract is that chlamydial infection may respond to certain antibiotics (see below).

  III. Diagnosis may be confirmed in untreated cases by the following approaches:

    A. A conjunctival scraping may be directly examined for the presence of inclusion bodies.

    B. More reliably, an attempt may be made to isolate the organism in cell culture from a vigorous conjunctival swab. Chlamydiae are intracellular parasites, and it is important that epithelial cells be present in the sample. Specialized transport media are required, and either rapid transport to the laboratory or $-70°C$ storage before collection.

  IV. In unvaccinated cats a positive serologic response (complement fixation test, or more reliably, indirect immunofluorescence) may also be helpful in diagnosis.

V. Recently, diagnostic test kits for human chlamydial infection have become available and some appear to be reasonably effective in detecting feline chlamydial infections as well.

Treatment

I. Although several antibiotics may have some effect on relieving the clinical signs of chlamydial infection, tetracyclines remain the drugs of choice.

II. There is no evidence that systemic tetracycline therapy is more effective than topical therapy, but in severe cases both routes of treatment may be indicated.

III. Oxytetracycline is more effective than chlortetracycline, the latter being unstable and requiring very frequent application.

IV. Erythromycin and tylosin may also be used and should replace systemic tetracyclines in pregnant queens and young kittens.

V. Treatment should continue for 4 weeks or at least 2 weeks after clinical signs have disappeared.

Prevention

I. Because chlamydial infection is thought to be transmitted in a manner similar to that for the feline respiratory viruses, similar control measures to stop the spread of infection should apply.

II. Because persistent or recurrent infection in a colony situation is common, it is important to treat all individuals in a cattery at the same time.

III. Vaccination against feline *C. psittaci* infection has been employed in the United States for some years, although there has been some discussion as to the efficacy of the vaccines. However, more recent studies have demonstrated significant (although not necessarily complete) protection against the disease and, in some studies, a reduced period of chlamydial shedding. Protection appears to last for at least 1 year.

SUGGESTED READINGS

FHV-1 and FCV Infections

Crandell RA: Feline viral rhinotracheitis (FVR). Adv Vet Sci Comp Med 17:201, 1973

Gaskell RM: An assessment of the use of feline respiratory virus vaccines. Vet Ann 21:267, 1981

Gaskell RM: Viral-induced upper respiratory tract disease. p. 257. Chandler EA, Gaskell CJ, Hilbery ADR (eds): Feline Medicine and Therapeutics. Blackwell Scientific Publications, Oxford, 1985

Gaskell RM, Wardley RC: Feline viral respiratory disease: a review with particular reference to its epizootiology and control. J Small Anim Pract 19:1, 1978

Gillespie JH, Scott FW: Feline viral infections. Adv Vet Sci Comp Med 17:163, 1973

Kahn DE, Hoover EA: Infectious respiratory diseases of cats. Vet Clin North Am 6:399, 1976

Lane JG: Pharyngostomy intubation of the dog and cat. Vet Annual 17:164, 1977

Povey RC: Feline respiratory disease—which vaccine? Feline Pract 7(5):12, 1977

Povey RC: A review of feline viral rhinotracheitis (feline herpesvirus I infection). Comp Immunol Microbiol Infect Dis 2:373, 1979

Scott FW: Virucidal disinfectants and feline viruses. Am J Vet Res 41:410, 1980

Feline *Chlamydia Psittaci* Infection

Cello RM: Microbiological and immunologic aspects of feline pneumonitis. J Am Vet Med Ass 158:932, 1971

Cello RM: Clues to differential diagnosis of feline respiratory infections. J Am Vet Med Ass 158:968, 1971

Hoover EA, Kahn DE, Langloss JM: Experimentally induced feline chlamydial infection (feline pneumonitis). Am J Vet Res 39:541, 1978

Kolar JR,, Rude TA: Duration of immunity in cats inoculated with a commercial feline pneumonitis vaccine. Vet Med Small Anim Clin 76:1171, 1981

Mitzel JR, Strating A: Vaccination against feline pneumonitis. Am J Vet Res 38:1361, 1977

Shewen PE, Povey RC, Wilson MR: Feline chlamydial infection. Can Vet J 19:289, 1978

Shewen PE, Povey RC, Wilson MR: A comparison of the efficacy of a live and four inactivated vaccine preparations for the protection of cats against experimental challenge with *Chlamydia psittaci*. Can J Comp Med 44:244, 1980

Studdert MJ, Studdert VP, Wirth HJ: Isolation of *Chlamydia psittaci* from cats with conjunctivitis. Aust Vet J 57:515, 1981

Wills, J., Gruffydd-Jones, TJ, Richmond S, Paul ID: Isolation of *Chlamydia psittaci* from cases of conjunctivitis in a colony of cats. Vet Rec 114:344, 1984

Wills JM, Gaskell RM: Feline chlamydial infection (feline pneumonitis). p. 304. Chandler EA, Gaskell CJ, Hilbery ADR (eds): Feline Medicine and Therapeutics. Blackwell Scientific Publications, Oxford, 1985

Wills JM, Gruffydd-Jones TJ, Bourne FJ, et al: Effect of vaccination on conjunctivitis due to feline *Chlamydia psittaci*. p. 416. In Chlamydial Infections: Proceedings 6th International Symposium on Human Chlamydial Infections, Cambridge University Press, 1986

14

Canine Transmissible Venereal Tumor

E. Gregory MacEwen

ETIOLOGY

I. Transmissible venereal tumor (TVT) is a naturally occurring tumor in the canine population, usually affecting the external genitalia and usually transmitted at coitus. The development of the TVT as a coitally transmitted neoplasm in the dog is probably facilitated by some unique characteristic of sexual intercourse in this species, which leads to injury of the vaginal and penile mucosae, providing a bed for tumor transplantation. Transmission of TVT occurs by transplantation of viable tumor cells from either sex to a susceptible host. The tumor has been reported to occur in most parts of the world but appears to be more prevalent in temperate climates. It is seen most often in young, roaming, sexually active dogs. Although metastasis has been reported, it is considered to be quite uncommon.

II. Transmissible venereal tumors are naturally transplanted tumors derived from a common origin; these tumors apparently have a cellular mode of transmission and have been maintained in the canine population of the world for many generations. This information is supported by karyotype studies, histocompatibility surface antigen studies, and labeled autoradiographic studies. Special staining and evaluation of TVT cell mitotic figures have demonstrated that most cells have a stemline chromosome number of 59 (range 57–64). Of these 59 chromosomes, 16 or 17 are metacentric and 43 or 42 acrocentric. These constant and highly specific chromosome aberrations are regarded as supportive of the cellular mechanism of transmission. The tumor consists of undifferentiated round cells, which are loosely packed and are believed to be of reticuloendothelial origin.

137

III. A viral etiology has been investigated but not verified. Virus particles have been observed but the tumor has not been transmitted by cell-free infiltrates. The TVT can be transmitted experimentally to other dogs. When injected into an adult dog, approximately 80% of tumors will regress within 180 days. When injected into very young dogs, the tumors will progress and fail to undergo any regression.

IV. It has been shown that the same histocompatibility complex (DL-A) antigens are expressed on the surface of TVT cells originating from different dogs from different locations.

V. The TVT possesses a tumor-associated antigen, as determined by immunodiffusion and enzyme-linked immunosorbent assay (ELISA), and the immune response plays a major role in inhibiting growth and spread of the neoplasm. The anti-TVT immune response is mounted, at least in part, against DL-A. Regression of the tumor is followed by development of immunity to subsequent reinfection. In addition, passive transfer of post-regression serum can inhibit the growth of experimentally transplanted tumors and can prevent the development of tumors if administered prior to transplantation.

VI. It has been observed that animals with a large TVT burden develop polycythemia and that TVT extracts contain erythropoietin. Thus, TVT cells probably synthesize and secrete erythropoietin.

CLINICAL SIGNS

I. Most cases of naturally occurring TVT are confined to the external genitalia. In the vagina TVTs may range in size from 0.5 mm to over 10 cm in diameter. They are usually cauliflower-like in appearance, friable, and flesh-colored. Areas of necrosis with superficial bacterial infection frequently are present, and hemorrhage is common.

II. In the male a serosanguineous discharge from the prepuce is often the presenting clinical sign. The TVTs are frequently located around the glans of the penis and therefore require total extension of the penis for visualization. Extremely large tumor masses may preclude total extension. These tumors can also be multicentric along the shaft of the penis and tend to be quite friable.

III. Transmissible venereal tumors have also been reported in the oral cavity, skin, sclera, and the anterior chamber. Intranasal TVTs frequently cause epistaxis and sneezing.

IV. In general, most TVTs will be localized to one particular area, especially the genitalia. They may metastasize to regional lymph nodes (inguinal and iliac), and in a few cases metastasis has been seen in the spleen, liver, brain, pituitary gland, and the lungs. Transmissible venereal tumors may also involve extragential sites owing to autotransplantation (e.g., by licking).

DIAGNOSIS

I. Histologically the TVT is composed of round, oval, or polyhedral cells. There is a large nuclear to cytoplasmic ratio. Nuclei show prominent chromatin clumping and usually contain a large nucleolus. Mitotic figures are common. Cytologically, the TVT has a very distinctive appearance: the cells appear round to oval, mitotic figures are common, and chromatin clumping and one or two prominent nuclei are obvious. Perhaps the most striking cytologic finding is the presence of multiple clear cytoplasmic vacuoles, frequently arranged in chains. The cytologic appearance of TVT is not readily confused with that of other neoplasms, such as mast cell tumors, histiocytomas, or malignant lymphomas.

II. Some oral TVTs have been misdiagnosed as amelanotic melanoma or poorly differentiated sarcoma. In some cases it is easier to make a definitive diagnosis by cytology than by histology. If one suspects that a tumor may be a TVT, it is advisable to make impression smears at the time of biopsy. In many cases cytologic examination may be more diagnostic than histopathologic examination.

TREATMENT

I. Transmissible venereal tumors will respond to many forms of therapy. Animals have been successfully treated by surgical excision, radiation therapy, chemotherapy, and immunotherapy. Surgery can be an effective therapy for small, localized TVTs. Usually, the TVT is too extensive for an adequate surgical excision, however, and other therapies must be considered. Another problem with surgical excision has been the high rate of recurrence associated with this treatment modality.

II. Radiation therapy is also effective in treating TVT. Radiation has been used both as a primary mode of therapy and following surgical failure or failure of both surgery and chemotherapy. Dosage recommendations range from 15 Gray divided over 5 days to 45 Gray divided over 3 weeks.

III. Chemotherapy appears to be the most effective treatment modality for TVT. A number of agents have been evaluated, including cyclophosphamide (Cytoxan, Bristol-Myers Oncology), vincristine (Oncovin, Lilly), methotrexate (Lederle), and doxorubicin (Adriamycin, Adria). Vincristine is reported to be one of the most effective agents in treating the TVT and can be given at a dosage of 0.5–0.7 mg/m^2 IV once weekly. An average of four to six treatments will be necessary to induce a complete remission. Complete cure can be expected in 90% of the cases treated. Another drug with significant activity against TVT is doxorubicin, which can be given at a dosage of 30 mg/m^2 IV every 21 days. It will usually take two courses of therapy with doxorubicin to induce a complete remission.

IV. Immunotherapy has been used experimentally to treat TVTs. Agents such as Bacillus Calmette-Guérin (BCG) and BCG cell walls, as well as immunoabsorption techniques, have been evaluated. Although responses have been noted with these treatments, the results have been inconsistent and recurrences more frequent. To date the use of immunotherapy must be considered investigational and certainly not as effective as chemotherapy.

PREVENTION

Because transmission of the disease requires direct transplantation of tumor cells from an infected dog to a susceptible host, avoiding exposure to infected dogs is required for disease prevention.

SUGGESTED READINGS

Brown NO, Calvert C, MacEwen EG: Chemotherapeutic management of transmissible venereal tumors in 30 dogs. J Am Vet Med Assoc 176:983, 1980

Calvert CA, Leifer CE, MacEwen EG: Vincristine for treatment of transmissible venereal tumor in the dog. J Am Vet Med Assoc 181:163, 1982

Cohen D: The transmissible venereal tumor of the dog—a naturally occurring allograft? Is J Med Sci 14:14, 1978

Cohen D: The canine transmissible venereal tumor: a unique result of tumor progression. Adv Cancer Res 43:75, 1985

Richardson RC: Canine transmissible venereal tumor. Compend Contin Ed Pract Vet 3:951, 1981

Yang TJ, Jones JB: Canine transmissible venereal sarcoma: transplantation studies in neonatal and adult dogs. JNCI 51:1915, 1973

15

Leptospirosis

Dawn Merton Boothe
George E. Lees

ETIOLOGY

I. All pathogenic leptospires are classified as *Leptospira interrogans.* This species includes 16 serogroups and more than 150 serovars. Conventionally, the species name is deleted when serovars are discussed.

II. Hosts

   A. Generally each serovar is enzootic in one or more wildlife hosts, which provide for the survival and transmission of the agent and become long-term carriers for it. Any mammal probably can be infected by any serovar, and a serovar may adapt to infect one or more animal species in a particular region.

   B. Primary reservoirs are mammalian wildlife hosts, particularly rodents. The dog is the natural carrier host for *Leptospira canicola* and *Leptospira bataviae* and serves as an accidental host for several other serovars.

   1. *Leptospira icterohaemorrhagiae* and *L. canicola* are the serovars most often isolated from dogs. *L. canicola* predominates in some canine populations, while *L. icterohaemorrhagiae* predominates in stray dogs. *Leptospira pomona* has been isolated from rural dogs, while *Leptospira grippotyphosa* and *Leptospira ballum* have been isolated from urban dogs. Other leptospires that have been isolated from dogs include *Leptospira australis, Leptospira autumnalis,* and *L. bataviae.*

   2. Serologic studies have found that approximately 5% of household dogs and 18–37% of stray dogs react in agglutination testing. However, the occurrence of clinical disease in dogs is much less than the prevalence of positive serologic results.

   3. Leptospires that have been identified in the cat include *L. bataviae, L. canicola, L. grippotyphosa,* and *L. pomona.*

III. Transmission

A. Initial exposure usually occurs by contact with water contaminated with leptospires that have been excreted in the urine of infected animals.

B. Transmission between animals may occur by direct contact, venereal and placental transfer, bite wounds, or ingestion of infected meat.

C. Indirect transmission may occur via fomites such as vegetation, soil, food, water, and bedding.

D. Leptospires have been isolated from invertebrates and nonmammalian vertebrates, but the role of these animals in transmission is not known.

IV. Distribution

A. Distribution is worldwide. Leptospires survive for several weeks under optimal conditions, which include a warm, wet environment and neutral or slightly alkaline (but not salt) water. Leptospires can survive in cold, but not freezing, water.

B. Accidental host infections

1. These are numerous throughout the year in tropical and subtropical regions.

2. They also occur in arid regions around water holes with high animal concentrations.

3. They occur in a seasonal pattern in temperate regions (such as the United States), where the incidence is higher in summer and early fall and infection is more common in southern states.

V. Disinfectant susceptibility includes iodine-based disinfectants.

CLINICAL SIGNS

I. Pathogenesis

A. Susceptible animals become infected through the mucous membranes or abraded skin. Local irritation does not occur at the site of penetration. Organisms invade vascular spaces and multiply rapidly.

B. Leptospiremia peaks after 4–12 days in natural infections and is associated with pyrexia. Internal organs are also invaded during this acute stage.

C. Pathologic lesions and clinical signs depend on virulence of the organism and on host susceptibility, which vary with the infecting serovar and with numerous other factors.

      1. Bacterial toxins that interfere with cell metabolism probably produce tissue necrosis and mediate virulence, but these toxins have not yet been identified.

      2. *L. canicola* and *L. icterohaemorrhagiae* are the serovars that produce the most severe signs in dogs.

      3. *L. pomona* usually causes subclinical infections and a chronic carrier state in dogs.

      4. Young dogs, particularly those without maternal antibodies or adequate immunization, are more susceptible to severe disease. Older dogs with an adequate antibody titer are minimally affected.

      5. Clinical disease is rare in cats.

  D. Recovery is characterized by increasing levels of neutralizing antibodies and decreasing numbers of organisms in the circulation, beginning as early as 7–8 days postinfection. The speed of recovery depends upon the extent of organ invasion.

  E. Localized infections may occur in renal, ocular, or genital tissues, where the organisms can persist despite the development of circulating antibodies. Localization depends upon host/serovar adaptation.

      1. Leptospires colonize renal tubules, leading to long-term shedding of the organism in the urine of natural hosts. Periodic pyrexia may result.

      2. In accidental hosts localization is transient, and shedding of the organisms does not occur.

  F. Natural infection in the cat is rare, and clinical signs usually are mild or inapparent even when leptospiremia, leptospiruria, and histopathologic changes in the kidney and liver can be documented.

II. Pathology

  A. The kidneys frequently are affected. *L. canicola* has the greatest potential for causing renal damage.

      1. Leptospires in renal tubular cells may not stimulate antibody production; consequently, infected animals may shed organisms for 1–3 years and remain seronegative.

      2. Organisms can also persist and multiply in renal tubular epithelial cells despite the production of antibodies.

      3. Spontaneous recovery may also occur.

  B. The liver is another major organ damaged during leptospiremia. *L. icterohaemorrhagiae* may cause hepatic necrosis and icterus more often than other serovars. *L. grippotyphosa* has been reported to cause chronic active hepatitis.

    C. Infection of miscellaneous organs may result in meningitis, uveitis, or possibly abortion.

    D. Necropsy findings depend upon the stage of disease in which death occurred.

        1. Acute changes may include focal oral ulcerations; tonsillar enlargement; an edematous respiratory tract; enlarged, pale kidneys; and an enlarged, friable liver with pronounced interlobar markings.

        2. Chronic changes may include shrunken, fibrotic kidneys and hepatic fibrosis.

III. Clinical course

    A. Peracute infections are characterized by pyrexia and generalized muscle tenderness, followed by vomiting, rapid dehydration, and peripheral vascular collapse. Renal failure and hepatic failure do not have time to develop in terminal cases. Vascular injury and disseminated intravascular coagulopathy (DIC) contribute to hemorrhage.

    B. Subacute infections

        1. Subacute infections are characterized by fever, anorexia, vomiting, and dehydration. Reluctance to move may be caused by muscular, meningeal, or renal inflammation.

        2. Vascular and platelet damage may cause widespread petechial and ecchymotic hemorrhages.

        3. The severity and outcome of subacute infections usually correlate with the degree of renal insufficiency. Azotemia usually occurs 4 days after infection and progressively increases with the severity of clinical illness. Renal function may deteriorate to oliguria or anuria, or it may return to normal in 2–3 weeks.

        4. Icterus may develop during *L. icterohaemorrhagiae* infections because of hepatic inflammation and intrahepatic cholestasis. Chronic hepatic fibrosis and liver failure may also develop.

    C. Chronic or subclinical infections

        1. Most canine infections are chronic or subclinical.

        2. A diagnosis of chronic leptospirosis should be investigated in dogs with fever or anterior uveitis of unknown origin.

IV. Clinical pathology

    A. Hematologic changes usually include an initial leukopenia, followed by leukocytosis with a left shift and an increased erythrocyte sedimentation rate.

    B. Biochemical changes depend upon the stage and severity of disease and upon the organs affected.

1. Renal involvement produces increased serum concentrations of blood urea nitrogen and creatinine.
2. Hepatic involvement causes an increase in serum alanine aminotransferase and serum aspartate aminotransferase activities. Intrahepatic cholestasis produces increased alkaline phosphatase activity and serum bilirubin concentration. Prolonged sulfobromophthalein clearance may precede hyperbilirubinemia.
3. Electrolyte and acid-base alterations will parallel the severity of renal and gastrointestinal dysfunction.

C. Coagulation abnormalities may be caused by direct damage to vascular tissue or platelets or by DIC. Coagulopathies are most likely to develop during infection with *L. icterohaemorrhagiae*.

D. Urinalysis may reflect renal disease (cylindruria, pyuria, hematuria, proteinuria, and/or altered specific gravity) or liver disease (bilirubinuria).

DIAGNOSIS

I. Culture
   A. Leptospires are aerobic organisms and require media containing serum or serum components for growth.
   B. The use of isolation and culture as a practical method of diagnosis is limited by the fastidious nature and slow growth of the organisms, as well as by their susceptibility to adverse environmental conditions. Proper timing and technique are essential to successful recovery.
   C. Selection of the appropriate tissues for isolation efforts is determined by the stage of disease. Dogs are leptospiremic in the first weeks of infection, but circulating organisms decrease as the antibody titer rises. Consequently, leptospires are best cultured from the blood during the acute stage of disease and from the urine after this stage is over.
      1. Kidney and liver tissue, blood, and aqueous humor should be collected from clinical and expired cases.
      2. Urine and kidney tissue should be collected from suspected carriers.
   D. Body fluids should be diluted with appropriate culture or transport media [1% bovine serum albumin (BSA) or polysorbate 80 media] at 1:10 dilution or 0.25–0.75 ml body fluid to 10 ml media. Dilution is necessary to negate the effects of natural inhibitors.

1. Blood specimens should be placed directly in the transport medium or may be heparinized prior to dilution.
2. Multiple urine samples should be collected. Cystocentesis is the preferred collection method because the number of bacterial contaminants that might overgrow the leptospires is reduced. Some sources suggest midstream collection of a second voided specimen following administration of furosemide. Alkalinization of the urine specimen may enhance survival of the organism.
3. Tissues should be placed aseptically in 100 ml of 1% BSA, homogenized for 1 minute and then diluted as described above.

    E. Overgrowth of contaminants can be minimized by using specimens obtained antemortem rather than postmortem.

II. Serology

    A. Titers should be interpreted in conjunction with the clinical signs and laboratory data. Titers usually peak 3–4 weeks following infection. Decline is gradual and animals may remain positive for months to years.

    B. The microscopic agglutination (MA) test is the method most frequently used for serologic diagnosis. Reactions are specific; therefore, several serovars must be used as antigens. The test effectively detects recent or past infections.

1. A single positive titer of 1:100 or higher indicates residual infection, response to current infection, or a vaccination titer.
2. Titers of 1:100–1:300 may be significant in unvaccinated animals.
3. While titers of 1:300 or higher usually indicate infection, titers of 1:1,000 or higher are most diagnostic. However, titers of 1:1,000 or higher are questionable when they are obtained within 2–3 months of repeated vaccination.
4. Paired serum specimens are helpful only when the initial sample is obtained during the acute stage of infection. A change from negative to positive or a fourfold or greater increase in titer is considered diagnostic. The initial specimen should be obtained as early in the course of disease as possible. Specimens should be collected at intervals of 7–10 days in clinically affected animals, 10–14 days in unvaccinated animals, and 14–21 days in vaccinated animals.
5. For the definitive diagnosis of leptospirosis, the MA test is 50% accurate if the second sample is taken within 10–14 days of infection and 100% accurate if a third titer is measured 7–14 days later.

6. Cross-reactions between serovars and the use of polyvalent vaccines have contributed to confusion in the interpretation of titers.

7. Confounding effects due to the inherent variability of the MA test procedure can be minimized by submitting all sequential samples at the same time.

8. Leptospires have been isolated from seronegative dogs.

9. The magnitude of the antibody response (titer) is not correlated with the prognosis or the development of a carrier state.

C. Macroscopic (rapid) plate agglutination tests are less sensitive than the MA test. Titers of 1:40 or higher should be considered positive.

D. The complement fixation test is less frequently used but is more valuable than the MA test. The complement fixation test can detect recent and chronic infections and effectively screens for several serovars because it has broader cross-reactivity.

E. A genus-specific enzyme-linked immunosorbent assay (ELISA) test is being developed.

F. Fluorescent antibody testing can be used to detect antibodies in tissues and is useful in lieu of culture to identify animals that are shedding organisms.

III. Other

A. Leptospires may be seen by light microscopy in tissues or in air-dried smears stained with Giemsa or silver stains.

B. Leptospires also may be seen with darkfield or phase-contrast microscopy. However, their concentration in blood is too low and survival in urine too short for practical diagnostic use of these methods.

TREATMENT

I. Supportive therapy depends upon the severity of disease.

A. Shock and dehydration should be treated with intravenous administration of balanced polyionic fluids.

B. Whole blood transfusions may be required when hemorrhage is severe. Blood transfusions necessary for the treatment of DIC should be given in conjunction with appropriate anticoagulant therapy.

  C. Oliguria and/or anuria associated with renal failure are treated initially by rehydration. Intravenous osmotic diuretics, tubular diuretics, and/or low-dose dopamine infusion may be used sequentially when oliguria persists despite rehydration. Peritoneal dialysis should be considered for patients that do not respond to these therapeutic maneuvers because impaired renal function is potentially reversible.

 II. Antibiotics

  A. Penicillin (40,000–80,000 units/kg, IM, sid or divided bid) is the antibiotic of choice for terminating leptospiremia. In the presence of renal dysfunction, penicillin should be given initially and continued until renal function improves. Tetracycline and chloramphenicol are less effective.

  B. Few drugs are capable of eliminating the organism from the interstitial tissues of the kidney and thus terminating the carrier state. However, dihydrostreptomycin (10–15 mg/kg, IM, bid for 2 weeks) or streptomycin are effective in this regard.

  C. Early appropriate antibiotic usage should lower the serum agglutination titer. Treated animals should be revaccinated in 6 months.

 III. The prognosis is guarded in severe cases because of widespread organ damage. Renal and hepatic damage may be permanent.

PREVENTION

 I. Elimination of the carrier state is unrealistic because wild animal reservoirs and subclinically infected domestic animals constitute a source of undetected infection.

 II. Environmental controls should include the following measures:

  A. Rodent control

  B. Eradication of environmental conditions conducive to survival of leptospires

  C. Isolation of infected animals

 III. Immunization

  A. Vaccines should contain serovars with a broad immunogenic spectrum. Multivalent vaccines should contain serovars enzootic for a given country.

  B. Bacterins available for dogs are bivalent, including *L. canicola* and *L. icterohaemorrhagiae*. The bacterins generally are marketed in a liquid form, and they are used as diluents for modified-live virus vaccines.

    C. Adequate primary immunization requires three to four injections given at 2- to 3-week intervals. Vaccination should be started at 9 weeks of age, and subsequent injections should be given at 12 and 15 weeks of age. Immunity will last 6–8 months and annual revaccination is recommended.

    D. Vaccinations should be given more frequently (every 4–6 months) to dogs at risk, such as those in enzootic areas, show dogs, and hunting dogs exposed to water.

    E. Immunization reduces the incidence and severity of canine leptospirosis, but it does not prevent the development of the carrier state following natural infection.

    F. Newer vaccines may provide immunity for 1 year and may reduce the development of the carrier state. Recently developed vaccines produced from the outer envelope of leptospires have produced maximal antibody titers 2 weeks following a single injection. These vaccines are less allergenic and less likely to cause anaphylactic reactions.

    G. Antibody titers following vaccination tend to be lower and more transient than titers following natural infection.

    H. Animals recovering from infection by one serovar are not immune to infection by another serovar.

PUBLIC HEALTH CONSIDERATIONS

    I. Leptospirosis is thought to be the most widespread zoonosis.

    II. Contaminated urine is highly infectious to humans and animals.

    III. Contaminated areas should be washed with detergent and treated with iodine-based disinfectants.

    IV. Animals that are shedding organisms should be treated with dihydrostreptomycin or streptomycin.

SUGGESTED READINGS

Alexander AD: Leptospira. p. 381. In Braude AI, Davis CE, Fierer J (eds): Infectious Diseases and Medical Microbiology. 2nd ed. WB Saunders, Philadelphia, 1986

Diesch SL: Leptospirosis vaccination and titer evaluation. Mod Vet Pract 61:905, 1980

Edwards GA: Leptospirosis. p. 1543. In Braude AI, Davis CE, Fierer J (eds):

Infectious Diseases and Medical Microbiology. 2nd ed. WB Saunders, Philadelphia, 1986

Greene CE: Leptospirosis. p. 588. In Greene CE: Clinical Microbiology and Infectious Diseases of the Dog and Cat. WB Saunders, Philadelphia, 1984

Hanson LE: Leptospirosis in domestic animals: The public health perspective. J Am Vet Med Assoc 181:1505, 1982

Larsson CE, Santa Rosa CA, Larsson MHMA, et al: Laboratory and clinical features of experimental feline leptospirosis. Int J Zoonoses 12:111, 1985

Marshal V: Efficacy of *Leptospira* vaccine (letter). J Am Vet Med Assoc 183:12, 1983

Thiermann AB: Leptospirosis: current development and trends. J Am Vet Med Assoc 184:722, 1984

16

Borreliosis (Lyme Disease)

Elizabeth C. Burgess

ETIOLOGY

I. Borreliosis is caused by infection of dogs with a spirochete, *Borrelia burgdorferi*. The infection can result in overt signs of disease, including erythema chronicum migrans, monoarticular and polyarticular arthritis or arthralgia, intermittent or migrating lameness, and generalized pain. The term *Lyme disease* is used to describe the specific syndrome resulting from infection of humans with *B. burgdorferi*.

II. The organisms have the phenotypic characteristics of the genus *Borrelia*. They appear as flexible helical cells with dimensions of 0.18–0.25 μm by 4–30 μm. They are motile and have regular coiling. The cells are gram-negative and stain with Giemsa and Warthin-Starry stains. Unstained cells are not visible by brightfield microscopy but can be visualized by phase-contrast or darkfield techniques. *B. burgdorferi* is microaerophilic, and optimal growth is obtained at 34–37°C.

III. Transmission

A. Arthropod

Arthropod transmission occurs primarily by the bite of an infected ixodid tick. The two principal vectors in the United States are *Ixodes dammini* (bear tick) on the East Coast and in the Midwest and *Ixodes pacificus* (western black-legged tick) on the West Coast. *B. burgdorferi* has also been isolated from other arthropods, including *Dermacentor variabilis* (American dog tick), *Amblyomma americanum* (Lone Star tick), *Haemaphysalis leporispalustris* (rabbit tick), *Ixodes scapularis* (black-legged tick), *Cuterebra fontinella* (botfly), *Aedes* spp. (mosquitoes), and *Orchopeas leucopus* (deer mouse flea); however, the vectoral capabilities of these arthropods is not known.

   B. Nonarthropod

      Transmission has also been shown to occur in dogs by direct contact in the absence of an arthropod vector. The spirochete has been isolated from the urine of infected *Peromyscus leucopus* (white-footed mice), and it is postulated that contact transmission occurs by exposure to infected urine.

IV. The epizootiology of the disease is primarily associated with the life cycle of *I. dammini,* a three-host tick. The principal vertebrate maintenance hosts for *B. burgdorferi* are *P. leucopus* and *Odocoileus virginianus* (white-tailed deer). *I. dammini* lives in grassy and wooded areas and feeds on small and large animals, including small rodents, birds, raccoons, opossums, deer, horses, dogs, cats, and humans. The preferred hosts of *I. dammini* are the white-footed mouse (for the larval and nymphal stages) and the white-tailed deer (for the adult stage). The spirochete has been recovered from the blood of both these species. All three stages of the tick will feed on humans, and nymphal and adult ticks are known to feed on dogs. Adult ticks are abundant in the spring and fall, the seasons during which the majority

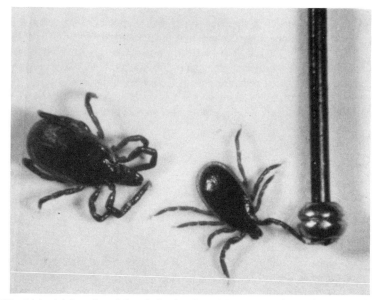

Fig. 16-1. Adult male and female *Ixodes dammini,* a vector of *Borrelia burgdorferi.*

of clinical cases in dogs occur (although cases have been reported from every month of the year). The life cycle of the tick from egg to adult may require as long as 2 years for completion. The adult ticks are small, about one-third of the size of the common dog tick *D. variabilis,* and the females have an orange body (Fig. 16-1). A significant number of *I. dammini* ticks may harbor the spirochete (10–65%), depending on the geographic area.

V. The geographic range of borreliosis has increased since 1970, when the disease was first recognized in the United States. The range now extends to 24 states, including the northeastern states, the Midwest (Wisconsin, Minnesota), California, Arkansas, North Carolina, and Texas.

VI. *B. burgdorferi* is susceptible to routine disinfecting procedures.

CLINICAL SIGNS

I. Pathogenesis

The exact mechanisms of pathogenesis in borreliosis are not completely understood. It is postulated that both direct and indirect effects of the spirochete are involved.

A. Direct effects
   1. Spirochetal lipopolysaccharide, producing a pyrogenic reaction
   2. Possible endotoxin
   3. Possibility that cell-wall peptidoglycans may induce persistent joint inflammation

B. Indirect effects
   1. Immune complexes are present in the serum and synovial fluid of infected humans in abnormal amounts, which suggests an immune-mediated inflammatory reaction. When these complexes localize in the joints, they may produce inflammatory joint disease.
   2. Interleukin-1 production by macrophages may produce increases in collagenase and prostaglandin E_2 secreted by synovial cells. Collagenase may play a role in the digestion of articular cartilage.
   3. Spirochetes may cause mast cell degranulation and the release of mast cell mediators.

C. Morbidity

The extent of morbidity in borreliosis is not known. Not all animals infected with *B. burgdorferi* develop clinical signs. Borreliosis is not known to cause mortality.

II. Clinical course
   A. All ages may be infected but the incidence is highest in dogs 0–5 years.
   B. All breeds are susceptible. Hunting and sporting breeds tend to have greater exposure to infected ticks and therefore have a higher incidence.
   C. The most common clinical signs are listed below in order of their observed frequency. Not all dogs will show every sign; some may have a combination of them.
      1. Fever (102.5–106°F)
      2. Inappetance (fever and inappetance often go undetected)
      3. Acute onset of lameness
         Onset is accompanied by severe pain with or without associated swelling. No history of trauma; usually it is difficult to pinpoint the affected area. The majority of dogs do not have swollen joints or arthritis but rather an arthralgia. Some dogs, however, will develop swollen joints and increased synovial fluid. Lameness may be intermittent and/or migrating from one leg to another.
      4. Recurrence of lameness weeks to months later
      5. Swollen lymph nodes (most commonly, popliteal and prescapular)
      6. Generalized pain
      7. Skin lesion
         Erythema chronicum migrans is an expanding skin lesion with an erythematous, circular border and a clear center. It differs from the localized swelling often seen as a reaction to a tick bite. The lesion is located at the site of a tick bite but usually can only be seen on the belly or other areas where the haircoat is thin.
      8. Chronic borreliosis
         This can occur in untreated patients. The signs in these dogs consist of a chronic or intermittent lameness or arthritis occurring over a period of several months to years.

DIAGNOSIS

Diagnosis is based on history, clinical signs, laboratory findings, and response to treatment.
   I. History

    A. The animal originates from, or has a history of travel to, a Lyme disease–endemic area.

    B. There is an acute onset of lameness with no history of trauma.

    C. There may be a history of current or past tick bites. The time of onset of disease following infection is dependent upon the spirochete dose (number of infected ticks feeding on the dog) and on the immunologic status of the dog. Erythema chronicum migrans has appeared as early as 4 days post-tick bite in a dog infested with hundreds of ticks. It has taken as long as a year for the arthralgia to develop in some dogs. The average incubation period appears to be about 1 month. Recurrences of disease and reinfections are both possible.

II. Serology

    A. Serology is the most commonly used diagnostic test. An indirect immunofluorescent antibody (IFA) test or an enzyme-linked immunosorbent assay (ELISA) can be used to determine antibody levels to *B. burgdorferi*.

    B. In experimentally inoculated dogs, IgM antibodies appeared within 1 month of infection, at the same time that specific IgG antibodies appeared. The IgG antibodies persist for months. Dogs presenting with acute lameness and pain have already developed high levels of IgG antibodies. The diagnostic serologic tests generally test for IgG antibodies.

    C. There is only a limited antigenic relationship to leptospires, and vaccination with *Leptospira* spp. will not interfere with a serologic diagnosis.

    D. Interpretation of serologic results must be made in conjunction with the history and clinical signs (not all infected dogs will show signs of illness). The majority of dogs showing clinical signs of borreliosis will have IgG antibody titers of 1:1024 or greater. If the dog is in the early stages of the disease, the IgG titer may be as low as 1:128. Any titer below 1:64 is considered negative. In dogs that have had a massive tick exposure and develop signs as early as 4 days postinfection, the antibody titer will be negative. A second titer should be taken on these dogs in 2 weeks. Convalescent serum titers may be of value. If the antibody titer persists for over 1 month post-treatment, it may indicate a persistent infection.

III. Culture

    Culture of *B. burgdorferi* from the blood or synovial fluid would give a definitive diagnosis; however, culture is very difficult and is usually unsuccessful. Spirochetes are rarely seen on direct examination of blood, urine, or synovial fluid.

IV. Clinical laboratory data
  A. A complete blood count (CBC) may be beneficial, although many infected dogs have a normal CBC. Some dogs have an increase in the white blood cell count, with increased numbers of segmented neutrophils and monocytes.
  B. The majority of infected dogs are radiographically negative and are antinuclear antibody–negative.
V. Response to treatment in acute cases of borreliosis is rapid and dramatic. Within 24 hours of initiation of antibiotic treatment, there is generally an almost complete relief of pain and lameness.

TREATMENT

  I. Tetracycline (25 mg/kg PO tid for a minimum of 14 days) is the drug of choice for the acute disease. Erythromycin or ampicillin is also effective. In human acute cases, tetracycline gave faster results, and there were fewer late complications of the disease than with use of penicillin or erythromycin.
 II. Intravenous penicillin G for 10 days has been effective in humans with chronic arthritis and might be beneficial in dogs with chronic borreliosis that does not respond to tetracycline (dose of 22,000 U/kg IV qid).
III. Treatment for pain in acute cases is generally not necessary because the response to antibiotic therapy is rapid and dramatic; the majority of patients are asymptomatic within 24 hours. If necessary, dexamethasone (0.25 mg/kg) may be used, but only in conjunction with antibiotic therapy.

PREVENTION

There is no vaccine for the prevention of borreliosis. Measures to limit tick exposure, the use of tick collars, and prompt removal of ticks are at present the only means of prevention.

PUBLIC HEALTH CONSIDERATIONS

  I. Infection with *B. burgdorferi* in humans (Lyme disease) can cause a wide variety of symptoms, including erythema chronicum migrans, arthritis, and neurologic disorders. The most common route of infection in humans is by the bite of an infected tick. Tick-infested dogs could bring infected ticks into close association with humans and indirectly contribute to human infection.

II. It is not known if humans can become infected by direct contact with infected animals.

III. *B. burgdorferi* has been isolated from the blood of infected dogs. Urine could also be a potential source of spirochetes.

IV. Care should be taken when handling blood and urine samples from any dog from a Lyme disease–endemic area.

SUGGESTED READINGS

Anderson JF, Johnson RC, Magnarelli LA, et al: Identification of endemic foci of Lyme disease: isolation of *Borrelia burgdorferi* from feral rodents and ticks (*Dermacentor variabilis*). J Clin Microbiol 22:36, 1985

Bosler EM, Ormiston BG, Coleman JL, et al: Prevalence of the Lyme disease spirochete in populations of white-tailed deer and white-footed mice. Yale J Biol Med 57:651, 1984

Bosler EM, Coleman JL, Benach JL, et al: Natural distribution of the *Ixodes dammini* spirochete. Science 220:321, 1983

Burgess EC: Natural exposure of Wisconsin dogs to the Lyme disease spirochete (*Borrelia burgdorferi*). Lab Anim Sci 36:288, 1986

Johnson RC: Lyme disease: a new, rapidly spreading spirochetosis. Norden News 60(2):14, 1985

Kornblatt AN, Urband PH, Steere AC: Arthritis caused by *Borrelia burgdorferi* in dogs. J Am Vet Med Assoc 186:960, 1985

Lissman BA, Bosler EM, Camay H, et al: Spirochete-associated arthritis (Lyme disease) in a dog. J Am Vet Med Assoc 185:219, 1984

Magnarelli LA, Anderson JF, Kaufmann AF, et al: Borreliosis in dogs from southern Connecticut. J Am Vet Med Assoc 186:955, 1985

Ryan CP: Lyme disease: an expanding health problem. Calif Vet 40(1):16, 1986

Schmid GP: The global distribution of Lyme disease. Yale J Biol Med 57:617, 1984

Spielman A, Wilson ML, Levine JF, et al: Ecology of *Ixodes dammini*–borne human babesiosis and Lyme disease. Ann Rev Entomol 30:439, 1985

Steere AC, Green J, Schoen RT, et al: Successful parenteral penicillin therapy of established Lyme arthritis. New Engl J Med 312:869, 1985

Steere AC, Hutchinson GJ, Rahn DW, et al: Treatment of the early manifestations of Lyme disease. Ann Intern Med 99:22, 1983

17

Salmonellosis and Yersiniosis

Craig E. Greene

SALMONELLOSIS

Etiology

I. Causative agent, *Salmonella* spp.
   A. These are motile, non-spore-forming, gram-negative bacilli belonging to the family Enterobacteriaceae.
   B. Certain species of pathogenic significance show an affinity for particular animals.
   C. Major species of pathogenic significance are: *Salmonella choleraesuis, Salmonella arizonae, Salmonella enteritidis,* and *Salmonella typhimurium.*
   D. Mucoid and encapsulated strains are more pathogenic.
II. Host range: a wide variety of vertebrates and invertebrates.
III. Life cycle
   A. *Salmonella* organisms are primarily intestinal parasites.
   B. Ingestion is the most common route of infection, although inhalation is possible.
   C. The parasites can survive for relatively long periods outside of host.
   D. They are ubiquitous in the environment; the aquatic biosphere is contaminated.
IV. Sources of infection include:
   A. Contamination of commercially processed foods during and after preparation
   B. Contamination of inanimate fomites, such as food dishes, endoscopic equipment, and bathing facilities
   C. Infected carriers, both human and animal, the latter being more persistent

    1. Dogs and cats infected with small numbers of organisms and those mounting an adequate defense have a milder clinical illness.

    2. Infected animals with mild illness or recovered animals may shed organisms for up to 6 weeks, usually in the absence of clinical signs.

  D. Prevalence of the carrier state may be in the 1–36% range in dogs and in the 0–14% range in cats.

  E. The predisposition to infection is affected by host resistance, which depends on:

    1. Age, nutritional state, and concurrent infections and other stresses

    2. Immunosuppressive phenomena, altered intestinal motility, or chronic antimicrobial therapy

Clinical Signs

  I. Pathogenesis

  A. Large numbers of organisms (more than 10^6) are needed to produce infection.

    1. Increased susceptibility to infection can be shown by increasing gastric pH.

    2. Organisms surviving gastric transit can reach the small intestine.

  B. The organisms become localized and persistent in intestinal lymph nodes.

  C. Chronic shedding occurs with persistent infections.

  D. Mucosal invasion and epithelial cell injury are common complications of acute infections.

    1. Enterotoxemia and bacteremia are more common with this organism.

    2. Once in the blood, the organism may localize in other organs.

  II. Gastroenteritis

  A. Clinical signs develop within 3–5 days.

  B. Fever and anorexia are followed by vomiting, abdominal pain, and diarrhea, which is watery to mucoid and bloody in most severe cases.

  C. Weight loss and dehydration are also seen.

  III. Bacteremia and endotoxemia

  A. These can develop in the most severely affected animals.

B. Usually they cause cardiovascular collapse and shock, with or without premonitory gastrointestinal (GI) signs.
IV. Other syndromes
   A. Abortions, stillbirths, or birth of weak neonates can occur.
   B. There may be abscess formation or infection in any system, including the eye, in which posterior uveitis or panendophthalmitis can result.

Diagnosis

I. Hematologic and biochemical findings
   A. Hematologic findings are nonspecific and can include:
      1. Nonregenerative anemia
      2. Leukopenia and leukocyte toxicity (in overwhelming infections)
      3. Mature neutrophilia and leukocytosis in less severely affected animals and in those with localized infections
   B. Biochemical alterations in animals with severe GI signs can include hypoproteinemia (with associated hypocalcemia) and prerenal azotemia.
II. Bacterial isolation
   A. This is the most definitive technique for diagnosing infection.
      1. Isolation of the organism does not necessarily indicate that it is responsible for the observed clinical signs.
      2. Isolation of the organism from GI secretions or feces may represent either an active infection or a carrier state.
      3. Culturing the organism from internal body fluids, such as urine, synovial fluid, transtracheal washings, or cerebrospinal fluid, or from organ tissues is specific for disseminated infections.
      4. Specimens from normally sterile tissues can be isolated on ordinary bacteriologic media.
   B. Because contaminants can interfere with isolation, the following steps should be applied to cultures from nonsterile tissues:
      1. The cultures should first be placed in enrichment broths, such as selenite or tetrathionate, to increase the yield.
      2. They should be cultured in selective media, such as deoxycholate, after 24 hours.
III. Serology
   A. Serology is relatively nonspecific because it cannot distinguish present from past exposure.

    B. Inconsistent increases in titers may be seen during clinical illness.

    C. Hence cultures are recommended over serologic methods because they are more definitive.

IV. Pathologic findings

    A. Gross lesions in animals with GI disease include a mucoid to hemorrhagic enteritis.

    B. The lesions usually are confined to the lower half of the bowel.

    C. Systemically infected animals that die as a result of sepsis have edematous or consolidated lungs and hemorrhagic intestinal and peripheral lymph nodes.

Treatment

I. Gastrointestinal illness

    A. Food and water should be withheld, but polyionic isotonic intravenous fluids should be given parenterally.

    B. Transfusions of fluid or plasma are indicated when mucosal disruption causes severe blood loss with resultant anemia and/or hypoproteinemia.

    C. Prostaglandin inhibitors, such as aspirin or flunixin, given early in the course of the disease may reduce the fluid loss from diarrhea by interfering with the hypersecretion induced by bacterial endotoxin.

    D. Antimicrobial therapy

        1. Antimicrobial therapy is not advocated for uncomplicated gastroenteritis.

        2. Parenteral therapy should be reserved for animals with systemic signs of endotoxemia.

        3. In acutely infected animals antimicrobial therapy may prolong the carrier state.

        4. In contrast, combined antimicrobial therapy has been helpful in resolving infection in animals that become chronic carriers.

        5. Organisms may acquire transferable drug resistance with indiscriminate antibiotic use.

II. Endotoxemia or bacteremia

    A. Intensive fluid replacement is needed.

    B. A mixture consisting of glucose, insulin, and potassium has been beneficial in treating endotoxic shock.

    C. Parenteral intravenous antibiotics are needed.

1. Chloramphenicol and trimethoprim are most effective.
2. Ampicillin and erythromycin show variable responses.

Prevention

I. Hygiene
   A. Routine cleaning and disinfection of tables, cages, and floors is an essential component in prevention. Phenolic disinfectants are best against salmonellae, but they can cause irritation when used near cats. Halogens can be used as an alternative.
   B. Food utensils should be machine-washed between use.
   C. Routine disinfection of hands and clothing should be instituted.
II. Isolation
   A. All animals developing acute diarrhea during hospitalization should be suspected of being infected.
   B. Fecal cultures should be submitted and the animal should be isolated.
   C. Long-term boarders or ill patients should not be housed in wards with short-term or day boarders.

Public Health Considerations

I. Dogs and cats have the greatest potential for infecting humans through contaminated feces.
II. Infected animals have been shown to shed the organisms either in the feces or in conjunctival secretions.
III. Unrestricted and indiscriminate use of antibiotics has selected for increasingly resistant animal strains of salmonellae, which are correspondingly more difficult to treat in infected humans.

YERSINIOSIS

Etiology

I. The causative agent is *Yersinia enterocolitica*.
   A. This is a motile gram-negative coccobacillus of the family Enterobacteriaceae.

B. Its unusual ability to replicate at 0°C makes selective culture possible.
II. Host range
   A. The bacterium is isolated worldwide from feces.
   B. There are a variety of wild and domestic animal reservoirs.
   C. Humans are unnatural hosts.
   D. The microorganism is thought to be a commensal of dogs and cats.

Clinical Signs

I. Signs usually are inapparent.
II. The diarrhea in those animals with clinical illness is characterized by:
   A. An increased frequency of bowel movements, with blood and mucus
   B. Absence of systemic illness

Diagnosis

I. Culture
   A. From feces of affected animals.
      1. Mere isolation of the organism is not definitive.
      2. Some animals may be carriers.
   B. Isolation from deeper tissues, such as blood or intestinal lymph nodes, is more meaningful for distinguishing asymptomatic carriers from clinically affected animals.
   C. Serotyping of strains is possible and can be used to determine common-source infections.
II. Pathologic findings
   A. Gross findings are nonspecific.
   B. Histologically a chronic enteritis with mononuclear infiltrates occurs.

Treatment

I. The response to therapy helps to confirm infection:
   A. In younger animals with clinical illness
   B. In animals in contact with humans

II. Drugs to which the organism is sensitive include chloramphenicol, tetracycline, gentamicin, cephalosporins, and trimethoprim-sulfonamides.

Prevention

I. It is difficult to employ treatment as a means for eliminating infection because many animals are carriers.
II. Good nursing care, to include warmth and good nutrition, will assist carriers in avoiding symptomatic illness.

Public Health Considerations

I. Humans develop a much more severe illness than do infected pets.
  A. Fever, diarrhea, and abdominal pain are seen.
  B. Generalized septicemia can develop.
II. The organism is often a commensal in animals, producing little clinical symptomology.
III. Very young or immunosuppressed animals may show diarrhea and are a source of infection for humans. They should be treated with appropriate antimicrobials when infection is suspected or diagnosed.
IV. Shedding of the organism by infected animals occurs primarily during diarrheic episodes.

SUGGESTED READINGS

Salmonellosis

Calvert CA: Salmonella infections in hospitalized dogs: epizootiology, diagnosis, and prognosis. J Am Anim Hosp Assoc 21:499, 1985

Greene CE: Enteric bacterial infections. p. 617. In Greene CE (ed): Clinical Microbiology and Infectious Diseases of the Dog and Cat. WB Saunders, Philadelphia, 1984

Ikeda JS, Hirsh DC, Jang SS, Biberstein EL: Characteristics of *Salmonella* isolated from animals at a veterinary medical teaching hospital. Am J Vet Res 47:232, 1986

Ketaren K, Brown J, Shotts EB, et al: Canine salmonellosis in a small animal hospital. J Am Vet Med Assoc 179:1017, 1981

Timoney JF: Feline salmonellosis. Vet Clin North Am 6:395, 1976

Yersiniosis

Farstad L, Landsverk T, Lassen J: Isolation of *Yersinia enterocolitica* from a dog with chronic enteritis. Acta Vet Scand 17:261, 1976

Papageorges M, Higgins R, Gosselin Y: *Yersinia enterocolitica* enteritis in two dogs. J Am Vet Med Assoc 182:618, 1983

18

Plague

John P. Thilsted

ETIOLOGY

I. Causative organism

Plague is caused by *Yersinia pestis* (formerly *Pasteurella pestis*), a gram-negative, rod-shaped bacterium belonging to the family Enterobacteriaceae. The bacterium has a bipolar "safety pin" appearance when stained with polychromatic stains such as Giemsa or Wayson. The organism grows readily on unenriched agar or blood agar, but the growth is slow. Colonies are pinpoint in size at 24 hours and only 1–2 mm in diameter at 48 hours. Large numbers of organisms are usually present in aspirates from enlarged lymph nodes and abscesses from infected animals.

II. Geographic distribution

A. Plague in the world

Presently plague is enzootic in a number of countries throughout the world. Countries reporting cases of human plague to the World Health Organization during the 10-year period 1975–1984 are listed in Table 18-1.

Plague is enzootic in areas of the Soviet Union, as well as in those countries listed in Table 18-1. Plague has apparently been eradicated from western Europe and Australia.

B. Plague in the United States

In the United States plague is restricted to the western states, where it is enzootic in wild rodents (so-called sylvatic plague). The states of Arizona, California, Colorado, Hawaii, Idaho, Nevada, New Mexico, Oregon, Texas, Utah, Washington, and Wyoming have accounted for all the human plague cases reported in the United States since 1927. Since 1976 New Mexico has reported more cases of human and feline plague than any other state.

TABLE 18-1. COUNTRIES REPORTING CASES OF HUMAN PLAGUE TO
THE WORLD HEALTH ORGANIZATION BETWEEN 1975 AND 1984

Africa	Americas	Asia
Angola	Bolivia	Burma
Lesotho	Brazil	China
Madagascar	Ecuador	Viet Nam
Namibia	Peru	
Uganda	United States	
Zaire		
Kenya		
Libya		
Mozambique		
South Africa		
Tanzania		
Zimbabwe		

III. Epizootiology

The cat is the only domestic animal in the United States that is both highly susceptible to *Y. pestis*–induced disease and likely to come into contact with the organism. Cats develop a severe febrile disease following infection, and the mortality in untreated cases is high. Experimental and seroepidemiologic studies indicate that dogs are susceptible to plague infection and do commonly come into contact with the organism in enzootic areas. However, dogs are very resistant to plague and develop only a transient mild febrile disease following infection. No mortality has been reported in dogs.

A. Reservoirs of plague

Wild rodents, primarily ground squirrels (*Spermophilus* spp.) and prairie dogs (*Cynomys* spp.), are the principal reservoir hosts for plague in the United States. Plague infection has also been documented in a number of other species of wild rodents and in rabbits, bobcats, and coyotes.

B. Vectors of plague

Rodent fleas are the principal vectors of plague. Virtually all species of rodent fleas are capable of transmitting plague; however, they vary considerably in their vector efficiency. *Xenopsylla cheopis* (the Oriental rat flea) is the highly efficient plague vector primarily responsible for plague transmission in several parts of the world outside the United States. In the United States the rodent fleas *Diamanus montanus* and *Hoplopsyllus anomalus* appear to be important plague vectors. Dog and cat fleas (*Ctenocephalides* spp.) are not considered to be vectors of plague.

C. Infection by direct contact

Although most plague infections in cats and dogs are thought to be acquired by the bite of an infected flea, a portion occur as the result of direct contact with, or ingestion of, *Y. pestis*–infected tissue. Cats and dogs rarely, if ever, contract plague by inhalation of the organism.

IV. *Y. pestis* does not survive long outside the mammalian host or the flea. It is rapidly killed by drying and by most commonly used disinfectants. Fomite transmission of plague rarely, if ever, occurs.

CLINICAL SIGNS

I. Three forms of plague—bubonic, septicemic, and pneumonic—are recognized in both humans and animals. Bubonic plague is the most common form of plague in cats. Cats become infected by a flea bite (the most common method) or by ingestion of plague-infected rodent tissue. The following comments apply to the disease in cats:

A. In bubonic plague the lymph node draining the site of inoculation becomes markedly enlarged (*bubo* formation) as the result of an acute inflammatory response to the plague organisms. An abscess often develops in the affected node and eventually ruptures. The exudate may be either serosanguineous or purulent. Submandibular nodes are most commonly affected, although any peripheral node may be involved. Bacteremia is almost always present in the acute stage of the disease. Affected cats are pyrexic (103°–106°F), depressed, and anorectic. The incubation period for all types of feline plague is short (2–4 days), and the duration of illness is variable. *Bubonic plague in cats cannot be differentiated clinically from fight wound abscesses caused by* Pasteurella multocida *and other pyogenic bacteria.* Plague should always be considered in any cat from a plague-enzootic area that presents with a high fever and either a lymphadenopathy or an abscess.

B. Septicemia without lymph node enlargement or abscess formation does occur occasionally in cats. This form of plague, if untreated, is more rapidly fatal than bubonic plague. Focal necrosis and suppurative inflammation in various organs may be seen in cats dying of septicemic plague. The clinical signs observed in this form of plague are similar to those that occur in bubonic plague, except that there is no lymphadenopathy.

    C. Primary pneumonic plague is very rare in both humans and animals. It results from the inhalation of plague organisms rather than from a flea bite. The incubation period for pneumonic plague is very short, and the disease progresses rapidly. The primary clinical sign present is dyspnea. This form of plague, unlike the previous two types, is highly transmissible from one individual to another.

II. Dogs can be infected with *Y. pestis,* however, they do not develop severe signs of disease and they recover from the infection without treatment. Lethargy, depression, a transient febrile response, and a localized swelling at the inoculation site have been reported in dogs experimentally infected with plague. The dogs were asymptomatic by the seventh day postinoculation. Naturally occurring cases of plague are very rare in dogs.

DIAGNOSIS

  I. Plague should be suspected in cats presented with the following history and clinical signs:
    A. From a plague-enzootic region
    B. Allowed to roam (often reported to be a hunter)
    C. Recent, sudden onset of lethargy and anorexia
    D. Pyrexia and lymphadenopathy/abscess found upon clinical examination
    E. Large numbers of gram-negative coccobacilli in aspirate of lymph node or abscess (in some cats with plague no lymphadenopathy or abscesses are present).

 II. The most definitive method of plague diagnosis is isolation and identification of the plague organism. *Y. pestis* is usually easily isolated from lymph node aspirates, exudate from abscesses, and peripheral blood. Samples for culture should always be taken prior to initiation of antibiotic therapy.
    A. Material aspirated from affected lymph nodes or abscesses should be submitted to the laboratory in a capped syringe or sterile tube. If there will be more than a 12-hour delay in culturing the specimen, it should be transferred from the syringe to a sterile swab and placed in a transport medium such as Stuart's or Cary-Blair.
    B. Blood samples for culture should be inoculated directly into a blood culture bottle containing trypticase soy broth, which is then submitted to the laboratory. If a blood culture bottle is not available at the time the blood sample is obtained, the blood should be aseptically drawn into an a tube containing ethylenediamine tetraacetate (EDTA) and submitted to the laboratory on ice.

C. Swabs or tissue samples should be taken from a dead animal and submitted to the laboratory on ice. The tissues that should be cultured are liver, spleen, lung, enlarged lymph nodes, and abscesses.

III. A fluorescent antibody (FA) test for *Y. pestis* is performed by some public health and veterinary diagnostic laboratories in plague-enzootic areas, as well as by the Plague Branch of the Centers for Disease Control in Fort Collins, Colorado. The FA test for plague is almost as reliable as culture, and results are obtained more quickly. It is recommended that two air-dried smears of exudate or lymph node aspirate be submitted to the laboratory along with samples for culture.

IV. The passive hemagglutination test utilizing the fraction 1A antigen is the most commonly used serologic test for plague. Cats and dogs both develop high passive hemagglutination titers 8–12 days postinfection, and the titers remain high for a year or longer following recovery. A single high titer may be due to active disease or to previous exposure. It is recommended that paired serum samples be drawn—an acute sample and, 10–14 days later, a convalescent sample. The titer of the acute sample is usually low or negative. The titer of the convalescent sample is typically greater than 1:128 (at least a fourfold increase over the acute titer) in an animal recovering from plague.

TREATMENT

I. All animals suspected of plague should be treated for fleas as soon as possible to minimize exposure to those handling the animal.

II. Systemic antibiotic therapy is indicated in all cases of plague except those in which there are signs of lung involvement. Animals with pneumonic plague are highly infectious and thus should be euthanized rather than treated. The antibiotics of choice for the treatment of plague are streptomycin, tetracycline, and chloramphenicol. Antibiotic therapy should be continued for 5 days after clinical signs disappear or a minimum of 10 days.

A. Streptomycin is commonly used to treat plague in humans because the plague organism is very sensitive to this antibiotic, it is bactericidal, and there are few adverse reactions. Streptomycin is less commonly used to treat plague in animals because it must be given parenterally rather than orally and because adverse reactions occasionally occur. The recommended streptomycin dosage in cats and dogs is 30–50 mg/kg/day IM divided bid.

B. Tetracyclines (including tetracycline, oxytetracycline, and chlortetracycline) are the antibiotics most commonly used to treat plague in cats. These antibiotics, although bacteriostatic rather than bactericidal, are very effective and have a low degree of toxicity. The recommended tetacycline dosage in dogs and cats is 75 mg/kg/day PO divided tid (parenteral dosage is 15 mg/kg/day divided bid). The effectiveness of doxycycline in the treatment of plague has not been determined, and thus this drug is not recommended for plague therapy.

C. Chloramphenicol is bacteriostatic, but it is very effective in treating plague and can be given orally. It has been used less commonly than either streptomycin or tetracycline. The recommended chloramphenicol dosage in cats and dogs is 100–150 mg/kg/day PO divided tid.

III. Other antibiotics and/or antibacterials that have been successfully used to treat plague in humans include gentamicin, kanamycin, and trimethoprim-sulfamethoxazole. Currently none of these drugs is recommended for plague therapy in animals unless there are contraindications to using any of the approved antibiotics.

IV. Penicillin and ampicillin *are not effective* in the treatment of plague. These antibiotics should not be used in suspect or confirmed cases of plague.

PREVENTION

I. Flea control and rodent control are the two primary measures used to prevent the spread of plague.

A. Cats and dogs in plague-enzootic areas should be routinely sprayed or dusted with an approved insecticide to reduce the likelihood of their becoming infected and to prevent them from carrying plague-infected fleas into the household. Insecticide spraying of the house and immediately adjacent areas may be indicated in some cases.

B. Food sources and harborage for wild rodents should be eliminated from areas near human habitations. Woodpiles, old tires, wrecked cars, discarded farm implements, and miscellaneous trash should be removed, and food sources such as grain and flour should be kept in rodent-proof containers. In some cases rodenticides may be necessary to reduce the rodent population. Rodent control should not precede flea control.

II. During seasons when plague is very prevalent in the rodent population (the summer in plague-enzootic areas of the western United States), cats and dogs should not be allowed to roam or to hunt rodents. Most cats and dogs contract plague directly from rodents or their fleas while hunting in rural and suburban areas.

III. Vaccines for plague are available; however, they are not used routinely in either humans or domestic animals. Plague vaccine has been used in humans in situations in which there was a known high risk of plague exposure. The vaccine currently available in the United States is a formalin-killed bacterin (Plague Vaccine, USP, Cutter). The protective antibody induced in humans by this vaccine is short-lived, which necessitates annual or biannual boosters. The efficacy of the vaccine in dogs and cats is presently unknown. Plague vaccination of dogs and cats is not currently recommended, and there are no vaccines licensed for use in these species.

PUBLIC HEALTH CONSIDERATIONS

I. Plague is a serious disease in humans. The mortality in untreated cases is greater than 50%, and in treated cases it is 5–15%. Early diagnosis and treatment are very important in reducing mortality.

II. Most human cases of plague result from the bite of an infected rodent flea. Two less common but important modes of contracting the disease are direct contact with infected animal tissues (such as dressing a plague-infected rabbit) and contact with a plague-infected cat. Within the last 10 years a number of cat-associated human plague cases have been reported. The human exposures in these cases occurred by a cat-inflicted scratch or bite, by the bite of a flea being carried on the cat, or by aerosol from a cat with plague pneumonia. These cases emphasize the necessity of taking precautions when treating cats from plague-enzootic areas. Public health officials should always be notified immediately when plague is suspected.

SUGGESTED READINGS

Butler TC: Plague and Other Yersinia Infections. Plenum Press, New York, 1983

Gregg CT: Plague: An Ancient Disease in the Twentieth Century. University of New Mexico Press, Albuquerque, N.M. 1985

Kaufmann AF, Mann JM, Gardiner TM, et al: Public health implications of plague in domestic cats. J Am Vet Med Assoc 179:875, 1981

Poland JD, Barnes AM: Plague. p. 515. In Steele JH (ed): CRC Handbook Series in Zoonoses. Vol. I, Sect. A. CRC Press Inc., Boca Raton, Florida, 1979

Rail CD: Plague Ecotoxicology: Including Historical Aspects of the Disease in the Americas and the Eastern Hemisphere. Charles C Thomas, Springfield, Ill. 1985

Rollag OJ, Skeels MR, Nims LJ, et al: Feline plague in New Mexico: Report of five cases. J Am Vet Med Assoc 179:1381, 1981

Rust JH, Cavanaugh DC, O'Shita R, Marshall JD: The role of domestic animals in the epidemiology of plague. I. Experimental infection of dogs and cats. J Infect Dis 124:522, 1971

19

Enteric Campylobacteriosis

James G. Fox

ETIOLOGY

I. The genus *Campylobacter* is now defined as a group of gram-negative, slender, curved, motile bacteria with a single polar flagellum and microaerophilic growth requirements. *Campylobacter jejuni* is the organism routinely associated with diarrheal disease in animals and humans. However *Campylobacter coli,* distinguished from *C. jejuni* on the basis of hippurate hydrolysis, is also occasionally isolated from diarrheic patients.

II. Enteritis due to *C. jejuni/coli* occurs in a variety of domestic animal species. Clinical diarrheal disease has been recognized in dogs, cats, cattle, sheep, chickens, ferrets, mink, and a number of laboratory animal species. The literature suggests that *C. jejuni* may be associated with proliferative bowel disease in hamsters and ferrets, but this has not been proved experimentally. The above-mentioned hosts can also serve as reservoirs of infection, as can a variety of other wild animals and birds.

III. *Campylobacter* spp. are distributed worldwide but are probably more prevalent in those areas in which hygiene and sanitation practices are suboptimal.

IV. As with most enteric pathogens, fecal-oral spread and foodborne or waterborne transmission appear to be the principal avenues of infection. One proposed source of infection for domestic pets, including ferrets, is ingestion of undercooked poultry and meat products. Animal hosts can be asymptomatic carriers and shed organisms in the feces for prolonged periods of time. The source of infection in many cases is, therefore, fecal contamination of food, water, milk, and fresh processed meats (including pork, beef, and poultry products).

V. Organisms can survive in vitro at 37°C for 2 months and can also survive in feces, milk, water, and urine. Wild birds also may be important sources for water contamination with *Campylobacter* spp. Unpasteurized milk has been cited as a principal source of infection in several diarrheal outbreaks among humans.

CLINICAL SIGNS

I. The diarrhea appears to be most severe in young animals. Typical clinical signs in dogs, cats, and ferrets include mucus-laden, watery, and/or bile-streaked feces (with or without blood and leukocytes) of 3–7 days' duration, partial anorexia, and occasional vomiting. Some animals may present with watery diarrhea, and fever and leukocytosis may also be present. Occasionally, an animal will present with acute-onset gastroenteritis, which in dogs must be differentiated from canine parvovirus infection. In certain other cases diarrhea may persist for more than 2 weeks (sometimes for several months) or may be intermittent.

II. Certain features of enteric campylobacteriosis seen in humans and animals—blood and leukocytes in the feces, congestion, edema, ulcerous lesions in various parts of the gastrointestinal tract, and occasional sepsis—suggest that the organisms are invasive. Experimental oral inoculation of *C. jejuni* in several animal species can result in bacteremia, which lends support to this idea. The rapid rise in circulating antibodies in infected animals and the isolation of organisms from the blood of some animals are indicative of the invasive capabilities of the bacteria.

   A. Gnotobiotic puppies inoculated with *C. jejuni* have been shown to develop malaise, loose feces, and tenesmus within 3 days postinoculation.

   B. Ferrets challenged orally with *C. jejuni* have been shown to develop a blood-tinged mucoid diarrhea within 5–7 days postinoculation.

   C. In other experiments, dogs and cats inoculated with *C. jejuni* have not developed diarrhea but instead have shed organisms in feces without showing clinical signs.

III. An enterotoxin has been identified in some strains of *C. jejuni*; its biologic role in the production of disease, while not completely elucidated, appears to involve the fluid loss associated with watery diarrhea. Specific strains appear to cause a secretory diarrhea, while others cause a bloody, mucoid diarrhea.

IV. Gross pathologic examination of dogs orally dosed with *C. jejuni* and killed 43 hours postinoculation has revealed primarily a congested and edematous colon; occasionally, hyperemia of the small intestine may be noted. Microscopically, there may be a reduction in epithelial height of colonic mucosa and reduced numbers of goblet cells in the colon and cecum. Incipient crypt abscesses may be present, with polymorphonuclear cell infiltration of the lamina propria. Focally, mucosal epithelial glands can be hyperplastic, which results in a thickened mucosa. This proliferative lesion is characterized by an immature, hyperchromatic, hyperplastic epithelium with a high mitotic index, deep and irregular crypts, and cystic glands. Lesions in the ileum can consist of focally shallow crypts and blunt, irregular villi, which occasionally are fused.

DIAGNOSIS

I. Direct examination of feces

Diagnosis is possible by using fresh feces and either darkfield or phase-contrast microscopy to identify the characteristic darting motility of *C. jejuni*. This technique can be especially useful during the acute stage of the disease, when large numbers of organisms are more likely to be shed in the feces. It is also helpful to ascertain if red or white blood cells are present in the feces.

II. Culture

Both *C. jejuni* and *C. coli* grow well at 42°C in a microaerophilic atmosphere of 5%–10% carbon dioxide and an equal amount of oxygen. The standard technique for diagnosis involves culture of feces on commercially available agars containing selective antibiotics. Cultures are incubated for 72–96 hours. Colonies are round, raised, translucent, and sometimes mucoid. Identification can be made by a series of biochemical tests that are readily available in any diagnostic laboratory.

III. Serology

A variety of techniques can be used to detect serum antibodies to various antigens of *Campylobacter*. A specific bactericidal assay has been employed using serially diluted serum samples to demonstrate a rising antibody titer; this is sometimes helpful in diagnosis of the disease. Other serologic assays such as enzyme-linked immunosorbent assay (ELISA) have been developed to survey human populations during outbreaks of campylobacteriosis and to ascertain previous exposure. It must be stressed that enteric viruses, as well as other enteric bacterial pathogens, must be ruled out in animals with *Campylobacter*-associated diarrhea.

IV. Serotyping

Various procedures have been employed to identify strain differences in *C. jejuni* and *C. coli* by utilizing thermostable and thermolabile surface antigens. Studies have shown that extensive serologic heterogeneity exists within these species of bacteria. The thermostable antigen used in the passive (indirect) hemagglutination assay (PHA) is comprised of lipopolysaccharide (LPS) O antigens that are structurally distinct from the LPS of the Enterobacteriaceae. At least 50 thermostable serotypes have been identified. Serotypes commonly isolated from diarrheic humans have also been isolated from dogs and cats with and without diarrhea.

TREATMENT

I. Isolation of *C. jejuni* from the diarrheic feces of animals does not always imply a need for antibiotic therapy. In certain cases in which animals are severely affected or present a zoonotic threat, however, antibiotic therapy may be indicated. Sensitivity patterns of *C. jejuni* isolates from animals are in general agreement with those from human populations. Erythromycin, the drug of choice for *Campylobacter* diarrhea in humans, is also effective at serum levels achievable in animals. Gentamicin, furazolidone, doxycycline, or chloramphenicol can also be used. Tetracycline and kanamycin usually demonstrate in vitro activity against *C. jejuni* and *C. coli*; however, plasmid-mediated resistance exists in certain *C. jejuni* strains and is transmissible within serotypes. It is generally accepted that the β-lactam antibiotic ampicillin is relatively inactive against most strains of *Campylobacter*. Penicillin also shows little activity, the majority of strains being resistant at therapeutically achievable drug levels. Sulfadimethoxine and sulfa combinations are variably efficacious in animals.

II. Before therapy for diarrhea in animals is instituted, isolation attempts should be made; if *C. jejuni* is identified, appropriate in vitro antibiotic sensitivity testing should be performed. To date the efficacy of antibiotic therapy in affected animals has been reported only infrequently. In humans if the disease is severe, *C. jejuni* diarrhea will respond to antibiotic therapy. It is important to note that some animals will continue to shed organisms in the feces despite antibiotic therapy. Alternative antibiotic therapy may be warranted; however, it is important to determine if other intercurrent disease states may exist in the affected animal. Careful attention to fluid and electrolyte balance is also important for successful treatment, particularly in young animals.

PREVENTION

Immunoprophylactic measures are currently unavailable for enteric campylobacteriosis in dogs and cats.

PUBLIC HEALTH CONSIDERATIIONS

It is now recognized that *C. jejuni* is a leading cause of diarrhea in humans. It is well established that dogs, cats, and captive nonhuman primates can serve as the source of infection for humans. Animals recently purchased from animal shelters or pounds are particularly suspect. Awareness of the potential for transmission of infection, particularly from dogs and cats to humans, and the utilization of reliable serotyping systems for identification of human and animal isolates will allow a more complete understanding of the epidemiology/epizootiology of *Campylobacter* infection and the exact role of animal hosts in the spread of organisms to human beings.

SUGGESTED READINGS

Blaser MJ, LaForce FM, Wilson NA, et al: Reservoirs for human campylobacteriosis. J Infect Dis 141:665, 1980

Fox JG, Ackerman JI, Newcomer CE: Ferret as a potential reservoir for human campylobacteriosis. Am J Vet Res 44:1049, 1983

Fox JG, Claps M, Beaucage CM: Chronic diarrhea associated with *Campylobacter jejuni* infection in a cat. J Am Vet Med Assoc 189:455, 1986

Fox JG, Krakowka S, Taylor NS: Acute-onset *Campylobacter*-associated gastroenteritis in adult beagles. J Am Vet Med Assoc 187:1268, 1985

Fox JG, Maxwell KO, Ackerman JI: *Campylobacter jejuni* associated diarrhea in commercially reared beagles. Lab Anim Sci 34:151, 1984

Fox JG, Moore R, Ackerman JI: Canine and feline campylobacteriosis: epizootiology and clinical and public health features. J Am Vet Med Assoc 183:1420, 1983

Fox JG, Moore R, Ackerman JI: *Campylobacter jejuni*-associated diarrhea in dogs. J Am Vet Med Assoc 183:1430, 1983

Klipstein FA, Engert RF, Short H, et al: Pathogenic properties of *Campylobacter jejuni*: assay and correlation with clinical manifestations. Infect Immun 50:43, 1985

Mills SD, Bradbury WC, Penner JL: Basis for serological heterogeneity of thermostable antigens of *Campylobacter jejuni*. Infect Immun 50:284, 1985

Prescott JF, Barker IK: Campylobacter colitis in gnotobiotic dogs. Vet Rec 107:314, 1980

Prescott JF, Karmali MA: Attempts to transmit *Campylobacter* enteritis to dogs and cats. Can Med Assoc J 119:1001, 1978

Prescott JF, Munroe DL: *Campylobacter jejuni* enteritis in man and domestic animals. J Am Vet Med Assoc 181:1524, 1982

20

Canine Brucellosis

Roy V. H. Pollock
Leland E. Carmichael

ETIOLOGY

I. Canine brucellosis is caused by *Brucella canis,* a small gram-negative aerobic coccobacillus.
II. Transmission occurs readily at breeding, but shedding of organisms in aborted fetuses and uterine discharges is probably the primary source of epizootic spread within kennels.
III. The disease appears to occur worldwide. The prevalence is estimated at approximately 1% among privately owned dogs and 5% among strays, although this varies greatly among geographic regions.
IV. The organism is relatively short-lived outside the dog and is readily inactivated by common germicidal disinfectants.

CLINICAL SIGNS

I. The principal clinical signs of canine brucellosis are associated with the reproductive tract.
II. In females the cardinal sign is abortion, which occurs after 45–55 days of gestation in about three-fourths of cases.
III. Early embryonic death and abortion 10–20 days after mating occur in some females. These may go unnoticed by the owner so that the bitch will be presented with a chief complaint of inability to conceive rather than abortion.
IV. The most common chief complaint in males is infertility.
   A. Physical examination usually reveals epididymitis; one or both epididymides will be swollen, firm, and tender. Testicular atrophy and a moist scrotal dermatitis may be present.
   B. Semen from infected males usually contains large numbers (80%–90%) of abnormal sperm and inflammatory cells, especially during the first 3 months postinfection.

    C. Chronically-infected males may be essentially azoospermic.
  V. Nonspecific clinical signs in both sexes include lethargy, loss of libido, premature aging, and generalized lymph node enlargement.
 VI. Rarely, *B. canis* is isolated from lesions of discospondylitis. Recurrent uveitis has been observed occasionally in infected dogs.

DIAGNOSIS

   I. The serologic diagnosis of canine brucellosis is difficult because surface antigens of this rough *Brucella* cross-react with antibodies to other nonpathogenic organisms commonly encountered by dogs.
  II. The *rapid slide agglutination test* is available commercially for use as an in-office screening test.
    A. Serum and fresh 0.2 *M* 2-mercaptoethanol are mixed and allowed to stand for 1 minute. The treated serum is then mixed with stained antigen (cross-reactive *Brucella ovis* organisms) and observed for evidence of agglutination.
    B. The test has a high *negative predictive value*. That is, over 99% of dogs negative by the slide test are truly free of infection.
    C. The *positive predictive value* of the slide test is relatively low, however; only half to two-thirds of dogs positive by the slide test are subsequently proved infected.
    D. Thus, dogs with positive slide test results should be categorized as suspect but they should *not* be considered infected until further tests are performed.
 III. The *tube agglutination test* and *agar gel immunodiffusion test* are two further serologic techniques available through diagnostic laboratories; they provide somewhat greater diagnostic specificity. Nevertheless, blood culture remains the definitive test for infection.
 IV. Dogs with canine brucellosis remain bacteremic for months to years. Hence, *blood culture* is the "gold standard" for infection.
    A. The laboratory should be familiar with bacteriologic methods for the diagnosis of *B. canis*.
    B. Blood should be collected aseptically into nutrient broth.
    C. The broth should be cultured aerobically for 3–5 days before a drop is transferred to solid media for identification.
    D. Since *B. canis* is relatively slow-growing, colonies may not become visible on agar media for 48–96 hours.

TREATMENT

I. Canine brucellosis is difficult and expensive to treat.
II. Repeated blood cultures are necessary to confirm effective treatment. Recrudescence of the infection after cessation of antibiotic therapy is common.
III. Even if the organism can be successfully eliminated, males frequently remain sterile owing to irreversible damage to the testes and epididymides.
IV. Neutering is believed to largely eliminate the risk of transmission from infected dogs, even if complete elimination of the organism is not obtained.
V. The best treatment results have been obtained with a combination of streptomycin and either high-dose minocycline or tetracycline hydrochloride administered during the first 3 months of infection.
   A. Streptomycin (10 mg/kg IM bid) is given for 7 days together with minocycline 25 mg/kg PO bid for 3 weeks or longer.
   B. There is one report in the literature of successful treatment with two 3-week regimens of tetracycline (250 mg PO tid) and streptomycin (250 mg IM bid) given 8 weeks apart.
   C. The cure rate is estimated to be approximately 80% in relatively recent infections (less than 3 months' duration). A cure is more difficult to achieve in long-standing infections.

PREVENTION

I. No vaccine is available.
II. Prevention depends upon elimination of infected dogs from the breeding program and screening of all dogs prior to mating or entry into a breeding colony.
III. Bitches should be screened by the slide test several weeks before their expected estrus. It is important to screen dogs prior to proestrus so that if a suspicious result is obtained, there is time to complete additional laboratory tests before the onset of estrus.
IV. Heavily used males should be bred only to test-negative females and checked twice yearly by the slide test.
V. Dogs introduced into a negative colony should be isolated until they are shown to be negative on two tests made 1 month apart.

PUBLIC HEALTH CONSIDERATIONS

I. Canine brucellosis is a zoonotic disease, although its transmissibility for humans appears to be low.

II. Signs in humans are nonspecific: generalized malaise, headache, joint pains, lymphadenopathy, intermittent fever, chills, and weight loss.

III. Tentative diagnosis can be made by serologic testing but should be confirmed by blood culture.

IV. Fortunately, the disease in humans (unlike dogs) responds readily to antibiotic therapy.

V. Veterinarians should use caution in handling suspected animals, particularly bitches with unexplained abortions.

SUGGESTED READINGS

Alton GG, Jones LM, Pietz DE: Laboratory Techniques in Brucellosis. 2nd Ed. World Health Organization, Geneva, 1975

Carmichael LE, Kenney RM: Canine abortion caused by *Brucella canis*. J Am Vet Med Assoc 152:605, 1968

Carmichael LE: Brucellosis (*Brucella canis*). p. 185. In Steele JH (ed): CRC Handbook Series in Zoonoses, Vol. I, Sect. A. CRC Press, Boca Raton, Fla, 1979

Flores-Castro R, Carmichael LE: Canine brucellosis: current status of methods of diagnosis and treatment. Cornell Vet 68: suppl. 7, 76, 1978

Greene CE, George LW: Canine brucellosis. p. 646. In Greene CE (ed): Clinical Microbiology and Infectious Diseases of the Dog and Cat. WB Saunders, Philadelphia, 1984

Jennings PB, Crumrine MH, Lewis GE, et al: The effect of a two-stage antibiotic regimen on dogs infected with *Brucella canis*. J Am Vet Med Assoc 164:513, 1974

Pollock RVH: Canine brucellosis: current status. Compend Contin Ed Pract Vet 1:255, 1979

Swenson RM, Carmichael LE, Cundy KR: Human infection with *Brucella canis*. Ann Intern Med 76:435, 1972

Zoha SJ, Carmichael LE: Serological responses of dogs to cell wall and internal antigens of *Brucella canis* (*B. canis*). Vet Microbiol 7:35, 1982

Zoha SJ, Walsh R: Effect of a two-stage antibiotic treatment regimen on dogs naturally infected with *Brucella canis*. J Am Vet Med Assoc 180:1474, 1982

21

Tyzzer's Disease

Kimberly S. Waggie

ETIOLOGY

I. The etiologic agent of Tyzzer's disease is *Bacillus piliformis,* a gram-negative, spore-forming bacterium. The organism has a length of 4–25 μm, with an average width of 0.5 μm. Spores are located terminally. Motility is conferred by peritrichous flagella.

   A. *B. piliformis* exhibits staining variability with basic aniline dyes. Individual bacteria may stain in a uniform manner or appear banded. The colorless segments of banded bacilli are periodic acid–Schiff (PAS)–positive. Organisms are stained only faintly by Gram stains. Methylene blue or thionine stains are effective for staining *B. piliformis* in smear preparations.

   B. *B. piliformis* is an obligate intracellular parasite that has not been propagated in cell-free media. Vegetative forms of the organism occur in characteristic bundles in the cytoplasm of hepatocytes, cardiomyocytes, and absorptive epithelial and smooth muscle cells of the intestinal tract. The bacterium has also been found in the cytoplasm of neurons and epithelial cells of the choroid plexus and leptomeninges of the brain in experimental infections.

II. Tyzzer's disease is thought to be transmitted through the ingestion of spores shed in the feces of infected or carrier animals. Contact with infected rodents has been implicated as, but not proved to be, a source of infection. Transplacental transmission has also been suggested as, but not proved to be, a route of infection.

   A. The disease was initially described in Japanese waltzing mice. It has since been reported in numerous rodents, rabbits, dogs, cats, horses, and primates. Cases have occurred in North America, Europe, and Asia.

   B. The incidence of Tyzzer's disease in dogs and cats is unknown; the disease tends to occur as sporadic isolated cases rather than as major epizootics. Experimental attempts at disease transmission to these species have failed. This suggests that dogs and cats are relatively resistant to infection.

III. Outside the host *B. piliformis* survives in the form of spores, which have been reported to survive in the environment for at least 5 years. Spores can survive repeated cycles of freezing and thawing but are killed by heating at 80°C for 30 minutes. A 0.3% solution of chlorine bleach is a rapidly effective sporicide, and iodophors are fairly effective after prolonged contact. Phenols, quaternary ammonium compounds, and ethanol are ineffective against *B. piliformis* spores.

CLINICAL SIGNS

I. The pathogenesis of *B. piliformis* infection is incompletely understood. Following ingestion of spores, the characteristic bacteria may be found in absorptive epithelial cells of the terminal ileum, cecum, and proximal colon. Dissemination to other organs probably occurs through the portal venous and lymphatic systems. After initial invasion of an organ, infection may spread via cell-to-cell contact.

II. Tyzzer's disease primarily affects weanling animals. Adult cats and dogs are occasionally affected. Clinical disease is often precipitated by concurrent infections such as canine distemper or feline leukemia. Other predisposing factors reportedly include poor sanitation, fluctuating environmental temperatures, shipping stress, sulfonamide administration, and treatment with immunosuppressive agents, such as cortisone.

III. Animals may die from acute *B. piliformis* infection without showing previous clinical signs of illness. When present, clinical signs are nonspecific. They include watery to pasty feces, which may be blood-tinged, dehydration, anorexia, vomiting, fever, and depression. The abdomen is generally painful on palpation. Illness may continue for several days. The disease course generally is longer in older animals. Neurologic signs, such as staring and convulsions, may occur immediately prior to death.

DIAGNOSIS

I. Tyzzer's disease is rarely diagnosed antemortem.

II. Elevation of serum alanine aminotransferase and aspartate aminotransferase levels occurs with involvement of the liver. Absolute neutropenia and hypoglycemia have occasionally been reported.

III. Warthin-Starry or Dieterle silver stains of liver biopsy specimens may reveal nests of *B. piliformis* within the cytoplasm of hepatocytes bordering foci of hepatocellular necrosis.

IV. No remarkable lesions may be present at necropsy. More frequently, multiple white to tan foci (from pinpoint size to several mm in diameter) are found in the liver. The mucosa of the ileum and/or proximal colon may be congested, and there may be patchy necrosis of the ileal mucosa. The mesenteric lymph nodes may be enlarged and edematous.

    A. Intestinal and liver lesions may occur independently.

    B. Bands of myocardial necrosis have been reported in numerous cases of Tyzzer's disease in other species. This lesion may be an as yet unrecognized lesion in the dog and cat.

V. Methylene blue–stained impression smears of suspect liver lesions may reveal clusters of typical rod-shaped bacteria in "pick up sticks" arrangement (Fig. 21-1). These clusters are diagnostic of *B. piliformis* infection. Singly occurring bacilli in the smears should be disregarded because terminal migration of intestinal flora to the liver frequently occurs.

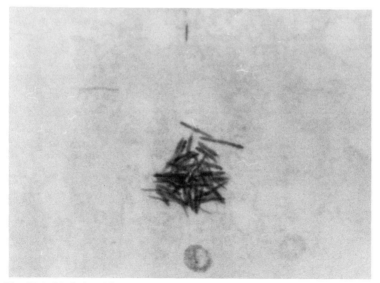

Fig. 21-1. Methylene blue–stained liver smear showing characteristic cluster of *Bacillus piliformis*, the causative agent of Tyzzer's disease.

VI. The best diagnostic method currently available for Tyzzer's disease in dogs and cats is the histologic demonstration of *B. piliformis* within hepatocytes bordering foci of liver necrosis or within absorptive epithelial cells of the distal ileum and/or colon.

    A. *B. piliformis* is rarely observed in hematoxylin-and-eosin– or Gram-stained tissue sections. The organism is well stained, even when present in low numbers, by silver impregnation techniques, such as Warthin-Starry or Dieterle.

    B. The vegetative phase of *B. piliformis* is highly unstable and begins to autolyze shortly after the death of the host. Therefore, tissue samples should be collected as soon as possible and placed in 10% buffered formalin.

TREATMENT

  I. Strategies for treatment of *B. piliformis* infection have not been thoroughly evaluated. Therapeutic measures reported in cases of canine and feline Tyzzer's disease have been ineffective owing in part to the rapidity of progression of the disease.

 II. *B. piliformis* has been found to be tetracycline- and cephaloridine-sensitive in antibiotic susceptibility tests. Oral tetracyline has also been reported to abate epizootics of Tyzzer's disease in rabbit and rodent colonies. The organism has been variably sensitive to penicillin, chloramphenicol, streptomycin, and erythromycin and resistant to sulfa preparations, neomycin, polymyxin, and colistin. Sulfa drugs have been reported to potentiate the disease in rabbit colonies.

III. Supportive therapy (replacement of fluids and electrolytes) may be attempted when appropriate.

IV. Prophylactic antibiotic treatment of littermates and the dam of affected animals may be considered if they inhabit the same area.

PREVENTION

  I. Many cases of Tyzzer's disease are associated with stressful environmental conditions or intercurrent disease. Therefore one of the best means of prevention is to follow standard preventive medicine procedures through routine vaccination, parasite control, and environmental maintainance.

   A. Exposure to wild rodents should be minimized because they have been suggested as a source of infection.
   B. Living areas and utensils should be frequently disinfected with a 0.3% solution of chlorine bleach where feasible.
II. Clinically ill animals should be physically isolated from healthy animals. Caretakers should not wear shoes or clothing previously worn in isolation areas when attending healthy animals. Utensils should not be exchanged between isolation and regular holding areas unless thoroughly sanitized and disinfected between uses.
III. A bitch or queen that has had more than one litter affected by Tyzzer's disease might be a *B. piliformis* carrier. Removing such an animal from the breeding program would be prudent even though the existence of carrier states has not been proved.

PUBLIC HEALTH CONSIDERATIONS

 I. No human cases of Tyzzer's disease have been documented. However, there has been one report of antibody to *B. piliformis* in sera of pregnant Danish women.
II. *B. piliformis* infection is of limited public health concern at present. Standard precautions for personal hygiene should be taken when handling animals suspected of having Tyzzer's disease.

SUGGESTED READINGS

Bennett AM, Huxtable CR, Love DR: Tyzzer's disease in cats experimentally infected with feline leukaemia virus. Vet Microbiol 2:49, 1977

Fries A: Antibodies to *Bacillus piliformis* (Tyzzer's disease) in sera from man and other species. p. 249. In Spiegel A, Erichsen S, Solleveld HA (eds): Animal Quality and Models in Biomedical Research. Gustav Fischer Verlag, Stuttgart, 1980

Fujiwara K: Tyzzer's disease. Jpn J Exp Med 48:467, 1978

Ganaway JR: Effect of heat and selected chemical disinfectants upon infectivity of spores of *Bacillus piliformis* (Tyzzer's disease). Lab Anim Sci 30:192, 1980

Ganaway JR,, Allen AM, Moore TD: Tyzzer's disease. Am J Pathol 64:717, 1971

Kovatch RM, Zebarth G: Naturally occurring Tyzzer's disease in a cat. J Am Vet Med Assoc 162:136, 1973

Poonacha KB, Smith HL: Naturally occurring Tyzzer's disease as a complication of distemper and mycotic pneumonia in a dog. J Am Vet Med Assoc 169:419, 1976

Qureshi SR, Carlton WW, Olander HJ: Tyzzer's disease in a dog. J Am Vet Med Assoc 168:602, 1976

Wilkie JSN, Barker IK: Colitis due to *Bacillus piliformis* in two kittens. Vet Pathol 22:649, 1985

22

Clostridial Diseases

Lea Stogdale

Clostridia are present in the soil and are part of the normal intestinal microbial flora. They are spore-forming, gram-positive, anaerobic bacteria that produce potent and specific disease–causing exotoxins. Dogs and cats are relatively resistant to the toxins produced by clostridia. Tetanus, botulism, clostridial enteritis, and gas gangrene occur occasionally in dogs. Tetanus and botulism occur rarely in cats; the signs are similar to those in dogs.

TETANUS

Etiology

I. Following infection with spores of *Clostridium tetani,* germination and neurotoxin production occur within necrotic, anaerobic wounds.
II. The incubation period is 5–10 days. The anaerobic conditions necessary for spore germination may develop within days or may result months later, from trauma in previously contaminated tissue.
III. Tetanus spores are distributed worldwide, but the disease, uncommon in dogs and rare in cats, is usually encountered only in tropical areas.
IV. The spores are extremely resistant to both disinfectants and environmental conditions.

Clinical Signs

I. Germinated spores produce the exotoxin responsible for the clinical signs. This exotoxin, tetanospasmin, travels along peripheral nerves and via the bloodstream to the central nervous system (CNS), where it binds to glycine-mediated interneural synapses.

II. Tetanospasmin inhibits the activity of spinal cord and brain stem interneurons. The resulting excessive lower motor neuron activity causes increased skeletal muscle tonus with intermittent clonus.

III. Clinical signs may commence a few days to several months after wound contamination. The incubation period is shortest with head and neck wounds. Rapid onset, within 4 days, is associated with high mortality.

IV. *Clostridium tetani* infection produces only minimal wound inflammation in dogs. In affected cats the wound is usually extensive and obvious.

V. Localized tetanus initially results in stiffness of a muscle group or limb near the infected area. The muscle contraction spreads bilaterally and then becomes generalized.

VI. Initially, the tonic muscle contraction results in stiffness of the hind legs and a stilted gait, giving the appearance of mild weakness or incoordination. Progressively, the tail becomes outstretched, and clonic convulsions, opisthotonus, and dyspnea occur.

VII. In dogs the muscle tonus causes the legs to be outstretched in a "saw-horse" appearance. In some cats all the legs extend caudally and the tail curves dorsally.

VIII. The head is noticeably affected. The ears become erect, the forehead wrinkled and the eyelids retracted, resulting in a "surprised" look. The lip commissures are retracted to produce a "grinning" appearance. The third eyelid prolapses, and there is enophthalmos. The animal demonstrates dysphagia, with salivation and difficulty in opening the jaws ("lockjaw").

IX. The patient is often hyperthermic owing to prolonged muscle contraction. Dysuria and constipation occur in severely affected animals. Alertness and appetite are maintained.

X. Hypersensitivity to touch and, to a lesser extent, to sound increases as the tetany worsens. The animal remains conscious; pain occurs during tetanic spasms.

XI. Death is due to respiratory complications with respiratory muscle paralysis.

Diagnosis

I. The clinical signs of progressive muscle tetany are distinctive. Prolapse of the third eyelid when the head is tapped is a characteristic sign.

II. A necrotic wound or history of previous tissue damage, including surgery (such as nonsterile castration), is suggestive.

III. Anaerobic culture of the organism, or mouse inoculation with the patient's serum or a wound extract, are usually unrewarding.

Treatment

I. Therapy and management of moderately affected animals are time-consuming and expensive. Improvement usually begins within 1 week after the start of treatment. Thereafter, gradual but complete recovery may take up to 3 weeks.

II. The prognosis depends on the distance of the infection from the brain, the speed of onset of clinical signs, the removal of the source of additional toxin (wound debridement), and the quality of nursing. Untreated animals usually die; treated patients generally recover.

III. Thorough wound debridement, irrigation, and drainage to remove all the necrotic tissue and expose the remaining tissue to air are *essential*.

IV. Penicillin must be administered systemically and locally into the wound area; 20,000 IU/kg bid for at least 5 days is recommended. It is advisable to use crystalline penicillin on the first day and procaine penicillin thereafter.

V. The use of tetanus antitoxin is controversial; the benefits are disputed. The antitoxin cannot penetrate the CNS and is ineffective in neutralizing the bound toxin. The antitoxin will neutralize the small amount of toxin still in the blood, however, and the small amount remaining in the wound area after debridement.

VI. Antitoxin should be administered prior to wound debridement. An initial test dose of 0.1–0.2 ml should be given subcutaneously and the patient observed for 30 minutes in order to check for hypersensitivity to equine serum (anaphylaxis). One or two vials of 10,000 U, given slowly IV, are considered more than adequate for the initial treatment.

VII. Good nursing care is most important. The animal should be placed on soft, dry, porous bedding in a darkened, quiet kennel. Disturbances should be kept to a minimum. Tranquilization with acetylpromazine or sedation with diazepam or phenobarbital should be used to control generalized tetany.

VIII. Atropine, glucocorticoids, and narcotics are contraindicated in animals with tetanus.

Prevention

I. Early and thorough wound irrigation with hydrogen peroxide followed by debridement and drainage will assist in preventing infection.
II. Systemic penicillin therapy for at least 3 days is advised for all patients with deep, contaminated wounds.
III. Immunization with tetanus antitoxin and toxoid is indicated only for dogs or cats living in a high-risk area that sustain deep wounds that are difficult to irrigate thoroughly.

BOTULISM

Etiology

I. Botulism is caused by ingestion of preformed neurotoxin produced in rotting carcasses and in food by *Clostridium botulinum*.
II. Under certain rare conditions, the toxin may be formed by organisms that have colonized the intestinal tract.
III. Dogs and cats are fairly resistant to the effects of the toxin. Dogs are occasionally affected, cats only rarely.

Clinical Signs

I. The toxin paralyzes the neuromuscular junctions, progressively causing muscle weakness, paresis, and flaccid paralysis.
II. The time course and severity depend on the amount of toxin absorbed. Signs may occur within hours of toxin ingestion or may require 1 week to become evident. The prognosis is poorest when a rapid onset of clinical signs is observed.
III. There is no sensory impairment; pain perception is normal.
IV. Some dogs will vomit early in the course of the disease.
V. Mildly affected animals show hind limb weakness, manifested as "bunny hopping" and an inability to climb steps or to jump.
VI. Moderately to severely affected animals show generalized paresis, progressing to flaccid paralysis. All reflexes are reduced or absent, but head and tail movements persist. Hypothermia is often evident.

VII. The cranial nerves are affected, with resulting facial muscle weakness, dysphagia, decreased pupillary light and palpebral blink reflexes, and mydriasis. Megaesophagus with regurgitation occurs in some dogs.

VIII. The toxin decreases cholinergic autonomic transmission, resulting in constipation, urinary retention, and diminished salivation and lacrimation. Bradycardia is an inconsistent sign.

IX. Paralysis of the respiratory muscles results in death.

Diagnosis

I. A high degree of suspicion is required to diagnose botulism. A suggestive history includes ingestion of a decomposing carcass and the involvement of other dogs.

II. The clinical signs of diffuse lower motor neuron dysfunction and muscle paralysis, with tactile and pain sensation remaining normal, strongly suggest botulism.

III. A confirmed diagnosis requires laboratory challenge of mice with the patient's gastric contents, feces, serum, or the remains of the suspected contaminated carcass. Poultry disease laboratories often can provide this service.

IV. Differential diagnoses include tick paralysis, snake envenomation, and polyradiculoneuritis, which are respectively suggested by the finding of an engorged tick, a snake bite, or muscle wasting and may also be suggested by the geographic region. A generalized flaccid paralysis, including the cranial muscles, suggests botulism. The other diseases produce an ascending paralysis that spares the head.

Treatment

I. Administration of *C. botulinum* antitoxin is of little or no value. The toxin type affecting dogs is not neutralized by commercial antitoxin. In addition, antitoxin cannot neutralize toxin already bound to the neuromuscular junctions.

II. Oral antibiotics will kill any clostridial organisms in the intestines. Laxatives and enemas will hasten removal of any toxin remaining in the alimentary tract.

III. Supportive therapy will prevent complications in moderately affected patients. The good nursing that is required includes a soft bed, laxatives, bladder catheterization, synthetic tears, and feeding of food and fluids by hand or via stomach tube.

IV. Improvement or death occurs within a week. Recovery is complete.

Prevention

Owners' preventing their animals from roaming unrestrained would eliminate many problems, including the ingestion of rotting carcases containing botulinum neurotoxin.

CLOSTRIDIAL ENTERITIS

Etiology

I. *Clostridium perfringens* or *Clostridium difficile,* along with other factors, can result in clostridial overgrowth and produce an enteritis. The unknown factors may allow an intestinal microbial imbalance, intestinal stasis, or both.

II. The clostridia produce exotoxins, some of which cause diarrhea. In addition, they may invade the intestinal mucosa.

III. Only dogs have been reported to be affected.

Clinical Signs

I. Melena, hematochezia, and rapid death result from peracute necrotizing hemorrhagic gastroenteritis or enteritis.

II. Chronic or recurrent diarrhea occurs most commonly in German shepherd dogs.

III. Viral enteritis due to canine distemper virus, parvovirus, coronavirus, or rotavirus may be complicated and worsened by clostridial proliferation and toxin production.

IV. Clostridial overgrowth secondary to antibiotic therapy results in pseudomembranous colitis. Clindamycin has been implicated in at least one dog, and other antimicrobial drugs have been suspected. The signs included a chronic watery diarrhea and abdominal pain, occurring within 1 day of administration of the drug.

Diagnosis

I. The necropsy diagnosis of clostridial enteritis requires the presence of tissue necrosis associated with the demonstration of clostridial organisms.
II. Anaerobic culture of small intestinal fluid, obtained at exploratory laparotomy or necropsy, generally is impractical. However, demonstration of large numbers of large gram-positive rods on smears made from the proximal small intestine is highly suggestive of clostridial enteritis.
III. Pseudomembranous colitis can be suspected when signs of enteritis and colitis appear soon after initiation of antimicrobial therapy and disappear when the antibiotic is withdrawn.

Treatment

I. Metronidazole, 60 mg/kg/day PO for 1 week, has been recommended.
II. A bland diet consisting of boiled rice with cottage cheese or chicken is helpful.
III. Pseudomembranous colitis is treated by withdrawal of the offending drug and its replacement with either metronidazole or vancomycin.
IV. Chronic or recurrent diarrhea may require long-term, low-dose metronidazole, 5 mg/kg/day PO for many months.

Prevention

Dogs suffering from hemorrhagic enteritis should be given broad-spectrum antimicrobials: penicillin and gentamicin, tetracycline, chloramphenicol, or metronidazole.

GAS GANGRENE

Etiology

I. This is produced by *C. perfringens* or *C. difficile* infection of devitalized tissue in wounds or fractures. The source of the organisms is the soil and fecal material.

II. Occasionally, other clostridial species are involved.

III. Owing to the resistance of dogs and cats to the effects of clostridial toxins, gas gangrene in these species is rare.

Clinical Signs

I. Infected wounds become edematous, crepitant, swollen, and foul-smelling.

II. The dog or cat is severely depressed and may have clinical signs resulting from splenic abscessation and pneumoperitoneum, cholecystitis, or discospondylitis.

Diagnosis

Diagnosis is based upon the history, signs of putrefactive tissue necrosis, and the results of anaerobic bacterial culture.

Treatment

I. Debridement of necrotic and infected tissue, with opening of the tissue to the air and surgical drainage, is mandatory.

II. High-dose penicillin therapy should be administered.

III. Death may occur within hours following debridement of an extensively necrotic wound owing to extensive absorption of toxin.

Prevention

I. Early and thorough wound irrigation with hydrogen peroxide, followed by debridement and drainage, is required.

II. Systemic penicillin therapy of contaminated wounds should be continued for at least 3 days.

GASTRIC DILATION

The cause of the gastric dilation-torsion (GDT) complex is unknown. The occasional "outbreaks" of GDT in kennels and the unequal distribution of this condition as seen by practitioners have led several veterinarians and many breeders to suspect an infectious etiology.

The bacterial groups primarily suspected are the clostridia and staphylococci although there is no concrete evidence that these infectious agents are significant contributors to the etiopathogenesis of GDT. However, the circumstantial cessation of cases concomitantly with the kennelwide use of antibiotics and clostridial antitoxin is both interesting and thought-provoking.

SUGGESTED READINGS

Barsanti JA: Botulism. p. 599. In Greene CE (ed): Clinical Microbiology and Infectious Diseases of the Dog and Cat. WB Saunders, Philadelphia, 1984

Berry AP, Levett PN: Chronic diarrhoea in dogs associated with *Clostridium difficile* infection. Vet Rec 118:102, 1986

Farrow BRH, Love DN: Bacterial, viral, and other infectious problems. p. 269. In Ettinger SJ (ed): Textbook of Veterinary Internal Medicine: Diseases of the Dog and Cat. Vol. I. 2nd Ed. WB Saunders, Philadelphia, 1983

Greene CE: Tetanus. p 608. In Greene CE (ed): Clinical Microbiology and Infectious Diseases of the Dog and Cat. WB Saunders, Philadelphia, 1984

Lorenz MD: Diseases of the large bowel. p. 1346. In Ettinger SJ (ed): Textbook of Veterinary Internal Medicine: Diseases of the Dog and Cat. Vol. II. 2nd Ed. WB Saunders, Philadelphia, 1983

Rothstein RJ, Baker FJ: Tetanus. Prevention and treatment. JAMA 240:675, 1978

Stogdale L: Canine tetanus. J S Afr Vet Assoc 47:299, 1976

23

Actinomycosis and Nocardiosis

Daria N. Love

ACTINOMYCOSIS

Etiology

I. Members of the genus *Actinomyces* are gram-positive branching, pleomorphic, rod-shaped bacteria.

II. They produce acetic, lactic, and succinic acids as products of metabolism. This distinguishes them from other bacteria of similar morphology (e.g., eubacteria, corynebacteria, and propionibacteria).

III. As a genus, *Actinomyces* is facultatively anaerobic. Most of the species that produce disease in cats and dogs grow well in an aerobic atmosphere (e.g., *Actinomyces viscosus, Actinomyces odontolyticus*), but others require reduced oxygen concentrations or strictly anaerobic conditions (e.g., *Actinomyces naeslundii, Actinomyces hordeovulneris*).

IV. Actinomycetes grow on blood agar plates or on other nutrient media that are supplemented with serum or with substances such as the Tween surfactants. Colonies are 1–2 mm in diameter at 48 hours and either are smooth, dome-shaped, and opaque or have a convoluted "molar tooth" shape, (e.g., *A. odontolyticus*). It is possible to speciate *Actinomyces* using biochemical tests once the fatty acid end products of metabolism have been analyzed. This is best done on a gas chromatograph, which is usually available in laboratories for accurately identifying anaerobic bacteria.

V. It is usually not possible to distinguish *Actinomyces* spp. from other similarly shaped anaerobic or facultative bacteria or from *Nocardia* spp. by Gram or other staining procedures, nor is it possible to differentiate them on the basis of the pathologic changes in affected animals.

VI. *Actinomyces* spp. are members of the normal flora of the respiratory and genital tracts of cats and dogs. Infection can occur at sites where they are normal residents (if there is a change in floral composition or in the normal balance of the microenvironment) or at sites where they are implanted, (e.g., by trauma).

    A. In situations in which disease occurs at a site such as the oral cavity or at sites adjacent to or contaminated by flora from the oral cavity, *Actinomyces* species generally are present as part of a mixed anaerobic and facultatively anaerobic bacterial population. For example, in feline pyothorax, *Bacteroides* spp., *Peptostreptococcus* spp., and *Pasteurella multocida* can be recovered along with members of the genus *Actinomyces*.

    B. A similar variety of organisms can be recovered from oral diseases such as gingivitis and periodontal disease of dogs and cats.

    C. Trauma or hematologic spread can result in osteomyelitis at various sites in the body.

    D. The most frequently encountered traumatic lesions from which *Actinomyces* spp. can be isolated are cat bite abscesses. *A. viscosus* and *A. odontolyticus* are most commonly isolated, along with *Bacteroides,* spp. *Peptostreptococcus anaerobius,* and *P. multocida*.

VII. *Actinomyces* spp. are susceptible to many disinfectants, including tincture of iodine, 70% alcohol, and chlorhexidine.

Clinical Signs

    I. Common clinical manifestations include subcutaneous tissue abscessation and draining sinus tracts from abscesses and osteomyelitic lesions.

   II. The contribution that *Actinomyces* spp. make to gingivitis and to periodontal lesions has not been assessed, but the organisms are frequently isolated from subgingival periodontal pockets and from deep gingival biopsy samples.

  III. Pyothorax in dogs and cats is now considered to be the result primarily of transplanted infections from the oral cavity.

    A. Disease production is thought to result from breakdown of the normal respiratory defense mechanisms, which ordinarily prevent contamination of the lower respiratory tract; viral infections, lung migration of parasite larvae, cold weather, and anesthetic gases all are known to affect the mucociliary escalator mechanism and can decrease the competence of alveolar macrophages.

B. Little credence can now be given to the idea that penetration of foreign bodies (e.g., grass seeds) is an important initiating factor in pyothorax. Early thoracic lesions present an airway pattern of pathology, and the bacterial species isolated in most conditions are known to originate in the oral cavity.

Diagnosis

I. Diagnosis is based on isolation and identification of *Actinomyces* spp. from purulent material, biopsy material, periodontal pockets, or osteomyelitic bone fragments.
   A. It is uncommon to find *Actinomyces* spp. alone in lesions, although the literature cites cases in which *A. viscosus* alone has been isolated.
      1. *A. viscosus* is a facultative species and would survive transport and inappropriate handling of specimens on the way to the laboratory.
      2. Likewise, conventional laboratory bacteriology may fail to grow many of the anaerobic organisms now known to be present in these lesions.
   B. Gram staining of purulent material is necessary to ensure that the true nature of the lesion is disclosed. Unless samples are taken and processed to preserve the viability of all anaerobic species, these species may not grow in the laboratory.
   C. Purulent material should be submitted in an anaerobic specimen collector or in a syringe from which all the air has been expelled. A thin, air-dried smear should be submitted along with the purulent material to permit accurate assessment of the lesion at the time of sampling.
   D. Samples taken from oral lesions will seldom yield anything other than facultative organisms unless the samples are cultured immediately onto anaerobic solid media or placed into anaerobic liquid media.

Treatment

I. *Actinomyces* spp., as well as most of the other anaerobes and facultative bacteria usually present, are susceptible to penicillin. Penicillin G should be given at a dosage of 20,000 IU/kg systemically bid or PO tid.

II. Treatment for uncomplicated subcutaneous bite wound abscesses should include extensive drainage and flushing of the wound cavity with sterile physiological saline for up to 5 days. It is usually not necessary to treat with antibiotics unless the animal is febrile.

III. Extensive curettage of affected bone is recommended for osteomyelitis, along with penicillin treatment for at least 2 weeks.

IV. Bilateral indwelling chest drains (with a three-way tap attached) should be inserted at the commencement of treatment of pyothorax cases.

    A. Purulent material must be removed every 12 hours until exudation ceases, a period that may last for as long as 2 weeks.

    B. Some practitioners find beneficial the instillation of crystalline penicillin (up to 500 mg in 10 ml of prewarmed physiological sterile saline) after each 12-hour drainage of the chest cavity. However, conscious animals sometimes find this procedure painful.

    C. The animal should be rehydrated as soon as therapy is commenced. Fluid therapy should be given until purulent exudate can no longer be drained from the thorax and the animal is in stable fluid balance.

    D. Penicillin should be administered systemically while the animal is hospitalized, and orally for at least 2 weeks after thoracic drains have been removed.

V. Treatment of oral lesions consists of extensive curettage, tooth removal, and penicillin therapy.

VI. The prognosis for recovery of animals with systemic manifestations of *Actinomyces* spp.–associated diseases is more favorable than for those with nocardiosis.

    A. Initial assessment of pyothorax should include the extent of lung pathology and the general systemic state of the animal.

        1. Severely dyspneic, dehydrated, emaciated animals generally respond poorly, while those presented before severe dyspnea is apparent may respond well to aggressive treatment.

        2. It is usual to have dogs presented at an earlier stage of the disease than cats, and the response of dogs is usually more predictable and more favorable.

    B. Osteomyelitis and oral diseases usually respond well if curettage is complete and penicillin therapy is continued for a sufficient period of time.

VII. Alternative antibiotics suggested in the literature should not be used unless there is a very good reason.

    A. Metronidazole, which is often recommended for anaerobes, does not work well for *A. viscosus* and other facultative bacteria that may be present.

B. The other anaerobes often found in mixed infections do not have predictable sensitivities to agents such as the tetracyclines, chloramphenicol, and lincomycin.

C. Long-term therapy with these agents can also lead to toxic side effects and the development of superinfections with other, more life-threatening bacteria.

D. Aminoglycosides are contraindicated for any disease process to which anaerobic bacteria contribute.

NOCARDIOSIS

Etiology

I. *Nocardia* spp. are gram-positive bacteria that form branching rods and filaments (hyphae).

II. Species of *Nocardia* that are frequently isolated from cats and dogs include *Nocardia asteroides, Nocardia braziliensis,* and *Nocardia caviae.*

A. These species have a growth cycle that results in late fragmentation of the filamentous bacterial forms; long, beaded rods are often seen in purulent exudate.

B. This late fragmentation gives rise to the very characteristic appearance of colonies of the organism grown on blood or other nutrient agar. The so-called aerial hyphae are obvious at 3–4 days, sitting above the surface of an otherwise conventional bacterial colony.

1. It was this colonial appearance that contributed to the original misclassification of *Nocardia* as a fungus.

2. This characteristic colonial appearance makes identification of *Nocardia* spp. very simple.

III. The cell wall of *Nocardia* spp. contains mycolic acids, which are similar to the mycolic acids found in the mycobacteria and which are partly responsible for the acid-fast staining characteristic of those species.

A. The literature states that *Nocardia* spp. are acid-fast and that this permits differentiation from members of the genus *Actinomyces*.

B. However, the nature of the mycolic acids and the cell wall of *Nocardia* spp. does not enable them to withstand the acid-fast stain used for the mycobacteria. Therefore, this staining reaction is not consistent and should not be relied upon to identify *Nocardia* spp.

IV. *Nocardia* spp. are soil saprophytes, whence the distribution of different species in different geographic areas (e.g., *N. asteroides* in temperate soils and *N. braziliensis* in tropical soils).

V. Despite the ubiquitous nature of *Nocardia* spp. in soils of the world, nocardiosis remains relatively uncommon.

    A. The disease is more common in dogs than in cats. The literature suggests introduction of organisms on grass awns or by inhalation of organisms in dust.

    B. The disease is thought to have a predilection for host tissues compromised by prior therapy with broad-spectrum antimicrobial agents. This is easily comprehended for infections initiated by inhalation, wherein the normal defensive flora of the respiratory tract has been depressed by antibiotics; it is less easily understood in cases of traumatic implantation of the organism. Animals with depressed immune systems are also considered to be at greater risk, although animals tested for defects in cellular or humoral immunity have not consistently demonstrated abnormal responses.

    C. Because the organism is a soil saprophyte and disease initiation requires a compromised host, nocardiosis does not spread from animal to animal or from animal to human.

VI. Organisms gain entry by inhalation, by ingestion, or by direct implantation via foreign bodies (e.g., grass awns).

    A. Multiplication is thought to occur in local tissues and lymph nodes prior to either confinement and abscess formation or dissemination via lymphatics and the bloodstream. Tissues and organs throughout the body may be involved in the inflammatory process, which is typically exudative in nature.

    B. Body cavities may also contain purulent effusions.

    C. Initially the inflammation is acute, but as the disease becomes more chronic, granulomatous tissue with central neutrophilic inflammatory foci predominates.

Clinical Signs

I. Typically, the disease has been divided into forms that are defined according to the site of the predominant lesions.

A. The subcutaneous form of the disease has been described in both dogs and cats, although much of the literature on this form is confounded by a lack of cultural identity. It is possible that many of these reports, especially those in which pharyngeal and cervical sinus tracts have been described, concerned *Actinomyces* rather than *Nocardia* spp.

　1. The lesions in the subcutis are characterized by cellulitis, abscessation, and draining sinus tracts.

　2. Occasionally, sinus tracts to the skin over limbs can be traced to osteomyelitis of long bones.

B. The thoracic form is characterized by early pyrexia followed by dyspnea, with extensive pleural effusion (empyemia or pyothorax).

　1. Radiography shows extensive fluid accumulation with destruction of normal pulmonary architecture.

　2. Extensive quantities of purulent material may be removed from one or both sides of the thorax by thoracocentesis.

　3. Clinically, this form cannot be distinguished from pyothorax caused by mixed anaerobic and facultative organisms, including *Actinomyces* spp.

C. In the systemic form of the disease purulent material often accumulates in the peritoneal cavity, and clinical signs may be referable to any of the organs and tissues involved (e.g., liver, kidney, brain, peritoneum).

Diagnosis

I. Diagnosis is dependent upon isolation and identification of *Nocardia* spp. from purulent exudate or biopsy material. It is not possible to differentiate *Nocardia* spp. from *Actinomyces* spp. by use of the Gram stain or of so-called acid-fast stains; neither is it possible to differentiate *Nocardia* spp. by pathologic features of the disease or by clinical signs.

A. Purulent material should be Gram stained to identify the presence of gram-positive branching and/or beaded rods and filaments.

B. Material should be plated to nutrient agar or blood agar plates and incubated aerobically at 37°C.

　1. Colonies (0.2 mm diameter) should be evident at 24 hours, and by 4 days the characteristic white aerial hyphae should be present on the surface of 2–3 mm colonies.

　2. Colonies may be cream, white, yellow, or orange, depending on the substrate on which they are growing.

C. If small numbers of organisms are present together with large numbers of inflammatory cells, pus should be inoculated also into a nutrient broth and incubated aerobically. Subculture to an agar plate at 3–4 days will then enable characteristic colonies to be seen.

D. Speciation of *Nocardia* is done by biochemical testing but is not necessary for routine identification.

E. It is not possible to give a definitive diagnosis of nocardiosis without culture and identification of the organism.

Treatment

I. The decision to treat an animal will depend on an assessment of the extent of the pathology and the underlying compromise to the host.

II. Antibacterial sensitivity tests should be carried out, although it is known that most *Nocardia* species are sensitive to sulfonamides but to few other antibacterial agents. Because nocardial lesions are highly exudative and the exudate will contain para-aminobenzoic acid (formation of which is the rate-limiting step in substrate inhibition by sulfonamides), removal of purulent material is mandatory before therapy can be contemplated.

III. In animals that appear to have no immunologic deficit and whose organ functions are adequate, it may be possible to attempt treatment if the affected tissue can be excised and adequate drainage instituted.

IV. Long-term therapy (a minimum of 4 weeks and up to 3 months) with sulfonamides (40 mg/kg sulfadiazine tid) is the antibacterial treatment of choice.

V. Localized lesions that receive adequate excision and/or drainage usually respond well to treatment.

A. The response of animals with thoracic pathology depends on the amount of damage and on the ability to maintain drainage until exudation ceases (this may last for up to 2 weeks or more).

1. In this form of the disease the general body condition and extent of clinical debility at presentation are reliable prognostic indicators.

2. Severely debilitated animals with cachexia on presentation usually do not survive the initial clinical work-up; others will survive for only a few days.

   B. It is usually inadvisable to give any reasonable prognosis to cases with extensive systemic involvement.

SUGGESTED READING

Hardie EM: Actinomycosis and nocardiosis. p. 663. In Greene CE (ed): Clinical Microbiology and Infectious Diseases of the Dog and Cat. WB Saunders, Philadelphia, 1984

24

Mycobacterial Infections
George T. Wilkinson

The mycobacteria (genus *Mycobacterium*) are members of the family Actinomycetaceae and can be divided into the following three groups according to their pathogenicity:

I. Classical pathogens—obligate parasites unable to multiply outside their vertebrate hosts (e.g., *Mycobacterium tuberculosis, Mycobacterium leprae*)

II. Facultative pathogens—normally existing as saprophytes in the environment but occasionally causing disease (e.g., *Mycobacterium fortuitum*)

III. Environmental saprophytes—very rarely causing disease (e.g., *Mycobacterium phlei*)

CLASSICAL PATHOGENS

Tuberculosis

Etiology

I. Canine and feline tuberculosis (TB) are caused by infection with either *Mycobacterium bovis,* the bovine tubercle bacillus, or *M. tuberculosis,* the cause of the human disease. Infection with *Mycobacterium avium,* more correctly called *mycobacteriosis,* has only rarely been reported in the dog or cat. The tubercle bacilli are morphologically similar, slender, acid-fast bacilli.

II. The cat is more susceptible to infection with *M. bovis,* whereas the dog is equally susceptible to either species. With the pasteurization of milk and the eradication of bovine TB from most developed countries, the disease is now rare in the cat, and uncommon in the dog as the incidence of human infection has also declined.

III. Tuberculosis has a worldwide distribution, but it is now especially prevalent among the human populations of developing countries, where overcrowded living conditions and poor standards of nutrition and hygiene are common. In such an environment pets are often the victims of transmission of the infection from their owners.

IV. The dog usually contracts the disease as an airborne infection, with lesions involving primarily the respiratory and alimentary tracts. The cat is most often infected by the ingestion of tuberculous milk, so that lesions are usually situated in the pharynx and alimentary tract.

V. Effective disinfectants include 3% formalin, phenol, or cresylic acid and 2% Lysol, provided they are applied for at least 30 minutes.

Clinical Signs

I. The outcome of infection depends upon several factors, including the resistance of the animal and the dose and virulence of the organism. The primary lesion at the site of infection is a tubercle, a granuloma formed mainly of epithelioid cells, which is the manifestation of a host allergic response to the tuberculoprotein of the organism. Depending upon the factors mentioned previously, the infection either may stabilize in the regional lymph node or may spread owing to proliferation of the mycobacteria. In an immunodepressed host the infection may become miliary or generalized, but this is rare in small animals.

II. In the majority of cases tuberculosis has an insidious onset. In the early stages affected animals may show little evidence of the infection apart from some loss of bodily condition. Such animals may harbor active and "open" lesions and consequently represent a danger to in-contact people and animals. There may also be an intermittent mild pyrexia.

III. In the respiratory form there is dyspnea, which is accompanied by exercise intolerance and which increases in severity as the disease progresses. Coughing, which may be productive, is also present. There may be an accumulation of tuberculous exudate in the pleural cavity, or, more rarely, a pneumothorax may result from breakdown of a subpleural pulmonary lesion.

IV. In the alimentary form there is progressive weight loss (often despite a reasonable appetite), and tuberculous peritonitis with the accumulation of exudate in the peritoneal cavity (tuberculous ascites) may develop. Abdominal masses may become palpable owing to involvement of various organs in the disease process—notably the liver, mesenteric lymph nodes, and kidneys.

V. Other systems may become involved. Occasionally lameness may result from infection of bone in tuberculous osteomyelitis. In the cat tuberculous metritis and chorioretinitis have been reported. Cutaneous lesions are uncommon and are manifested chiefly as indolent ulcers following breakdown of the skin overlying an infected lymph node. Granulomatous nodules and plaques can also occur and may ulcerate, leaving a raw granular surface that fails to heal. Skin lesions occur most frequently on the head, neck, and limbs.

Diagnosis

I. Diagnosis can be difficult because similar clinical signs can occur in neoplasia and in some of the deep mycotic infections of the dog and cat.

II. Radiography of the thorax and abdomen may detect enlarged organs and lymph nodes and thoracic or abdominal effusions.

III. Examination of Ziehl-Neelsen–stained smears of needle aspirates from lymph nodes or examination of the centrifuged deposits of transtracheal washes or thoracic and abdominal effusions often is unrewarding because the bacilli are few in number and difficult to detect. Culture of such specimens may yield a positive diagnosis but requires several weeks, as does guinea pig inoculation.

IV. Intradermal tuberculin tests give generally inconsistent results in the dog and cat, but in dogs injection of bacillus Calmette-Guérin (BCG) vaccine is reported to be a sensitive and reliable test. The vaccine (0.1–0.2 ml) is injected intradermally and the inoculation site examined 48 and 72 hours later. Positive reactions show erythema and induration, and central necrosis may occur. The test is not without danger because infected dogs may experience an acute hypersensitivity reaction. The test is not recommended for use in cats.

Treatment

In view of the serious risks to public health posed by tuberculous dogs and cats, treatment is not recommended.

Prevention

I. The diminishing incidence of the disease renders prophylactic vaccination unnecessary.

II. Cats and dogs should be fed meat that is intended only for human consumption or that has been well cooked, and any milk offered should be pasteurized.

Public Health Considerations

Animals with open lesions constitute a serious hazard to human contacts and should be euthanized as soon as a definitive diagnosis has been made. Local public health authorities should be notified once suspicions of tuberculosis have been aroused.

Cat Leprosy

Etiology

I. Cat leprosy has usually been ascribed to infection with the rat leprosy bacillus, *Mycobacterium lepraemurium,* but recently it has been suggested that the causal organism may be *Mycobacterium leprae,* the human leprosy bacillus. Experimental studies have shown that while it is possible to transmit the infection from cat to cat and from cat to rat, attempts to infect cats with *M. lepraemurium* have failed. The causative organism is morphologically similar to the tubercle bacillus. In lesions the organisms are usually found in massive numbers (lepromatous leprosy), often arranged in parallel bundles within macrophages. In about one-third of cases, however, bacilli are few in number and difficult to find (tuberculoid leprosy). These differences have been ascribed to the varying quality of the immune response in infected cats.

II. The bacillus cannot be cultured in vitro except in very complex media and it causes only localized lesions when inoculated into guinea pigs; these findings constitute two important points of differentiation from the tubercle bacillus.

III. Cat leprosy has a worldwide distribution but is uncommon in tropical and subtropical areas. This may be due to a preference for lower temperatures, which could also account for the rarity of systemic infections, lesions in the majority of cases being confined to the skin. The disease was originally reported from New Zealand, which has an unusually high incidence of the infection (179 cases having been diagnosed over a 4-year period by New Zealand Animal Health Laboratories), with most cases occurring in the North Island and in the winter months.

IV. The mode of transmission is unknown, but the predilection sites on the head and limbs suggest contaminated fight wounds as a possible route of entry. However, a survey of the teeth and claws of 100 cats conducted by the author failed to reveal any acid-fast organisms.

V. One case presenting with cutaneous nodules similar to those of cat leprosy was found to be infected with *M. xenopi,* an acid-fast bacillus originally isolated from toads. This organism has the distinction of growing optimally at an incubation temperature of 42°C.

Clinical Signs

I. The cat leprosy organism possesses the ability to multiply within macrophages, evoking a granulomatous reaction similar to that seen in the formation of tubercles.

II. In the New Zealand survey most cases occurred in cats under 4 years of age, and the majority were males. The lesions take the form of single or multiple, rapidly developing fawn-colored hemispherical nodules, up to 2 cm in diameter. The infection shows a predilection for the head and limbs, but lesions may occur on any part of the body. The lesions are painless, fleshy, but not fluctuant to palpation and are freely movable over the underlying tissues. They have a tendency to ulcerate, leaving a finely granular pink surface, which fails to heal and which often exudes a scanty, glairy discharge. The regional lymph nodes may or may not be enlarged. Apart from the cutaneous lesions the cat appears to be in good health. In rare cases there is systemic involvement, with granulomatous foci appearing in the liver, spleen, lungs, and other internal organs; the cat may show signs of general malaise and loss of condition, with an intermittent, mild pyrexia. A primary ulcerative condition in which there are multiple shallow, granulating ulcers, again especially on the head, has been seen occasionally.

III. A similar condition has occurred in the dog. The canine disease has a predilection for the boxer breed and the lesions are most common on the pinnae, where they occur as granulomatous nodules similar to those seen in the cat. Histopathologic features are similar to those of the feline lesions, only the lepromatous form having been seen to date. Attempts to culture the organism have been unsuccessful. Unlike the feline lesions, the nodules tend to resolve spontaneously.

Diagnosis

I. In the lepromatous form diagnosis is easily made by examining a Ziehl-Neelsen–stained smear of an ulcerated lesion or a biopsied nodule. Sometimes the number of organisms is so great that the stained smear or section appears pink to the naked eye. The tuberculoid form can be very difficult to differentiate histologically from skin tuberculosis, and it may be necessary to resort to culture or guinea pig inoculation.

II. The nodules must be differentiated from those of cryptococcosis, feline eosinophilic granuloma complex, mast cell tumor, lymphosarcoma, and chronic cat bite granuloma. This can usually be accomplished by histopathologic examination of a biopsy specimen.

Treatment

I. When only a few nodules are present, surgical excision is probably the treatment of choice because the lesions seldom recur at the same site.

II. The antileprosy drug dapsone (Avlosulfon, ICI) has been recommended for use in cat leprosy (1 mg/kg/day PO), but in the author's experience has proved ineffective and toxic. Some atypical mycobacteria are sensitive to tetracyclines, so this group of antibiotics may be worth trying.

Prevention

No prophylactic measures are available.

Public Health Considerations

In view of the possibility that the causal organism may be the human leprosy bacillus, it would be prudent to avoid prolonged close contact with an infected animal.

FACULTATIVE PATHOGENS

These so-called atypical or anonymous mycobacteria are ubiquitous in nature and are normally harmless. However, when introduced into the body by trauma or injection or when the host is immunocompromised, they may become pathogenic, usually producing a chronic pyogranulomatous inflammation. For this reason they are often referred to as the "opportunist" mycobacteria. Runyon classified them into four groups, the first three constituting the "slow growers" and group IV constituting the "fast growers." Members of the latter group reported to have caused disease in small animals include *Mycobacterium fortuitum, Mycobacterium chelonei,* and *Mycobacterium smegmatis.*

Mycobacterium Fortuitum/Chelonei Complex Infection

Etiology

I. Because *M. fortuitum* and *M. chelonei* share several characteristics and produce similar lesions, they may be considered to form a single infection complex (MFCC).

II. The causal organisms are long, slender, slightly pleomorphic, aerobic, gram-positive, acid-fast bacilli. Both appear to have a worldwide distribution and are found mainly in soil and water. Occasionally they can be isolated from the sputum and saliva of healthy humans.

III. *M. fortuitum* has been incriminated as a cause of bovine mastitis associated with the use of oil-based intramammary antibiotic preparations. In humans infection with this organism has become an important complication of lipid pneumonia, and the author has seen a similar case in a cat. Most reported small animal patients have had a history of trauma, usually either a bite wound or a skin laceration following a road accident. It seems probable that soil contamination of such wounds is an important factor in the establishment of the infection.

IV. Susceptibility to disinfectants is similar to that of the tubercle bacillus.

Clinical Signs

I. Experimental studies have shown that the pathogenicity of some mycobacteria is enhanced by the presence of oil, lipid, or fat. For example, severe mastitis is produced when *M. fortuitum* is injected into the bovine udder in an oil suspension but not in an aqueous vehicle. The mechanism of such enhancement is not yet fully understood, but mechanical protection of the bacilli by the oil may be important. This is supported by the observation that the bacilli in the lesions are found only within what appear to be extracellular fat vacuoles, which are surrounded by polymorphs and macrophages, as if kept "at bay" by the vacuole. In the dog and cat only cutaneous infections with this complex have been described, the patients otherwise appearing healthy and usually afebrile. In such cases it is thought that the subcutaneous fat of the panniculus is disrupted by the initiating trauma, thus providing the lipid necessary to establish an infection.

II. In dogs and cats there is usually a history of trauma (e.g., bite wounds, lacerations, surgery) preceding the development of lesions. The infection usually presents as a rapidly developing subcutaneous nodule which extends to form a mass, with subsequent formation of draining sinus tracts and a granulomatous reaction. There may be variable degrees of regional lymph node involvement. Sometimes the cutaneous nodules are painless and freely movable over the underlying tissues. In other cases the lesions are warm and tender to the touch.

III. Infections are resistant to routine antibiotic therapy and become chronic with a prolonged clinical course, which may extend over several months or even years. Surgical excision may be followed by recurrence and extension of the infection or by dehiscence and the formation of large open wounds, with thickened, draining, granulomatous margins. Such lesions generally fail to heal.

Diagnosis

I. Any chronic abscess or granulomatous lesion with draining fistulous tracts or any nonhealing wound should raise the suspicion of a mycobacterial infection.

II. It is difficult to identify the causative organisms in smears or swabs of exudates from the lesions. However, culture from homogenized biopsy tissue is relatively easy, with colonies appearing on blood agar at 37°C within 2–5 days. It is important to request the laboratory to look for mycobacteria; otherwise, cultures may be discarded before mycobacterial growth has occurred, or a concurrent staphylococcal infection may be reported as the cause of the condition. The bacilli may be absent from exudates by virtue of their intravacuolar situation. Homogenization of infected tissue may disrupt the vacuoles and liberate the organisms.

Treatment

I. The fast-growing mycobacteria are resistant in vitro to all the standard anti-TB drugs and also to most other antibacterial agents. The most active of the latter are amikacin, kanamycin, gentamicin, and tetracycline. Despite in vitro sensitivity, however, antibiotic treatment of these infections is often unrewarding; possibly this again might be due to the protective intravacuolar situation of the bacilli.

II. Repeated surgical excision and drainage have proved successful in some cases and constitute the treatment of choice in humans. It is important to remove as much subcutaneous fat as possible from the margins of the surgical wound in order to deny the organisms fertile soil for persistence of the infection. In some cases, however, excision may result in large, unsightly, nonhealing wounds.

III. In humans infection with opportunistic mycobacteria may persist for long periods (sometimes several years) and then heal. There is one report of a cat with a large open lesion that had remained unchanged for over 4 years, so perhaps the same situation exists in animals.

Prevention

Prophylactic measures are not available or necessary.

Public Health Considerations

The zoonotic potential of these infections is unknown. However, because the atypical mycobacteria can be pathogenic for humans, care should be taken in handling infected animals, discharges, and tissues.

Mycobacterium Smegmatis Infection

Etiology

I. *M. smegmatis* is a fast-growing atypical mycobacterium, which is found in soil and water and is usually saprophytic. It is a long, slender bacillus and is strictly aerobic, pleomorphic, nonmotile, gram-positive, and variably acid-fast.

II. Transmission of the infection appears to follow penetrating wounds of the skin, particularly those involving subcutaneous fat.

III. The organism probably has a worldwide distribution, although the only reports of small animal infections have emanated from subtropical Queensland, Australia, with a possible additional case from Florida.

IV. In animals, apart from being a rare cause of bovine mastitis, *M. smegmatis* infection has only been reported in the cat, in which species it causes a specific disease entity.

Clinical Signs

I. Affected cats usually are fairly obese, neutered adults of either sex up to about 5 years of age, often with prominent inguinal fat pads. Almost invariably there is a history of trauma to the ventral abdominal skin as a result of a cat fight or a road accident a few months prior to presentation. Such trauma, resulting primarily from claw wounds, facilitates soil contamination of the damaged skin. As in MFCC infection, the pathogenicity of the organism is enhanced by the presence of lipid material, which is amply provided in the site of predilection by the inguinal fat pads.

II. Typically, infection results in the formation of large areas of hairless, firm to hard, sometimes boardlike thickening of the skin of the caudal ventral abdomen. These areas may be up to 2 cm in thickness and are firmly attached to the underlying tissues. The infected areas are warm and variably painful to the touch. Over the surface are scattered sinus openings discharging a thin pus, along with small, focal, purplish depressions, imparting an appearance reminiscent of the top of a pepper pot; these depressions appear to be due to thinning of the epidermis over sinuses or pockets of pus. The affected area often involves the whole of the ventral abdomen and may extend into the perineal area or track into the lumbar region, where large, nonhealing, open lesions may be present.

III. Severely affected cats become depressed and inappetent, and lose weight, possibly from chronic pain. They may be reluctant to walk owing to involvement of the inguinal area in the inflammatory process.

Diagnosis

I. As in MFCC infection, diagnosis is most easily made by culture of homogenized tissue obtained by biopsy.

II. Histopathology reveals a pyogranulomatous panniculitis, the bacilli being found only within extracellular lipid vacuoles, as in MFCC infection.

Treatment

The condition is very refractory to treatment and the prognosis is poor. The organism has a spectrum of antimicrobial sensitivity similar to that of MFCC, but, as in the latter infection, therapy is generally unrewarding. Repeated surgical excision of all infected tissue, paying particular attention to removal of all fat from the wound margins, offers the best hope of success.

Prevention and Public Health Considerations

These are the same as for MFCC infections.

SUGGESTED READINGS

Gross TL, Connelly MR: Nontuberculous mycobacterial skin infections in two dogs. Vet Pathol 20:117, 1983

Jennings AR: The distribution of tuberculous lesions in the dog and cat, with reference to the pathogenesis. Vet Rec 61:380, 1949

Kunkle GA, Gulbas NK, Fadok V, et al: Rapidly growing mycobacteria as a cause of cutaneous granulomas: report of five cases. J Am Anim Hosp Assoc 19:513, 1983

Orr CM, Kelly DF, Lucke VM: Tuberculosis in cats. A report of two cases. J Small Anim Pract 21:247, 1980

Robinson M: Skin granuloma of cats associated with acid-fast bacilli. J Small Anim Pract 16:563, 1975

Snider WR: Tuberculosis in canine and feline populations. Am Rev Respir Dis 104:877, 1971

Thompson EJ, Little PB, Cordes DO: Observations of cat leprosy. NZ Vet J 27:233, 1979

White SD, Ihrke PJ, Stannard AA, et al: Cutaneous atypical mycobacteriosis in cats. J Am Vet Med Assoc 182:1218, 1983

Wilkinson GT, Kelly WR, O'Boyle D: Cutaneous granulomas associated with *Mycobacterium fortuitum* infection in a cat. J Small Anim Pract 19:357, 1978

Wilkinson GT, Kelly WR, O'Boyle D: Pyogranulomatous panniculitis in cats due to *Mycobacterium smegmatis*. Aust Vet J 58:77, 1982

25

Dermatophilosis

Donna Walton Angarano

ETIOLOGY

I. Dermatophilosis was first described in 1915 as a specific dermatologic disease of cattle in the Belgian Congo. The causative organism was thought to be a fungus and was named *Dermatophilus congolensis*. Reports of the disease in the United States first appeared in the veterinary literature as late as 1961. At that time the disease was recognized primarily in cattle and horses.

II. More recently the organism has been classified as a bacterium (specifically, an actinomycete) and is believed to have worldwide distribution. The disease is seen frequently in horses and occasionally in cattle and sheep in the United States. It has been reported in numerous other species including wildlife, small animals, and humans. Experimental infections have been produced in laboratory animals.

III. In early reports three species of *Dermatophilus* (*D. congolensis, D. dermatonomus* and *D. pedis*) were described on the basis of the occurrence and variability of clinical lesions in different animal hosts. When the reports were examined more closely, however, it was found that the causative organism was the same in all species; hence *D. congolensis* was retained as the original name.

IV. *Dermatophilus congolensis* is an aerobic to facultatively anaerobic actinomycete, which is gram-positive and non-acid-fast. In culture *Dermatophilus* grows best on blood agar or brain-heart infusion agar. It does not grow well on Sabouraud dextrose agar, dermatophyte test medium, or on most agars containing antibiotics. When it is cultured, 3–4 days may be required for bacterial growth to become evident.

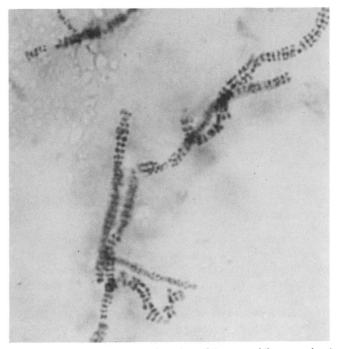

Fig. 25-1. Giemsa-stained, oil-immersion view of *Dermatophilus congolensis.* Division in both longitudinal and transverse planes produces the characteristic parallel rows of coccoid cells ("railroad tracks"). (Courtesy J. R. Saunders, University of Saskatchewan.) (Timoney JF, Gillespie JH, Scott FW: Hagan and Bruner's Infectious Diseases of Domestic Animals. 8th Ed. Cornell University Press, 1987.)

V. The exact habitat of the organism is not known. Attempts to isolate it from the soil have been unsuccessful. The organism is thought to survive on carrier or subclinically affected animals as an obligate parasite. Viable organisms have been found in crusts and scabs on affected animals for as long as 42 months after infection. An increased incidence of clinical disease occurs following the rainy season, when moisture causes a release of the infective zoospores present on the animal. These motile forms are thought to be chemotactically responsive to carbon dioxide diffusing out from the surface of the skin. The zoospores invade the living epidermis and proliferate, dividing both longitudinally and transversely to produce parallel rows of coccoid cells ("railroad tracks") (Fig. 25-1).

VI. Predisposing factors are thought to include moisture as well as injury to the skin. Skin defects may be microscopic and can be caused by insects bites, trauma, or maceration due to prolonged exposure to moisture.

VII. Transmission may be achieved by direct contact with affected animals, fomites, or insect vectors. Experimentally, flies have been found to be capable of transmission.

CLINICAL SIGNS

I. Diseases such as dermatophilosis are intriguing in that a single organism is capable of producing not only a variety of clinical manifestations in a number of species but also a diverse number of clinical signs even within a single species. The number of published reports concerning dermatophilosis in small animals is limited, but the diversity of lesions is evident. (Table 25-1).

II. Canine dermatophilosis

A. Dermatophilosis has been described as an exudative dermatitis, and this is generally the case in large animals and in the dog. In dogs the lesions are apparent most often as thick, adherent crusts resulting from exudation. The early, suppurative lesions are usually superficial and located primarily within the epidermis. Intact hairs are present within the crusts. When the crusts are removed, the underlying surface may disclose a yellowish pus, erythema, or virtually normal skin, depending upon the stage of the lesion. In the normal course of the disease the crusts will dry and fall off, pulling the adherent hair out with them and producing another clinical sign, focal alopecia.

B. Canine cutaneous lesions have been found to occur on various parts of the body, or they may be more generalized. Extracutaneous lesions have not been reported.

C. Pruritus is not usually associated with the disease but may occur with excessive crust buildup.

D. Pain may be associated with acute lesions.

E. Dermatophilosis appears to be of rare occurrence in the dog. Explanations for why and how it occurred in the few reported clinical cases are speculative. In the only published group of naturally occurring cases, 15 dogs with culture-confirmed dermatophilosis were noted to have had contact with affected cattle; this was suggested as the origin of the infections. One other reported ca-

TABLE 25-1. DERMATOPHILOSIS IN SMALL ANIMALS

Author	Species	Lesion	Location	Method of Diagnosis	Treatment	Follow-up	Other
O'Hara (1963)	F	G	Tongue	H	None	E	Farm cat[d]
O'Hara (1963)	F	G	Urinary bladder	H	Surgical excision	D	
Baker (1972)	F	G	Tongue	H	Surgical excision and antibiotics	R	
Jones (1976)	F	G	Popliteal LN	Cu and H	Surgical excision	R	
Miller (1983)	F	G	Popliteal LN	H	None	E	
Miller (1983)	F	G	Popliteal LN	H	Surgical excision	R	Farm cat
Carakostas (1984)	F	G	Popliteal LN	Cy	Antibiotics	R	
Blancou (1973)	C[a]	Cr	Generalized	Cy and Cu	None	Remission 20–30 days	Contact with affected cattle
Blancou (1973)	C[b]	Cr	Generalized	Cy and Cu	None	D	Contact with affected cattle
Chastain (1976)	C	Cr	Back	Cy and Cu	Antibiotics and topicals	R	
Chastain (1976)	C	Cr	Shoulder	Cy and Cu	Antibiotics	R	
Richard (1973)	C[c]	Cr	Trunk	H	None	E	Experimentally induced

F = Feline
C = Canine

[a] 13 cases
[b] 2 cases
[c] 4 cases
[d] feather foreign body

G = Granuloma
Cr = Crusts

LN = Lymph node

H = Histopathology
Cy = Cytology
Cu = Culture

E = Euthanized
D = Died
R = Recovered

nine case occurred in a debilitated dog with a 6-month history of nonspecific systemic illness. In this case underlying disease was suggested as a factor in the development of dermatophilosis.

III. Feline dermatophilosis

A. Naturally occurring lesions in the cat have been reported to be granulomatous rather than exudative. Exudative cutaneous lesions have been produced experimentally, however, by applying *Dermatophilus* organisms isolated from a feline granuloma to scarified skin of another cat.

B. The pathogenesis of feline dermatophilosis is unknown.

C. Two feline cases have been reported in which granulomatous lesions were present on the dorsal surface of the tongue. The granulomas had necrotic centers and contained *Dermatophilus* organisms, which were identified by histopathologic examination. In one of these cases a feather was present within the granuloma. This led to speculation that foreign body penetration may introduce the organism, with resultant granuloma formation.

D. Four other feline cases have been reported in which the popliteal lymph node (or its general area) has been the site of a *Dermatophilus* granuloma. Two of these lymph node granulomas were discharging seropurulent material at the time of presentation. One animal also had draining lesions on a distal extremity. The diagnosis was based on histologic examination in three of the cases, one of which was confirmed by bacterial culture. In one case cytology alone was used to establish the diagnosis.

E. Experimentally, subcutaneous injection of *Dermatophilus* has resulted in abscess formation in the cat.

F. The most unusual published report of feline dermatophilosis concerned a granulomatous mass on the serosal surface of the urinary bladder. The pedunculated mass was surgically removed, and *Dermatophilus* organisms were identified histologically within the necrotic center of the granuloma. The cat died shortly thereafter, but no postmortem examination was performed.

DIAGNOSIS

I. Clinical signs

A. Dermatophilosis should be considered in cases of exudative dermatitis.

B. Granulomas may result from *Dermatophilus* infection.

II. Cytology

    A. Crusts may be removed from the animal and a small section placed on a glass slide and macerated in water.

    B. Smears may be stained with Diff-Quik (Harleco), Giemsa, or new methylene blue. Giemsa has been suggested as the easiest to interpret; however, Diff-Quik is readily available and quite satisfactory.

    C. Examination under oil immersion will reveal the filaments composed of parallel rows of cocci (Fig. 25-1).

III. Bacterial culture

    A. Bacterial culture should be performed to confirm the diagnosis.

    B. The organism grows well on blood agar or brain-heart infusion agar.

IV. Histopathology

    A. Skin biopsies from exudative lesions should include the crust because it is the best area in which to locate and identify the organism.

    B. All excised granulomatous lesions should be submitted for histopathologic examination.

    C. Samples for histologic examination should be preserved in 10% formalin. These samples are not suitable for bacterial culture.

    D. *Dermatophilus* organisms stain basophilic with routine hematoxylin and eosin (H&E) staining.

TREATMENT

I. Canine dermatophilosis

    A. The main goal of treatment is to minimize the predisposing factors of moisture and skin trauma.

    B. Cases have been reported to clear spontaneously.

    C. Daily bathing with antibacterial shampoos, such as tamed iodines or chlorhexidine (Nolvasan Shampoo, Fort Dodge), should be helpful in removing the infective crusts. After the crusts have been removed, it has been suggested that weekly topical treatment should be continued for 3–4 weeks.

    D. Affected animals should be housed in dry quarters.

    E. Systemic antibiotics (e.g., penicillin, streptomycin, or tetracycline) may be needed in severe cases.

    F. The prognosis for canine dermatophilosis is good. Affected animals should be quarantined to prevent spread to other animals.

II. Feline dermatophilosis
   A. Treatment in the cat includes surgical excision of the granuloma-tous lesion. This is usually done also in order to establish the diagnosis.
   B. Systemic antibiotic therapy may be beneficial.

PREVENTION

   I. Prevention is aimed at reducing exposure to prolonged moisture and minimizing skin trauma.
   II. Ectoparasite control may be a major factor in avoiding minor skin trauma.
   III. Contact with affected animals should be avoided.

PUBLIC HEALTH CONSIDERATIONS

   I. Dermatophilosis in humans has been reported but is relatively un-common. The majority of the reported cases have occurred in people handling affected large animals.
   II. Lesions consist most often of a pustular eruption, which frequently clears spontaneously.
   III. Care should be taken to avoid direct contact with crusts, which con-tain infective organisms. Gloves should be worn when bathing or grooming affected animals. Once removed, the crusts should be dis-posed of properly.

SUGGESTED READINGS

Baker GJ, Breeze RG, Dawson CO: Oral dermatophilosis in a cat: a case report. J Small Anim Pract 13:649, 1972

Blancou J: Infection du chien par *Dermatophilus congolensis* (Van Saceghem, 1915). Rev Elev Med Vet Pays Trop 26:289, 1973

Carakostas MC, Miller RI, Woodward MG: Subcutaneous dermatophilosis in a cat. J Am Vet Med Assoc 185:675, 1984

Chastain CB, Carithers RW, Hogle RM, et al: Dermatophilosis in two dogs. J Am Vet Med Assoc 169:1079, 1976

Jones RT: Subcutaneous infection with *Dermatophilus congolensis* in a cat. J Comp Pathol 86:415, 1976

Lorenz MD: Integumentary infections. p. 189. In Greene CE (ed): Clinical Microbiology and Infectious Diseases of the Dog and Cat. WB Saunders, Philadelphia, 1984

Miller RI, Ladds PW, Mudie A, et al: Probable dermatophilosis in 2 cats. Aust Vet J 60:155, 1983

Muller GH, Kirk RW, Scott DW: Small Animal Dermatology. 3rd Ed. WB Saunders, Philadelphia, 1983

O'Hara PJ, Cordes DO: Granulomata caused by *Dermatophilus* in two cats. NZ Vet J 11:151, 1963

Richard JL, Pier AC, Cysewski SJ: Experimentally induced canine dermatophilosis. Am J Vet Res 34:797, 1973

26

Mycoplasma Infections
James W. Crissman

ETIOLOGY

I. In common usage the term *mycoplasma* refers to members of the order Mycoplasmatales, which includes three genera of importance to veterinarians: *Mycoplasma, Acholeplasma,* and *Ureaplasma* (T strains). Mycoplasmas, the smallest free-living form of life, are wall-less organisms: essentially membrane-bound bags of protoplasm. Because they possess limited biosynthetic abilities, they require close association with host cells for a supply of complex biological substrates. Mycoplasmas tend to be host-specific and to have highly adaptive interactions with the colonized tissues and immune system of the host. Thus, mycoplasmas are often commensals or persistent agents of chronic disease. Less commonly, they may cause acute disease.

II. Most mycoplasma species identified in cats and dogs are present as normal flora. Therefore, when they are identified in a disease state, their pathogenic role may be difficult to assess, especially because they are often seen in mixed infections. In studies of mycoplasma flora in the conjunctiva, upper respiratory tract, and urogenital tract of animals, the frequency of colonization generally is marginally higher in diseased than in normal animals. Often, however, disease cannot be reproduced by the organism alone, which leaves Koch's postulates unfulfilled. Frankly pathogenic mycoplasmas, similar to those causing pneumonia and arthritis in food and laboratory animals, have not been identified in dogs and cats.

III. Mycoplasmas may cause disease of uncharacteristic severity in immunodeficient hosts.

CLINICAL SIGNS

I. Feline conjunctivitis caused by *Mycoplasma felis*
   A. This species occurs on the conjunctivae of normal cats but is much more frequent in conjunctivitis and may be seen in mixed infections with *Chlamydia.*

   B. Clinical signs can include:
      1. Uni- or bilateral epiphora, blepharospasm, and conjunctival hyperemia
      2. Lymphoid follicles and papillary hypertrophy of conjunctival surfaces (the latter finding observed with a slit lamp)
      3. Mucopurulent conjunctivitis with pseudomembrane formation but not corneal ulceration
      4. Upper respiratory signs
   C. The disease is usually self-limiting after 10 days.
  II. Urinary tract disease in dogs
   A. A survey of 60 mycoplasma-positive urine cultures from 41 dogs with urinary tract infection (from a total of 2,900 urine samples) revealed that two-thirds were pure cultures; of these, two-thirds of the affected dogs showed clinical signs of disease.
   B. The most common urinary isolate (24 of 29 speciated) was *Mycoplasma canis*. *Mycoplasma spumans* and *Mycoplasma cynos* also were isolated.
 III. Canine respiratory disease
   A. Experimentally, *M. cynos* has produced a relatively mild pneumonia in endobronchially inoculated puppies. It has not been recorded as the sole agent of natural disease. However, it may be present in mixed infections, as in distemper pneumonia or canine tracheobronchitis.
   B. *Ureaplasma* spp. were isolated from dog lungs in three cases of pneumonia; however all were mixed infections (one with *Mycoplasma edwardii*, others with eubacteria), and one was associated with paraquat poisoning. Therefore the role of mycoplasmas and ureaplasmas in canine respiratory disease remains unresolved.
  IV. Feline respiratory disease
   A. Most healthy and diseased cats have mycoplasmas in the oropharynx.
   B. In one study mycoplasmas were isolated from lungs of 17% of cats with respiratory disease.
   V. Canine reproductive disease
   A. Mycoplasmas are common vaginal and uterine flora of normal dogs.
   B. Experimental intrauterine inoculation of *M. canis* has resulted in a purulent endometritis.
   C. Ureaplasmas are commonly isolated from the vaginas of normal bitches and marginally more often from those with a mucopurulent vulvar discharge and infertility problems.

    D. Mycoplasma isolations are very common from the prepuce and semen of normal dogs but even more common when the dogs are afflicted with balanoposthitis and infertility.

    E. Ureaplasmas are present on the prepuce and in semen significantly more often in infertile dogs, usually as part of a mixed mycoplasma infection. Ureaplasmas in semen are associated with subnormal sperm motility, low sperm counts, and/or a high percentage of midpiece and tail abnormalities.

VI. Feline reproductive disease

    A. Experimental intrauterine inoculation of *Ureaplasma* has produced abortion and neonatal death.

    B. Mycoplasma isolations are common from the genitals of normal cats but are more common from those of cats with genital disease.

VII. Arthritis

    A. There is a single report of isolation of *M. spumans* in a case of polyarthritis in a greyhound.

    B. In cats *M. gateae* was isolated in a single case of intractable polyarthritis and tenosynovitis. Experimentally, an acute polyarthritis, which was self-limiting, was consistently produced by intravenous injection of the organism.

    C. Several natural cases of polyarthritis attributed to unspeciated mycoplasmas have been recorded in immunosuppressed cats.

VIII. Granulomatous colitis in boxer dogs

    A. Mycoplasmas were isolated from four of six affected animals. The disease experimentally reproduced with the isolates lacked granulomas.

    B. Mycoplasmas have been isolated from the colon and draining lymph node in about one-third of normal dogs sampled.

IX. Chronic abscesses in cats

    A. Mycoplasma-like organisms were isolated in two of three cases of treatment-refractory abscesses. No eubacteria were isolated. The abscesses responded to tetracycline therapy.

DIAGNOSIS

I. Feline conjunctivitis

    A. Giemsa-stained conjunctival scrapings may reveal organisms at the periphery of epithelial cells. They may also be found in normal eyes.

    B. *Mycoplasma felis* may be a synergistic pathogen with *Chlamydia*.

    C. Differential diagnoses should include all the causes of feline upper respiratory disease.

II. Arthritis

    A. Diagnosis is by culture of joint aspirates.

    B. Differential diagnoses should include feline chronic progressive polyarthritis in adult male cats and chlamydial arthritis or neonatal septicemia in kittens.

TREATMENT

I. Antibiotics with spectra covering the mycoplasmas are commonly available and include the tetracyclines, chloramphenicol, erythromycin, and tylosin. Site-specific formulations, such as tetracycline ophthalmic ointments, may be appropriate.

II. Tylosin has been effective for canine urinary tract infection.

III. Dogs with respiratory infections and systemic signs should be treated with an antibiotic that is effective against *Bordetella bronchiseptica*. Tetracycline and chloramphenicol also qualify and, as stated above, are also effective against mycoplasmas.

PREVENTION

Although vaccines have been and are being developed for several mycoplasmal diseases of humans and animals, the relative insignificance of mycoplasmal diseases in dogs and cats makes it unlikely that such products will be available in the foreseeable future.

SUGGESTED READINGS

Ball HJ, Bryson DG: Isolation of ureaplasmas from pneumonic dog lungs. Vet Rec 111:585, 1982

Bowe PS, Van Kruiningen HJ, Rosendal S: Attempts to produce granulomatous colitis in boxer dogs with a mycoplasma. Can J Comp Med 46:430, 1982

Campbell LH, Snyder SB, Reed C, et al: *Mycoplasma felis*-associated conjunctivitis in cats. J Am Vet Med Assoc 163:991, 1973

Doig PA, Ruhnke HL, Bosu WTK: The genital mycoplasma and ureaplasma flora of healthy and diseased dogs. Can J Comp Med 45:233, 1981

Jang SS, Ling GV, Yamamoto R, et al: Mycoplasma as a cause of canine urinary tract infection. J Am Vet Med Assoc 185:45, 1984

Keane DP: Chronic abscesses in cats associated with an organism resembling mycoplasma. Can Vet J 24:289, 1983

Moise NS, Crissman JW, Fairbrother JF, et al: *Mycoplasma gateae* arthritis and tenosynovitis in cats: case report and experimental reproduction of the disease. Am J Vet Res 44:16, 1983

Razin S, Freundt EA (eds): Biology and pathogenicity of mycoplasmas. Isr J Med Sci 20:749–1028, 1984

Rosendal S: Canine and feline mycoplasmas. p. 217. In Tully JG, Whitcomb RF (eds): The Mycoplasmas, Vol. 2. Academic Press, New York, 1979

Rosendal S: Canine mycoplasmas: their ecologic niche and role in disease. J Am Vet Med Assoc 180:1212, 1982

Tan RJS, Lim EW, Ishak B: Ecology of mycoplasmas in clinically healthy cats. Aust Vet J 53:515, 1977

Tan RJS, Miles JAR: Incidence and significance of mycoplasmas in sick cats. Res Vet Sci 16:27, 1974

Tan RJS, Miles JAR: Possible role of feline T-strain mycoplasmas in cat abortion. Aust Vet J 50:142, 1974

27

Canine Ehrlichiosis

Miodrag Ristic
Cynthia J. Holland

ETIOLOGY

I. Canine ehrlichiosis is a tickborne rickettsial blood disease of domestic and wild canids. The disease may be presented as acute, subclinical, chronic, or severe chronic in form. The latter form is often referred to as tropical canine pancytopenia (TCP).

II. The etiologic agent of canine ehrlichiosis is *Ehrlichia canis,* which is classified within the tribe Ehrlichieae, family Rickettsiaceae, order Rickettsiales.

III. *E. canis* is a gram-negative, small coccoid, ellipsoid, or often pleomorphic microorganism, which occurs within intracytoplasmic vacuoles of monocytes and lymphocytes (Fig. 27-1). The agent may occur singly (elementary bodies) or in the form of small clusters (initial bodies) or large, tightly packed clusters (morulae). The size of elementary bodies is in the range 0.2–0.4 μm, initial bodies from 0.5–4 μm, and morulae from 3–6 μm.

IV. The brown dog tick, *Rhipicephalus sanguineus,* is the sole biologic vector involved in the transmission of *E. canis.* Trans-stadial but not transovarial transmission has been demonstrated in the tick.

V. The microorganism may also be transmitted from infected to susceptible dogs by whole blood inoculation. Accordingly, potential blood donor dogs should be confirmed free of *E. canis* infection prior to their use.

VI. Canine ehrlichiosis has been diagnosed worldwide wherever the vector tick exists. The majority of cases in the United States have been reported to occur in the western, southwestern, and southeastern regions.

VII. The disease may often be diagnosed in regions where the brown dog tick is not found; however, case histories usually reveal that such infections were imported from enzootic areas.

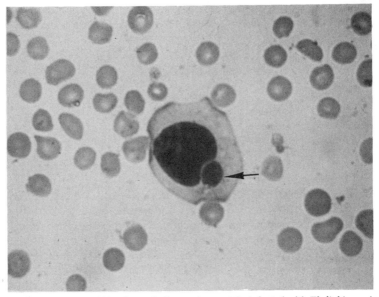

Fig. 27-1. Peripheral blood sample from a dog acutely infected with *Ehrlichia canis*. An inclusion body, a cluster of tightly packed elementary bodies referred to as a *morula,* is evident in the cytoplasm of a monocyte (arrow). (Wright-Giemsa, × 1,600).

CLINICAL SIGNS

I. Clinical course
   A. The onset of the acute phase of the disease generally occurs within 8–16 days following the bite of an infected tick or after inoculation of infected blood. This stage lasts 2–4 weeks and is usually characterized by fever (104–106°F), depression, anorexia, and occasionally corneal opacity. Edema of the limbs and ataxia may also be present.
   B. The acute stage is generally followed by a subclinical phase of varying duration. During this period, the dog may appear clinically normal; however, all blood values remain at subnormal levels when compared with values recorded prior to infection. The disease may remain at a mild chronic level with occasional episodes of fever or develop into the severe chronic phase known

as TCP. Certain breeds of dogs, such as the German shepherd, appear to be predisposed to acquiring the more severe manifestations of the disease.

C. Typically, TCP is characterized by fever, corneal opacity, regenerative or nonregenerative anemia, and a severe leukopenia and thrombocytopenia. During the early phase of the disease bone marrow hyperplasia is evident. However as the disease progresses, cellular elements in the marrow become exhausted, producing a state of hypoplasia. Owing to the severe thrombocytopenia, epistaxis, petechiation of mucous membranes, hemorrhagic skin lesions, and peripheral edema are often observed. Death during this phase of the disease is generally due either to extensive mucosal and serosal hemorrhages or to secondary bacterial infections prompted by the dog's debilitated condition.

II. Clinical pathology

A. The most prominent clinicopathologic manifestations of ehrlichiosis are a greatly increased erythrocyte sedimentation rate, thrombocytopenia, and a slight to severe pancytopenia. In recovering animals there is a gradual to spontaneous improvement in thrombocyte levels. The appearance of bone marrow specimens obtained by aspiration cytology during the acute phase of the disease may range from normal cellularity to various degrees of hypopcellularity.

B. Thrombocytopenic dogs may develop severe chronic ehrlichiosis subsequent to surgery or chemotherapy. Consequently, the severe chronic phase of ehrlichiosis may be precipitated by stress or by immunosuppression after a prolonged subclinical infection.

C. Hypergammaglobulinemia that develops during the acute febrile phase persists during the subclinical and the subsequent terminal phase of the disease. These excessive γ-globulins, however, are not all specific for *E. canis*. Such manifestations are often misdiagnosed and attributed to an autoimmune process rather than to canine ehrlichiosis.

III. Immunopathology

A. Among various prominent pathologic manifestations of fatal ehrlichiosis are extensive plasmacytosis and perivascular cuffing in most parenchymal organs, particularly the lung, meninges, kidneys, and spleen, suggesting an immunopathologic phenomenon.

B. Such a phenomenon has been further substantiated by the finding that lymphocytes from infected dogs exert a cytotoxic effect upon autologous monocytes. This monocytotoxicity was shown to bear a temporal relationship to the thrombocytopenia.

C. A further indication that the thrombocytopenia in canine ehrlichiosis is immunologically mediated has been provided by evidence that serum from diseased dogs inhibits platelet migration
in vitro. Scanning electron microscopy has indicated that the
platelet migration inhibition factor (PMIF) interferes with platelet
migration by inhibiting platelet pseudopod formation. Affected
platelets become rounded and show evidence of clumping and
leakage.

DIAGNOSIS

I. A diagnosis of acute ehrlichiosis by microscopic detection of the organism in Giemsa-stained blood smears or buffy coat preparations is
generally difficult, if not impossible, because the percentage of infected monocytes within the peripheral blood is extremely low.

II. An indirect fluorescent antibody test (IFA) is currently the only available specific means for detection and titration of antibodies to *E.
canis*. The organism generated by in vitro culture techniques serves
as an antigen in the test. The IFA test is applicable to both experimental laboratory and field diagnosis of canine ehrlichiosis. In experimentally infected dogs the period prior to detection of antibodies
at a beginning 1:10 serum dilution varies from 11 to 24 days. Analysis
of the inoculation data indicates that this variation is apparently due
to individual animal responses rather than to the volume of inoculum
used. The serum titer in the IFA test may vary from 1:10 to 1:10,240
or greater, depending on the stage of infection, immune involvement
of a given dog with the agent, and breed of the dog. In the acute stage
of infection there is generally a spontaneous and rapid increase in
titer, which usually reaches high levels during early convalescence.
Thereafter, the titer is generally maintained at variable levels for long
periods of time.

III. More recently, a new plate latex agglutination test has been developed
for diagnosis of canine ehrlichiosis. This simple and rapid test is designed for on-the-spot diagnosis of the disease. It is considered a
screening test to be followed by the laboratory IFA test.

IV. Infection-immunity (premunition) seems to be a functional protective
mechanism in infections with *E. canis*. In vitro studies of protective
immunity have demonstrated that the interaction between humoral
and cellular immune responses exerts an anti-*E. canis* effect.

TREATMENT

I. Recommended therapeutic regimens consist of 33 mg/kg PO tid. of oxytetracycline given for 2–4 weeks, depending on the individual case. If this treatment is effective in totally eliminating the organism from the affected dog, the IFA titer should gradually subside to a nondetectable level within 6–12 months post-treatment. If this is not the case, the clinician may decide to repeat the treatment. For this reason periodic serologic screening is recommended.

II. Supportive therapy (blood transfusions, electrolytes, vitamins) should be administered as needed.

PREVENTION

I. The only preventive therapeutic measure for canine ehrlichiosis thus far available is administration on a continuous basis of tetracycline at a low dosage (6.6 mg/kg/day). This may be highly effective for dogs traveling to enzootic areas.

II. The routine use of commercially available acaracides for the control of tick infestation is strongly recommended.

III. Preliminary studies using an inactivated *E. canis* immunogen coupled with an appropriate adjuvant suggest the possibility that a degree of vaccinal protective immunity to challenge can be induced.

SUGGESTED READINGS

Buhles WC, Huxsoll DL, Ristic M: Tropical canine pancytopenia: clinical, hematologic, and serologic responses of dogs to *Ehrlichia canis* infection, tetracycline therapy, and challenge inoculation. J Infect Dis 130:357, 1974

Greene CE: Rocky Mountain spotted fever and ehrlichiosis. p. 1080. In Kirk RW (ed): Current Veterinary Therapy. Vol. 9. WB Saunders, Philadelphia, 1986

Hibler SC, Hoskins JD, Greene CE: Rickettsial infections in dogs. Part II. Ehrlichiosis and infectious cyclic thrombocytopenia. Compend Cont Ed Pract Vet 8:106, 1986

Lewis GE, Ristic M, Smith RD, et al: The brown dog tick *Rhipicephalus sanguineus* and the dog as experimental hosts of *Ehrlichia canis*. Am J Vet Res 38:1953, 1977

Price JE, Sayer PD: Canine ehrlichiosis. p. 1197. In Kirk RW (ed): Current Veterinary Therapy. Vol. 8. WB Saunders, Philadelphia, 1983

Ristic M: Pertinent characteristics of leukocytic rickettsiae of humans and animals. p. 182. In Leive L, Bonzentre PS, Morello JA, et al (eds): Microbiology 1986. Am Soc Microbiology, Washington, 1986

Ristic M, Huxsoll DL, Weisiger RM, et al: Serological diagnosis of tropical canine pancytopenia by indirect immunofluorescence. Infect Immun 6:226, 1972

Smith RD, Ristic M: Ehrlichiae. p. 295. In Kreier JP (ed): Parasitic Protozoa. Vol. 4. Academic Press, New York, 1977

Stephenson EH: Canine rickettsial diseases. p. 143. In Scott FW (ed): Contemporary Issues in Small Animal Practice, Vol. 3: Infectious Diseases. Churchill Livingstone, New York, 1986

28

Salmon Disease Complex

Richard L. Ott

ETIOLOGY

I. The salmon disease complex (SDC) is caused by one or both of two helminth-transmitted rickettsiae that are coccoid to coccobacillary in shape and approximately 0.3 μm in diameter. These gram-negative organisms stain purple with Giemsa stain (Fig. 28-1) or pale blue with hematoxylin and eosin. The organisms resist freezing ($-20°C$ to $-80°C$) for 31–158 days; however, they are rapidly destroyed by heating above 60°C (140°F).

   A. *Neorickettsia helminthoeca* is the agent of salmon poisoning disease. This agent is rarely found alone in naturally infected dogs. Untreated, the disease is usually fatal.

   B. *Neorickettsia elokominica,* a possible strain variant of *N. helminthoeca,* is the etiologic agent of Elokomin fluke fever. This agent may be found alone or in combination with *N. helminthoeca* in naturally infected dogs. The disease associated with *N. elokominica* infection results in high morbidity but is less frequently fatal than is salmon poisoning disease.

II. The SDC rickettsiae are transmitted naturally by ingestion of infected metacercariae of the trematode *Nanophyetus salmincola*. Infected metacercariae are found in salmonid fish (salmon, steelhead, trout), certain nonsalmonid fish, and the Pacific giant salamander.

   A. *N. salmincola* harbors the rickettsiae throughout its life cycle, from eggs to adult fluke.

   B. Three different hosts are required for the completion of the life cycle of *N. salmincola*—snails, fish, and mammals.

      1. Undeveloped ova are passed in large numbers in the feces of infected mammals. The light brown, indistinctly operculated ova are approximately 87–97 μm by 35–55 μm in size. There is a small blunt point on the end of the egg opposite the indistinct operculum (Fig. 28-2). In approximately 3 months' time, ova deposited in water develop into free-swimming miracidia.

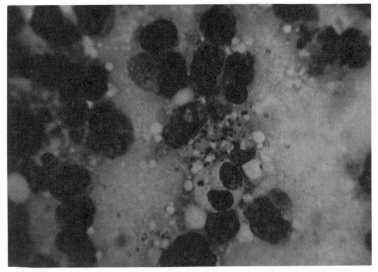

Fig. 28-1. Giemsa-stained lymph node aspirate, showing *Neorickettsia helminthoeca* organisms within the cytoplasm of a reticuloendothelial cell. (Courtesy N. L. Shatto, Astoria, Oregon.)

2. Miracidia penetrate the snail intermediate host, *Oxytrema silicula*. Within the snail cercariae develop through rediae—a replicative cycle.
3. Cercariae, following emergence from the snail, penetrate the skin of the second intermediate host, a susceptible fish, and encyst as metacercariae in various tissues. The metacercariae usually localize in large numbers in the kidneys or gills of infected fish; however, they can be found in any tissue. Fish are infected in fresh water; however, they retain the metacercariae (and the rickettsiae) through their ocean migration or for at least 3 years.
4. The final host—dog, coyote, cat, fox, bear, or mink—becomes infected by eating fish infected with metacercariae. Although any of the aforementioned mammals can serve as definitive hosts for the fluke, clinical signs of the SDC are usually shown only by members of the family Canidae, particularly domestic dogs and coyotes.

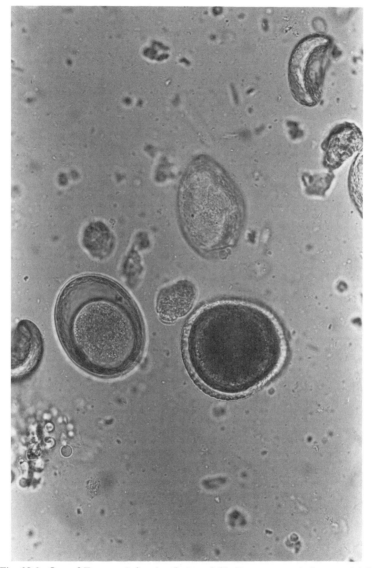

Fig. 28-2. Ova of *Toxascaris leonina* (bottom left), *Toxocara canis* (bottom right), and *Nanophyetus salmincola* (top). Note the relative sizes of the eggs and, in *N. salmincola,* the small, blunt point on the end of the egg opposite the operculum. (Courtesy W. J. Foreyt, Washington State University.)

5. The metacercariae develop rapidly to adult flukes in the intestinal tract of the definitive host. The adult fluke is white in color and approximately 0.5 mm wide by 1.1 mm long; it is barely visible on the surface of the intestinal epithelium without magnification. Ova may be passed in the feces of the infected host within 5–8 days after ingestion of infected fish.

C. The agents of the SDC can be transmitted by parenteral injection of blood, spleen, or lymph node suspensions from infected canids. Other, experimental, means of transmission of these agents have been attempted; however, the ingestion of infected fish is the most common means of transmitting the organisms under natural conditions.

D. Both diseases of the SDC occur predominantly on the western slopes of the Cascade Range, from northwestern California to southwestern Washington. This corresponds to the distribution of the snail intermediate host, *O. silicula*. Rickettsiae-infected salmon and steelhead may be found toward the eastward origin of the rivers in the enzootic area. Inadequately frozen or smoked salmon containing metacercariae, transported anywhere, are capable of producing SDC when fed to susceptible dogs.

CLINICAL SIGNS

I. After ingestion of raw, metacercariae-infected fish by a susceptible dog, the fluke matures, attaches to the intestinal mucosa, and injects the rickettsiae. The organisms replicate in the intestinal epithelium or, more likely, in the lymphoid tissue of the intestine. Rickettsiae enter the circulation early in the course of the infection and spread to the lymph nodes, spleen, tonsils, thymus, liver, lungs, and brain of the infected host.

II. After an incubation period of 5–7 days (occasionally as long as 33 days), the infected dog develops fever, depression, anorexia, lymphadenopathy, vomiting, diarrhea, dehydration, emaciation, occasionally mucoid nasal and ocular discharges, and, rarely convulsions.

A. The sudden onset of fever, which may reach 40°–42°C (104°–107.6°F), is the first sign of disease in infected dogs. After the febrile peak, the temperature gradually declines to normal or subnormal in dogs infected with *N. helminthoeca*. The fever may plateau for 4–7 days before returning to normal in dogs infected with *N. elokominica*. In either infection patients are usually hypothermic at the time of death.

B. Enlarged peripheral lymph nodes (mandibular, prescapular, etc.) can often be palpated as early as 5–7 days postinfection, at the time of the onset of fever.

C. Anorexia and depression occur at the onset or immediately following the onset of fever. Patients will frequently drink copious amounts of water.

D. Vomiting is an early sign of disease, particularly in the anorectic patient that drinks copious amounts of water. The vomitus usually consists of a slightly brown-tinged fluid.

E. A watery diarrhea occurs shortly after the onset of fever. The diarrhea increases in severity during the course of the disease, becoming foul-smelling and hemorrhagic prior to death.

F. Dehydration and emaciation become progressively more severe throughout the course of the disease.

G. Slight, serous oculonasal discharges, which may become mucopurulent, occasionally occur during the course of the disease.

H. Terminal grand mal seizures occur rarely in SDC.

DIAGNOSIS

I. The diagnosis of SDC is based on the characteristic clinical signs, the finding of *N. salmincola* ova in fecal samples, and, if necessary, the identification of rickettsiae in Giemsa-stained aspiration biopsies obtained from a swollen peripheral lymph node.

A. The history of ingestion of uncooked salmonid fish and the characteristic clinical signs are highly suggestive of SDC in an ezootic area.

B. The detection of undeveloped, operculated eggs of *N. salmincola* (Fig. 28-2) in the patient's feces, combined with the history and signs of disease, is usually sufficient to confirm a clinical diagnosis of SDC.

1. *N. salmincola* ova can be detected in feces on a direct smear or by using the detergent-washing-sedimentation technique.

2. The use of flotation techniques involving high-density solutions *is to be discouraged* because such solutions distort the eggs.

C. Cytologic examination of Giemsa-stained peripheral lymph node aspirates reveals purple staining rickettsiae in the cytoplasm of reticuloendothelial cells. This technique is seldom necessary for the clinical diagnosis of SDC. If lymph node aspirates are used, the stained smear should be examined by an experienced technician. Artifacts may easily be confused with rickettsiae by inexperienced personnel.

    D. Hematologic findings in cases of SDC are extremely variable and hence are unreliable for diagnosis. Total leukocyte counts in SDC vary from leukopenia to leukocytosis. A neutrophilic leukocytosis is the most common finding in dogs that have been ill more than 1–2 days.

II. The severe gastrointestinal signs of the SDC must be differentiated from those produced by a variety of canine ailments—parvovirus or coronavirus infections, canine distemper, giardiasis, and intussusception, for example. Although the peripheral lymphadenopathy in addition to the finding of large numbers of fluke eggs in the feces tends to characterize SDC, appropriate laboratory tests may be indicated to determine if other diseases are present concurrently.

TREATMENT

  I. The treatment of SDC is directed toward eliminating the rickettsiae, correcting the dehydration, and providing supportive nursing care.

    A. Food and water should be withheld during the acute, severe stages of the disease. As the patient responds to therapy, a bland, high-caloric diet may be provided.

    B. The rickettsiae of SDC are susceptible to sulfonamides, penicillin, chlortetracycline, chloramphenicol, oxytetracycline, and tetracycline. Streptomycin is ineffective.

       1. The severe vomiting that occurs early in the course of the disease precludes the use of oral medication.

       2. Intravenous oxytetracycline (Terramycin, Pfizer) or tetracycline (Achromycin, Lederle) are the drugs of choice. They are administered at the rate of 7 mg/kg bid for at least 3 days or until the vomiting has ceased.

       3. Once the vomiting has ceased, oral tetracycline is administered at the rate of 22 mg/kg tid for 14–21 days.

    C. A polyionic, isotonic fluid should be administered intravenously.

       1. The amount of fluid given must be sufficient to provide for the patient's daily water needs and to correct the existing dehydration.

       2. The transfusion of whole blood may be necessary for patients that are anemic as a result of severe hemorrhagic diarrhea.

    D. Keeping the dog dry, clean, and warm is essential for successful therapy. The patient should be placed on a wire mesh or similar rack, which is raised above the cage floor in order to reduce contact with the vomitus and fluid excreta. Frequent cleaning of the patient and the cage is mandatory.

    E. Control of the rickettsial infection usually results in control of the vomiting and diarrhea. Continuing diarrhea, should it occur, may be controlled by the judicious use of preparations containing bismuth subsalicylate (Pepto-Bismol, Norwich-Eaton), at a dose of approximately 2.2 ml/kg PO as needed.

II. Fenbendazole (Panacur, American Hoechst) may be administered after the patient has recovered from the SDC in an attempt to eliminate the residual *N. salmincola* infestation. It is administered orally at a dose of 50 mg/kg once daily for 10–14 days. This treatment is seldom warranted, however, because the fluke infestation seldom produces clinical signs once the rickettsial infection has been controlled, and because the efficacy of fenbendazole in treating *N. salmincola* infections is still questionable.

PREVENTION

    I. Recovered animals are usually immune to reinfection with the same rickettsia that caused the original infection. For all practical purposes it is safe to assume that a dog that has survived a natural case of SDC is immune for life.

  II. Preventing dogs from eating metacercariae-infected fish is the best method of preventing infection with the rickettsiae of SDC.

    A. Metacercariae and the rickettsiae can survive for months in raw or inadequately cooked or frozen fish carcasses; therefore, all rotten fish or fish viscera should be disposed of in a manner that precludes ingestion by dogs.

    B. Freezing fish at $-20°C$ ($-4°F$) for 24 hours will destroy the metacercariae and thus prevent the natural transmission of the rickettsiae that may survive such freezing.

    C. Thorough cooking [above $60°C$ ($140°F$)] of infected fish will destroy both the metacercariae and the rickettsiae.

    D. Smoked or kippered salmon can be infective for dogs if the brine is of insufficient strength or if the smoking temperature was low. Such improperly smoked and kippered salmon have been responsible for the spread of SDC outside the normal enzootic area.

III. Dogs can be immunized by feeding them infected fish and treating them with appropriate antibiotics at the first sign of disease. Although this technique has been used for farm dogs in the enzootic area, it is not widely accepted as a preventive measure.

SUGGESTED READINGS

Farrell RK, Ott RL, Gorham JR: The clinical laboratory diagnosis of salmon poisoning. J Am Vet Med Assoc 127:241, 1955

Farrell RK: Canine rickettsiosis. p. 985. In Kirk RW (ed): Current Veterinary Therapy Vol. 5. WB Saunders, Philadelphia, 1974

Farrell RK: Rickettsial diseases. p. 65. In Catcott EJ (ed): Canine Medicine. Vol. I. 4th Ed. American Veterinary Publications, Santa Barbara, 1979

Gorham JR, Foreyt WJ: Salmon poisoning disease. p. 538. In Greene CE (ed): Clinical Microbiology and Infectious Diseases of the Dog and Cat. WB Saunders, Philadelphia, 1984

Hibler SC, Hoskins JD, Greene CE: Rickettsial infections in dogs. Part III. Salmon disease complex and haemobartonellosis. Compend Contin Ed Pract Vet 8:251, 1986

Knapp SE, Millemann RE: Salmon poisoning disease. p. 376. In Davis JW, Karstad LH, Trainer DO (eds): Infectious Diseases of Wild Mammals. 2nd Ed. Iowa State University Press, Ames, 1981

29

Rocky Mountain Spotted Fever

Edward H. Stephenson

ETIOLOGY

I. Rocky Mountain spotted fever (RMSF) is a tickborne rickettsial disease that occurs in many areas throughout the United States. Although the significance of the disease among dogs has not been fully clarified, the occurrence of natural as well as experimental infections is recognized.

II. *Rickettsia rickettsii,* the causative agent, is an obligate intracellular parasite that replicates in the cytoplasm and nucleus of infected cells. Dogs are readily susceptible to infection. Two other spotted fever–group rickettsiae, *Rickettsia montana* and *Rickettsia rhipicephali,* are antigenically related to *R. rickettsii* and are known to infect dogs. Neither of these two species induces overt disease, however.

III. Transmission of infections rickettsiae to the dog or other vertebrate hosts occurs during the feeding of an infected tick. Principal vector ticks are *Dermacentor variabilis* (American dog tick) and *Dermacentor andersoni. Rhipicephalus sanguineus* (brown dog tick) is considered a prime vector in Mexico but has not been found in the United States to be naturally infected with *R. rickettsii.* Transmission of rickettsiae from infected ticks to a susceptible host is an inefficient process; several days are required for ticks to become engorged.

IV. Either sodium hypochlorite (bleach) at a concentration of 2,000 to 5,000 ppm or 5% (vol/vol) Lysol is an effective disinfectant.

CLINICAL SIGNS

I. The incubation period is variable; it can be 2–10 days depending on the rickettsial dose received.

II. Fever as high as 40.6°C (105°F), anorexia, and lethargy are exhibited by all infected dogs. Other clinical signs can include lymph node enlargement, weight loss, dehydration, edema of the limbs, and, in male dogs, edema of the sheath and scrotum. Petechial and ecchymotic hemorrhages in the ocular, oral, and genital mucous membranes and nonpigmented skin may develop following the subacute illness. Severe experimental infections proceed to death.

III. Definite changes occur in the hemogram. There is a marked thrombocytopenia ($< 100,000/\mu l$), and a leukopenia precedes leukocytosis, as is also seen in canine ehrlichiosis. Biochemical abnormalities include increases in serum alkaline phosphatase and cholesterol and decreases in serum sodium (hyponatremia) and chloride (hypochloremia). Variable prolongation of the prothrombin time, activated partial thromboplastin time, and thrombin time, with elevated fibrin degradation products, are consistent with overt disseminated intravascular coagulopathy.

IV. Primary gross pathologic alterations in terminal cases are petechiae and ecchymoses on the mucous membranes, unpigmented skin, and various organs. These lesions are attributable to the necrotizing vasculitis that occurs.

DIAGNOSIS

I. The clinical diagnosis of RMSF in dogs only can be made after consideration of the history, physical examination, and laboratory analyses.

II. A preliminary diagnosis of *R. rickettsii* infection during the acute phase of the disease can be confirmed by the primary monocyte culture technique. However, the procedure requires tissue culture expertise and supporting equipment and supplies.

III. Humoral antibodies to *R. rickettsii* develop 7–14 days after infection and can be used to make a definitive diagnosis. Preferred procedures for measuring antibody titers are the indirect fluorescent antibody (IFA) test and the enzyme-linked immunosorbent assay (ELISA). Other serologic tests (complement fixation, microagglutination, indirect hemagglutination, latex agglutination) have been used, but each of these is much less sensitive. Regardless of the test procedure employed, control antigens must include, at a minimum, the other two spotted fever rickettsiae (*R. montana, R. rhipicephali*) that infect dogs. Dogs with RMSF consistently will exhibit antibody titers 2- to 16-fold greater against *R. rickettsii* than against the other rickettsiae.

IV. Isolation of *R. rickettsii* in susceptible species of laboratory animals, although most definitive, is not a useful procedure in support of clinical cases because the time required for isolation of rickettsiae can approach 30 days.

V. Direct fluorescent antibody (FA) staining of skin biopsy specimens can yield a rapid diagnosis of RMSF. Extensive laboratory equipment and expertise are required to carry out the procedure, however.

VI. The differential diagnosis must include canine ehrlichiosis and babesiasis. These diseases present with acute clinical signs similar to those of RMSF.

TREATMENT

I. Tetracycline hydrochloride is the drug of choice and is given at a minimum oral dosage of 22 mg/kg/day divided bid or tid for 14 days. The dosage can be increased to 66 mg/kg/day divided tid in severe cases, as for canine ehrlichiosis therapy. Since this drug is rickettsiostatic only, total recovery is dependent on the host's immune response for ultimate elimination of the rickettsiae.

II. Dogs treated during the acute phase of the disease will show definite improvement within hours of tetracycline administration. The fever will begin to abate within 24 hours; improved physiologic parameters develop more slowly and may require several days for a return to normal levels. Relapses may occur if chemotherapy is discontinued before the host's immune response has effected a complete resolution of the infection.

III. Supportive therapy is required as an adjunct, especially in severely ill, debilitated patients. Fluid therapy must be used with caution, however, because of the increased vascular permeability that could produce an expanded extracellular volume and give rise to pulmonary and cerebral edema.

PREVENTION

I. Prevention is limited to avoidance of tick-infested areas whenever possible and maintenance of strict tick control programs for both dogs and premises. Ticks should be removed from dogs as soon as possible to decrease the potential for transmission of rickettsiae.

II. Rocky Mountain spotted fever is a zoonotic disease. Dogs remain rickettsemic for at least 14 days; therefore, extreme care must be taken to prevent exposure of persons obtaining blood samples or performing necropsies.

III. Ticks should not be removed from dogs with bare fingers, as *R. rickettsii* can be transmitted via tick feces or hemolymph. Remove ticks instead by applying constant traction close to the point of insertion, using tweezers or fingers protected with surgical gloves.

IV. In highly endemic areas, a seroassay program can be beneficial in detecting inapparent cases of RMSF.

PUBLIC HEALTH CONSIDERATIONS

I. Humans are exceptionally sensitive to infection with *R. rickettsii*. The infectious dose of rickettsiae for humans approximates one viable, virulent organism. Care must be taken to maintain aseptic technique when handling suspect, as well as confirmed, cases of RMSF. Infection has been known to occur in humans when infectious materials come into contact with the conjunctivae or with abraded skin.

II. Handling of ticks should be avoided after removal from dogs; the feces and hemolymph of infected ticks contain large numbers of rickettsiae.

SUGGESTED READINGS

Breitschwerdt EB, Meuten DJ, Walker DH, et al: Canine Rocky Mountain spotted fever: a kennel epizootic. Am J Vet Res 46:2124, 1985

De Shazo RD, Boyce JR, Osterman JV, et al: Early diagnosis of Rocky Mountain spotted fever. Use of primary monocyte culture technique. JAMA 235:1353, 1976

Feng WC, Murray ES, Rosenberg GE, et al: Natural infection of dogs on Cape Cod with *Rickettsia rickettsii*. J Clin Microbiol 10:322, 1979

Greene CE, Burgdorfer W, Cavagnolo R, et al: Rocky Mountain spotted fever in dogs and its differentiation from canine ehrlichiosis. J Am Vet Med Assoc 186:465, 1985

Gordon JC, Gordon SW, Peterson E, et al: Rocky Mountain spotted fever in dogs associated with human patients in Ohio. J Infect Dis 148:1123, 1983

Kelly DJ, Osterman JV, Stephenson EH: Rocky Mountain spotted fever in areas of high and low prevalence: survey for canine antibodies to spotted fever rickettsiae. Am J Vet Res 43:1429, 1982

Keenan KP, Buhles WC, Huxsoll DL, et al: Pathogenesis of infection with *Rick-*

ettsia rickettsii in the dog: a disease model for Rocky Mountain spotted fever. J Infect Dis 135:911, 1977

Keenan KP, Buhles WC, Huxsoll DL, et al: Studies on the pathogenesis of *Rickettsia rickettsii* in the dog: clinical and clinicopathologic changes of experimental infection. Am J Vet Res 38:851, 1977

Lissman BA, Benach JL: Rocky Mountain spotted fever in dogs. J Am Vet Med Assoc 176:994, 1980

Magnarelli LA, Anderson JF, Philip RN, et al: Antibodies to spotted fever–group rickettsiae in dogs and prevalence of infected ticks in southern Connecticut. Am J Vet Res 43:656, 1982

Norment BR, Burgdorfer W: Susceptibility and reservoir potential of the dog to spotted fever–group rickettsiae. Am J Vet Res 45:1706, 1984

Sexton DJ, Burgdorfer W, Thomas L, et al: Rocky Mountain spotted fever in Mississippi: survery for spotted fever antibodies in dogs and for spotted fever group rickettsiae in dog ticks. Am J Epidemiol 103:192, 1976

Smith RC, Gordon JC, Gordon SW, et al: Rocky Mountain spotted fever in an urban canine population. J Am Vet Med Assoc 183:1451, 1983

Thornton JT: Rocky Mountain spotted fever in dogs and man. Mod Vet Pract 62:313, 1981

30

Haemobartonellosis

John W. Harvey

ETIOLOGY

I. Feline haemobartonellosis is more important as a disease entity and has been studied in much greater detail experimentally than has canine haemobartonellosis. For these reasons, most of the emphasis in this chapter will be on the disorder in cats, with comments concerning dogs made where appropriate.

II. The causative agents of haemobartonellosis in cats (*Haemobartonella felis*) and dogs (*Haemobartonella canis*) are rickettsial parasites that attach to the external surface of erythrocytes. Both agents appear to be worldwide in distribution.

III. Transmission
  A. Both organisms can be transmitted by injection of susceptible animals with infected blood; consequently, iatrogenic transmission can occur via blood transfusions.
  B. Transmission of infection by blood-sucking arthropods, such as fleas, is considered likely in cats. Transmission of *H. canis* by the brown dog tick (*Rhipicephalus sanguineus*) has been demonstrated experimentally.
  C. Severe disease has been reported in nursing animals, and *in utero* transmission is considered possible.

CLINICAL SIGNS

I. The severity of disease varies from inapparent infection in some animals to marked depression and death in others. Generally, the severity of clinical signs correlates with the severity of the anemia. Without therapy, it is estimated that approximately one-third of cats with uncomplicated haemobartonellosis will die of severe anemia. In contrast, adult dogs generally do not become ill when inoculated with *H. canis* unless they have been splenectomized.

II. Pathogenesis of anemia

   A. Generally 1 to 3 weeks are required following inoculation with infected blood before significant numbers of parasites appear on erythrocytes. Thereafter parasites generally appear in the blood in a cyclic manner as discrete parasitemic episodes, with days between episodes when parasites cannot be seen. In most cases several weeks of repetitive parasitemia are required for anemia to become severe.

   B. Erythrocytes may be damaged directly by attached parasites; however, most erythrocyte injury is immune-mediated. Phagocytosis is much more important than intravascular hemolysis in erythrocyte destruction.

   C. Role of the spleen

      1. The spleen is a blood filter that is rich in lymphocytes and macrophages; consequently, it is of primary importance in the defense against bloodborne infectious agents.

      2. In cats the spleen is important for removal of *Haemobartonella* organisms, but splenectomized cats do not appear to be more likely to develop life-threatening disease than intact cats. At times the spleen appears to selectively sequester parasitized erythrocytes without destroying them. Once parasites are released or removed from erythrocytes, the cells may reenter the circulation.

      3. In dogs, in contrast to cats, splenectomy is clearly predisposing to the development of more severe disease, and a substantial proportion of clinical cases of canine haemobartonellosis have been associated with splenectomy or impairment of splenic function.

   D. Predisposing factors to development of disease

      1. While prior or concurrent disease conditions, such as abscesses or feline leukemia virus infections (FeLV), may contribute to the occurrence and/or severity of disease, approximately half of all cases of feline haemobartonellosis do not have demonstrable concomitant diseases.

      2. In addition to splenectomy or splenic dysfunction, concurrent infections with *Babesia, Ehrlichia,* viruses, and bacteria may predispose dogs to the development of haemobartonellosis. Rarely, nonsplenectomized dogs with no concurrent disease condition are found with clinically significant haemobartonellosis.

III. Physical findings
   A. Common findings in cats include depression, weakness, anorexia, pale mucous membranes, and a rapid heart rate. Weight loss is usually recognized unless the anemia has developed acutely. Splenomegaly can be palpated at times. Icterus is seldom appreciated on physical examination, even though the plasma may appear yellow.
   B. The rectal temperature is increased approximately 50% of the time in acutely ill cats. Temperatures may be subnormal in moribund animals.
   C. Unless other diseases are also present, clinical signs are rarely apparent in nonsplenectomized dogs infected with *H. canis*. Signs attributable to anemia may be recognized in those with severe disease.

DIAGNOSIS

I. A definitive diagnosis of haemobartonellosis in cats and dogs requires that parasites be observed on a stained blood film. Unfortunately, organisms occur in cyclic parasitemias (especially in cats) and are not always identifiable in blood, even in animals that are severely ill. The synchronized disappearance of organisms from the blood of experimentally infected cats has been observed to occur within 2 hours or less. Because haemobartonellosis is a common cause of hemolytic anemia in cats, it should always be considered in the differential diagnosis of cats with regenerative anemias.
II. Identification of organisms
   A. *H. felis* organisms appear as small, blue-staining cocci, rings, or rods on erythrocytes in routinely stained (e.g., Wright-Giemsa) blood films (Fig. 30-1A). By their attachment parasites may appear to indent the surface of erythrocytes, a feature that aids in differentiating low numbers of parasites from staining artifacts.
   B. *H. canis* differs from *H. felis* in that it more commonly forms chains of organisms within grooves in the erythrocyte surface (Fig. 30-1B). Although composed of multiple individual organisms, chains may appear as beaded, branching, filamentous structures when examined by light microscopy.
   C. Organisms must be differentiated from precipitated stain, refractile drying or fixation artifacts, poorly staining Howell-Jolly bodies, and basophilic stippling.

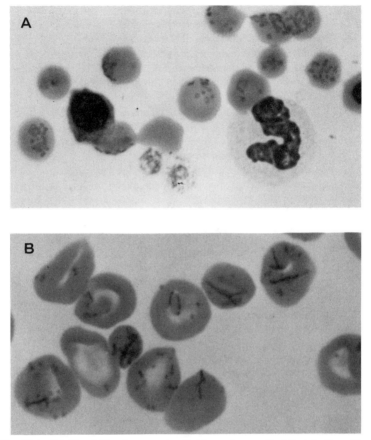

Fig. 30-1. (A) Blood film from a cat with *Haemobartonella felis* infection. Ring, rod, and coccoid forms of the parasite are present on erythrocytes. A metarubricyte and a neutrophil are also present. Wright-Giemsa. (B) Blood film from a dog with *Haemobartonella canis* infection. Epicellular parasites appear as single coccoid forms and in chains. Wright-Giemsa.

      D. Blood films must be examined for organisms before therapy is begun because parasites are absent while animals are being treated with tetracycline antibiotics.

III. Hematologic findings

      A. Animals should be anemic before a diagnosis of haemobartonellosis is made. While organisms may be observed in low numbers in the blood of nonanemic animals with latent infections, these animals will not appear ill unless other concurrent diseases are present. In uncomplicated haemobartonellosis, the severity of clinical signs generally correlates with the degree of anemia.

B. In most cases there is considerable evidence (polychromasia and reticulocytosis) of a regenerative response to the anemia. The mean corpuscular volume is frequently increased (above 50 fl), the mean corpuscular hemoglobin concentration may be decreased (below 32%), and nucleated erythrocytes are generally present. The anemia may appear poorly regenerative if a precipitous decrease in packed cell volume (PCV) has occurred early in the disease and there has not been sufficient time for a strong response. The anemia may also appear nonregenerative if other concurrent disorders (e.g., FeLV infection in cats) are present.

C. Autoagglutination may be seen in blood collected for hematology.

D. Total and differential leukocyte counts are variable and of little diagnostic assistance. Absolute monocyte counts are increased in nearly half the cases in cats, and erythrophagocytosis by monocytes may be observed.

IV. Other laboratory findings

A. Slight hemoglobinemia is rarely observed, but hemoglobinuria has not been reported in either species.

B. Plasma and serum sometimes appear yellow, and hyperbilirubinemia may be measured in some cases but is seldom severe. Substantial bilirubinuria has been recognized in some canine cases.

C. Clinical chemistry profiles may demonstrate abnormalities related to anemic hypoxia, but profiles can be normal.

D. Hypoglycemia may be present in moribund cats.

E. Plasma protein concentrations are usually normal but may be increased in some cats owing to increased globulin concentrations.

F. The direct Coombs test is usually positive in cats and may be positive in dogs.

V. Differential diagnosis

A. If organisms are not found, it may be difficult to differentiate haemobartonellosis from other causes of regenerative anemia.

B. Blood-loss anemias generally show a less dramatic regenerative response than do hemolytic anemias.

C. Autoimmune hemolytic anemia in cats cannot be easily differentiated from haemobartonellosis, because both disorders are Coombs test–positive and the parasites are not always identifiable in the blood. Because haemobartonellosis is more common than primary autoimmune hemolytic anemia in cats, Coombs test–positive animals generally are treated with tetracycline antibiotics as well as glucocorticoids.

D. Feline leukemia virus may cause transient regenerative anemia, even though most anemias associated with this virus are nonregenerative. These regenerative anemias may be Coombs test–positive. While a negative FeLV test tends to rule out FeLV as the cause of the anemia, a positive test does not eliminate the possibility that the animal has concurrent haemobartonellosis.

E. Heinz-body hemolytic anemia can be differentiated by the appearance of Heinz bodies on reticulocyte stains.

F. Other potential causes of hemolytic anemia in cats are uncommon; they include snake and arthropod venom, bacterial toxins, burns, and microangiopathic disease.

TREATMENT

I. Drug therapy

A. Oxytetracycline is effective against *H. felis* infections and is given at a dosage of 20 mg/kg PO tid for 3 weeks. Relapses may occur at times in animals treated for shorter periods. Some tetracycline products appear to produce a fever and/or evidence of illness in cats as adverse side effects. A lower dosage or a different tetracycline product may be used, or the drug may be discontinued altogether. Oxytetracycline at 40 mg/kg, given PO bid or tid for 9–14 days, has been efficacious in treating dogs.

B. Two IV injections, given 48 hours apart, of thiacetarsamide sodium (Caparsolate, CEVA) 1 mg/kg has been recommended for use in cats; however, this drug is not approved for use in this species, and relapses may occur.

C. Chloramphenicol has been recommended in the past for treatment of feline haemobartonellosis, but this drug would seem to be contraindicated because the recommended therapeutic dosage is toxic to cats. In addition to various signs of illness, chloramphenicol produces a dose-dependent bone-marrow erythroid hypoplasia, a feature obviously counterproductive to recovery from anemia.

D. Glucocorticoids such as prednisolone (1–2 mg/kg given PO bid) may be used in severely anemic animals to decrease erythrophagocytosis. The glucocorticoid dosage should be decreased gradually as desired increases in PCV are measured.

II. Supportive therapy
   A. Intravenous blood transfusions are required when the anemia is considered life-threatening.
   B. Intravenous fluid containing glucose is recommended in moribund animals.
   C. Hypothermic patients should be warmed.

PREVENTION

   I. Blood-sucking arthropod vectors should be eliminated from dogs and cats.
   II. A seldom employed method to minimize the possibility of iatrogenic transmission is to use as blood donors splenectomized animals that are shown to be free of blood parasites (latent infections) for a period of 10 days postsplenectomy. Because splenectomy makes dogs more susceptible to the development of haemobartonellosis, this potential sequela should be considered before splenectomy is performed in this species.

SUGGESTED READINGS

Benjamin MM, Lumb WV: *Haemobartonella canis* infection in a dog. J Am Vet Med Assoc 135:388, 1959

Donovan EF, Loeb WF: Hemobartonellosis in the dog. Vet Med 55:57, 1960

Harvey JW: Haemobartonellosis. p. 576. In Greene CE (ed): Microbiology and Infectious Diseases of the Dog and Cat. WB Saunders, Philadelphia, 1984

Harvey JW, Gaskin JM: Experimental feline haemobartonellosis. J Am Anim Hosp Assoc 13:28, 1977

Harvey JW, Gaskin JM: Feline haemobartonellosis: attempts to induce relapses of clinical disease in chronically infected cats. J Am Anim Hosp Assoc 14:453, 1978

Maede Y: Studies on feline haemobartonellosis. V. Role of the spleen in cats infected with *Haemobartonella felis*. Jpn J Vet Sci 40:141, 1978

Maede Y, Hata R: Studies on feline haemobartonellosis. II. The mechanism of anemia produced by infection with *Haemobartonella felis*. Jpn J Vet Sci 37:49, 1975

Pryor WH, Bradbury RP: *Haemobartonella canis* infection in research dogs. Lab Anim Sci 25:566, 1975

Venable JH, Ewing SA: Fine structure of *Haemobartonella canis* (Rickettsiales: Bartonellacea) and its relation to the host erythrocyte. J Parasitol 54:259, 1968

31

Dermatophytosis

Stephen D. White

ETIOLOGY

I. Dermatophytosis ("ringworm") is a fungal infection of keratinized tissues (stratum corneum, nail, hair) caused by a dermatophyte. In the dog and cat virtually all the causative dermatophyte species belong to either the *Microsporum* or *Trichophyton* genus.

II. Dermatophytes are found in various reservoirs in the environment, depending upon the species. Of the three species responsible for the overwhelming majority of cases in small animals, *Microsporum canis* and *Trichophyton mentagrophytes* are zoophilic (commonly found on animal reservoirs), whereas *Microsporum gypseum* is geophilic (commonly found in soil). Classically, *M. canis* has been described in an asymptomatic carrier state on the cat, whereas rodents have been the suspected carriers of *T. mentagrophytes*.

III. The actual incidence of dermatophytosis in dogs and cats is unknown. Because of the many clinical presentations, the disease may be underdiagnosed. On the other hand, many inflammatory skin diseases are incorrectly diagnosed as "fungal" infections.

IV. Pathophysiology

A. The dermatophytes live on the host only in keratinized tissues. Except in very rare instances they are not found in living tissue. Dermatophytes cannot survive in areas of intense inflammation. Most dermatophyte infections in animals are *ectothrix* infections, with conidia ("spores") found on the outside of the hair shaft and hyphae penetrating and invading the shaft.

B. When dermatophytes invade resting phase (telogen) hairs, the infection results in hair breakage. When growth phase (anagen) hairs are invaded, the fungi grow down to the uppermost border of mitotic activity (fringe of Adamson), where they can multiply and keep pace with the hair's own growth.

C. The involvement of the hair shaft within the follicle warrants a diagnosis of folliculitis.

D. As previously infected hair shafts break and fall off the host, new hair shafts adjacent to the infection are invaded, leading to an outward enlargement of the lesion with a central area of alopecia and broken hair shafts.

E. Occasionally the folliculitis caused by the dermatophyte produces a weakening of the follicular wall, with subsequent rupture into the dermis. This is accompanied by an inflammatory foreign-body response to both the hair shaft keratin and the dermatophyte, leading to furunculosis.

F. Severe inflammatory reactions of folliculitis or furunculosis are termed *kerions*. These are believed to represent a hypersensitivity reaction to the dermatophytes or to their by-products. The generalized hypersensitivity to localized dermatophytosis that occurs in humans (the *id* reaction) has not been well documented in animals.

G. In general, most dermatophyte infestations are felt to occur in a host which is in some way immune-compromised. Thus it is not unusual to find dermatophytosis among very young animals; it may occur in those animals secondary to hyperadrenocorticism or hypothyroidism; as a side effect of immunosuppressive or antineoplastic therapy; in animals in poor nutritional states; or in feline leukemia virus–positive cats.

H. In addition, the role of the environment must be taken into account. Factors that may favor dermatophyte infection include the following:
1. Crowded or unclean conditions
2. Warmth and humidity
3. Lack of adequate sunlight

DIAGNOSIS

I. History
A. Age, breed, sex
1. Younger animals are more likely to have dermatophytosis, although animals of any age may be affected. The young animal may be more succeptible owing both to an immature immune system and a greater likelihood of exposure to suboptimal housing conditions (pet stores, animal shelters, etc.)
2. No breed or sex predilection has been noted.
B. Environmental history

1. Nutritional status of the affected animal
2. Housing of the animal
   a) Crowded conditions
   b) Recent acquisition of the animal from an animal shelter, pet shop, etc.
3. Other animals in the household
   a) Although usually thought of as contagious, dermatophytes may be carried asymptomatically by some pets, especially cats. Therefore, the *lack* of lesions on other animals does *not* preclude a diagnosis of dermatophytosis.
   b) Recent introduction of another animal into the household
4. Skin lesions in any of the human occupants of the house

C. Most commonly, dogs and cats present with a history of alopecia. The owners may also note
   1. Scaling
   2. Pruritus
   3. Erythema
D. Less commonly, in cases of furunculosis or kerion, the owners' complaint may be of swellings, tumors, or draining tracts.
E. Dermatophytes affecting the feet may lead to owners' noticing splitting or malformed nails or, in severe cases, lameness.
F. Occasionally the animal may be asymptomatic but the owners (or their children) may have been diagnosed as having dermatophytosis, and the family pet may be suspected of being a carrier.
G. Probably, dermatophytosis usually is a slowly progressive disease of insidious onset; however, owner awareness of the condition (particularly in long-coated, nonpruritic animals) limits the usefulness of knowledge of duration.

II. Physical examination
   A. Clinical signs usually include the following:
      1. Alopecia (localized or generalized)
      2. Seborrhea sicca
      3. Pruritus
      4. Papules and crusts (miliary dermatitis)
      5. Erythema
      6. In cases of dermatophytosis involving the nails (onychomycosis), cracked nails or purulent exudate draining from the nail beds may be seen.
   B. Less commonly, particularly in cases of kerion, furunculosis, or granulomatous reaction to dermal dermatophytosis, clinical signs may include:
      1. Fistulous tracts

    2. Cutaneous or subcutaneous nodules

    3. Plaques

    4. Pain on palpation of lesions

III. Clinicopathologic evaluation

  A. Hematologic or biochemical parameters are rarely altered by dermatophytosis unless another disease process is present.

    1. If secondary bacterial infection or furunculosis is present, leukocytosis and neutrophilia may be seen.

    2. Concurrent hypothyroidism may produce a nonresponsive anemia and/or elevated serum cholesterol levels.

    3. Concurrent hyperadrenocorticism may produce a stress response leukogram and/or elevated serum alkaline phosphatase levels.

IV. Specific diagnostic techniques

  A. Fungal culture is the most accurate method of diagnosis and the one offering the greatest possibility of success.

    1. In general, abnormal hair should be used for culture. Broken or split hair shafts, whether from the periphery or from the center of the lesion, are preferred. The area to be cultured should be *lightly* swabbed with alcohol (to reduce the likelihood of saprophyte contamination) and allowed to air-dry before plucking the hair. The hair may be placed into a sterile tube with or without culture medium (requirements vary with different laboratories) and sent to a diagnostic laboratory.

    2. When nails are affected, a portion of the nail should be removed and ground into tiny pieces for inoculation onto culture media. If dewclaws are present and infected, their removal and submission to the laboratory is a relatively easy method of obtaining sufficient amounts of nail and nail bed.

    3. An alternative (and generally less expensive) method of culture is the use of in-house fungal culture assays (Dermatophyte Test Medium, Pitman-Moore; Derm-Duet, Bacti-Lab). In general, these consist of culture vials or plates containing a fungal growth medium, antibiotics to reduce bacterial contamination, and a color indicator (usually phenol red). The latter operates on the principle that dermatophytes will preferentially digest proteins in the medium, changing the pH (by producing alkaline metabolites) to produce a red color change. Saprophytes, on the other hand, will preferentially utilize carbohydrates in the medium (producing acidic metabolites), thus keeping the pH acidic and the color of the medium its original yellow.

4. Interpretation of the results of in-house assays should be made according to the manufacturer's instructions. Because most saprophytes will eventually utilize the proteins in the medium (and dermatophytes will eventually utilize the carbohydrates), the significant color change to red *must occur with the first growth noted* in order to be indicative of a dermatophyte. In addition, colony morphology must be taken into account. Generally, dermatophyte colonies will be cottony or powdery in texture, white or buff-colored, and relatively flat. Dark, nodular, or stalagmite-type growths are probably saprophytes.

5. Identification of the type of dermatophyte may be made by gently applying a piece of clear cellophane tape to the colony, then placing the tape on a microscope slide over a drop of lactophenol cotton blue stain. Examination of the hyphae and especially the macroconidia will enable the clinician to identify the fungus (Fig. 31-1). This technique works best when a culture medium favoring sporulation is used (Derm-Duet, Bacti-Lab).

6. If kerions or fistulous tracts are to be cultured, the area should be swabbed with alcohol and a sterile biopsy taken. The biopsy sample should be sent to a diagnostic laboratory. Because povidone-iodine may suppress fungal growth, its use as a preparation swab solution should be avoided.

B. Histopathology
1. Histopathology of suspected lesions may give a diagnosis of dermatophytosis, although not as frequently as fungal culture.
2. Multiple biopsies should be obtained from both central and peripheral areas of lesions.
3. Any histopathologic report of folliculitis and/or furunculosis, especially in a cat, should prompt an investigation for dermatophytosis.
4. While usually visible with hematoxylin and eosin, dermatophyte spores and hyphae are better distinguished by using other stains, such as periodic acid–Schiff (PAS) or Grocott's methenamine silver.

C. Direct microscopic examination
1. Direct microscopic examination of affected hair shafts can provide a rapid diagnosis of dermatophytosis. However, proficiency in distinguishing spores and hyphae from cutaneous debris requires practice, and the procedure itself is time-consuming and does not lend itself to speciation of the dermatophytes.

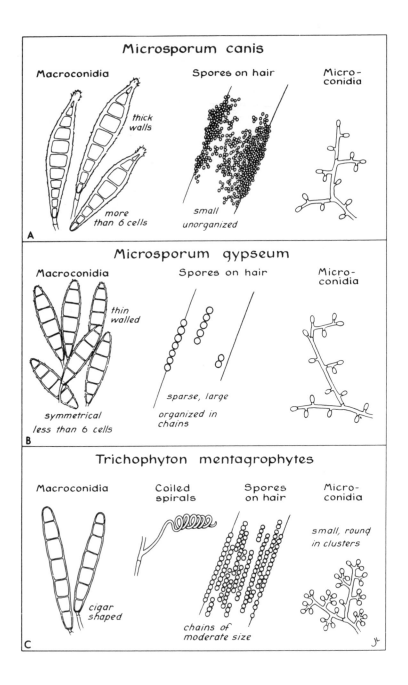

Microsporum canis

Macroconidia — thick walls — more than 6 cells

Spores on hair — small, unorganized

Microconidia

A

Microsporum gypseum

Macroconidia — thin walled — symmetrical, less than 6 cells

Spores on hair — sparse, large, organized in chains

Microconidia

B

Trichophyton mentagrophytes

Macroconidia — cigar shaped

Coiled spirals

Spores on hair — chains of moderate size

Microconidia — small, round in clusters

C

2. The hair shafts to be examined should be cleared with 20% potassium hydroxide (KOH) and 15–20 seconds of *gentle* heating (avoid boiling). Alternatively, the KOH hair mount may be left on the microscope stage with the lamp turned on for 15–20 minutes and then examined.

D. Ultraviolet (UV) light examination

   1. Use of a UV light such as a Wood's lamp may be of some use in diagnosing dermatophytosis.

   2. Of the common dermatophytes in veterinary medicine, only *M. canis* will fluoresce. This effect is caused by a tryptophan metabolite produced by the fungus. Typically, the fluorescence will be bright apple–green, resembling that of a watch dial. The fluorescence often will be noted along the hair shafts.

   3. However, only approximately 40–60% of *M. canis* isolates will fluoresce. In addition, epidermal scale and topical medications will also fluoresce, although not usually with an apple green color.

   4. Therefore, a *negative* (nonfluorescent) UV light examination does *not* eliminate a diagnosis of dermatophytosis. A *positive* (fluorescent) UV examination should always be confirmed by fungal culture. Culturing of the fluorescent hairs is recommended.

V. Differential diagnosis

A. Expansive, centrally alopecic lesions will commonly occur in superficial pyodermas. Because of the ringlike nature of the surrounding epidermal collarette crust, such lesions lend themselves to misdiagnosis as ringworm. Collarettes are seldom seen surrounding dermatophyte lesions.

B. Fistulous-tract lesions may be caused by bacteria, foreign bodies, intermediate or deep mycoses (such as sporotrichosis or blastomycosis), or neoplasia.

C. Kerions, with their nodular, erythematous, circular appearance, resemble neoplasms, particularly canine histiocytomas.

D. Demodicosis may cause irregular alopecic areas, which can mimic "classic" ringworm.

←——————————

Fig. 31-1. Characteristic microscopic morphology of (**A**) *Microsporum canis,* (**B**) *Microsporum gypseum,* (**C**) *Trichophyton mentagrophytes.* (Muller GH, Kirk RW, Scott DW: Small Animal Dermatology. 3rd Ed. WB Saunders, Philadelphia, 1983, p. 256.)

    E. Seborrheic dermatitis due to other causes (endocrine, idiopathic, etc) should also be included in the differential diagnosis.

TREATMENT

I. Systemic treatment
    A. The treatment of choice is oral griseofulvin. Griseofulvin comes in two forms, microsize (Fulvicin-U/F, Schering), and ultramicrosize in a formulation of polyethylene glycol (PEG) (Gris-PEG, Dorsey). The dosage range is 50–100 mg/kg for the microsize, and 5–10 mg/kg for the ultra microsize, given once daily. If vomiting occurs, the dose may be divided bid. The concurrent feeding of fat or a slightly oily meal may enhance absorption. The author begins at the low end of the dosage scale when treating cats.
    B. Side effects are uncommon but can include vomiting, anorexia, lethargy, diarrhea, pyrexia, icterus, neurotoxicity, neutropenia, and angioedema.
    C. Griseofulvin should be given to all animals with lesions in the household. Treatment should be continued for at least 2 weeks past clinical resolution of the lesions on all animals.
    D. When griseofulvin is used properly with the doses and regimen described and is combined with proper topical and environmental therapy, treatment failure is highly unusual. Failure usually is due to inadequate doses or durations of therapy, failure to treat other animals in the environment, or, occasionally, an underlying immune defect in the animal.
    E. When a griseofulvin-resistant fungus is suspected, oral ketoconazole (Nizoral, Janssen Pharmaceutica) may be used. The recommended dosage varies, but 5–30 mg/kg once daily has been suggested. Ketoconazole may cause vomiting and anorexia and has not been approved for use in dogs and cats.

II. Topical therapy
    A. All the hair in affected lesions and at least a 2-cm border should be clipped off and thrown out. In long-haired animals, particularly cats, a general body clip is recommended. This reduces the dermatophyte "load" on an animal and thus the potential for contagion.
    B. All in-contact animals, whether showing lesions or not, should be treated topically. Dips, which are sponged on an animal, permitted to air-dry, and not washed off, are superior to shampoos for their residual action and to ointments and lotions for their ability to cover large areas.

    C. The author prefers 45% captan (Blue Ribbon Products) wettable powder (a rose fungicide) as a dip. The suspension is made by mixing two tablespoons of the powder in a gallon of water. Owners are instructed to wear gloves because captan may be a contact irritant in humans. Because the powder forms a suspension, the preparation should be shaken intermittently. Captan is available at most garden supply stores.

    D. An alternative dip is 2% lime sulfur (Lym Dyp, DVM), which is safe but odoriferous and will alter the color of metal jewelry.

    E. If a small area is affected, topical lotions containing clotrimazole (Veltrim, Haver) or miconazole (Conofite, Pitman-Moore) may be used. In solitary, severely inflamed kerions, thiabendazole combined in a lotion with an antibiotic and a corticosteroid (Tresaderm, MSD AGVET) may be helpful. Any of these topicals can occasionally produce a contact dermatitis, and they are ineffective in treating asymptomatic areas of fungal presence on the coat. Tolnaftate cream (Tinavet, Schering) is not effective in small animal dermatophytosis.

III. Environmental therapy

    A. Because fungal spores may persist in the environment, rigorous vacuuming of the premises and cleaning (or preferably, disposal) of bedding is of prime importance. In persistent or multiple animal involvement, vacuuming of air ducts and filters may be necessary.

IV. Prognosis

    A. When adequate topical, systemic, and environmental therapy is used, the prognosis for recovery from dermatophytosis is very good to excellent. In addition, a certain number of cases are self-limiting, owing to the host's ability to mount an adequate defense.

    B. In multiple-animal households, particularly in catteries and kennels, the prognosis may be more guarded, owing to the technical and financial constraints involved in dipping, treating, and clipping the animals.

V. Public health aspects

    A. Dermatophytosis is a zoonosis. If the owners of infected animals have suspect lesions, they should seek advice from a physician, preferably a dermatologist. This is not only for their sake but to prevent them from becoming a reservoir for the animals.

    B. Occasionally the veterinarian will be confronted with owners who have been diagnosed as having dermatophytosis but whose pet or pets have no clinical signs. In these cases it is important that the physician attempt to substantiate the diagnosis and speciate the dermatophyte; if it is not *Microsporum* or *Trichophyton,* then it is highly unlikely that the animal has contributed to the human infection.

C. In addition, a sterile brush (a new toothbrush will do) should be run through the animal's coat and the bristles or debris cultured for dermatophytes.

D. If the same dermatophytes are cultured from the pet and the affected humans(s), the animal should be dipped as noted above. The author recommends that griseofulvin be administered to the pet for 3–4 weeks in these instances even if the animal has no lesions.

E. It is important for the owner, the veterinarian, and the physician to realize that treating the pet does not eliminate the need for treating the environment, particularly clothing and bedding. The animal may not even be a carrier per se but may have contracted the dermatophyte from the affected human(s).

SUGGESTED READINGS

Muller GH, Kirk RW, Scott DW: Small Animal Dermatology. 3rd Ed. WB Saunders, Philadelphia, 1983

Foil CS: Antifungal agents in dermatology. p. 560. In Kirk RW (ed): Current Veterinary Therapy. Vol. 9. WB Saunders, Philadelphia, 1986

Foil CS: Diagnosis and management of dermatophytosis. Am Anim Hosp Assoc Sci Proc: p. 174. 1986

Helton KA, Nesbitt GH, Caciolo PL: Griseofulvin toxicity in cats: literature review and report of seven cases. J Am Anim Hosp Assoc 22:453, 1986

32

Subcutaneous Mycoses

Marie H. Attleberger

The subcutaneous mycoses involve a miscellaneous group of fungi that infect skin and subcutaneous tissue primarily but that may invade other organs. With the exception of *Sporothrix schenckii*, they are opportunistic invaders.

RHINOSPORIDIOSIS

Etiology

I. Rhinosporidiosis is a chronic infection of the mucocutaneous tissues of the nasal cavity characterized by the formation of polyps. Other tissues may also be involved. The etiologic agent, *Rhinosporidium seeberi*, is found worldwide, frequently in association with bodies of water, but has been seen in humans living in drier regions.

II. The infecting organism is a small spore (6–10 μm), which penetrates the mucosal epithelium and begins to mature in the subepithelial tissue. The spherule (sporangium) continues to grow and undergoes nuclear division until thousands of spores are present. The spherules may reach 350 μm in size upon maturity but spherules of all sizes may be present. Spores are released through a pore in the wall of the spherule.

III. Although *Rhinosporidium seeberi* has recently been cultured in vitro, its saprobic existence remains unknown, and it has not been experimentally transmitted to animals or humans.

IV. Although the natural method of transmission is unknown, cases have been reported in humans, dogs, horses, mules, cattle, geese, ducks, and goats.

V. The infection occurs more frequently in males than in females.

Clinical Signs

I. A bloody nasal discharge, frequent or occasional, and usually from a single nostril, is the most frequent sign.
II. Sneezing for weeks to months may occur. In one case seen by the author exposure of a dog to cold temperatures caused sneezing, which ceased when the dog was placed in warm quarters.
III. Sessile or pedunculate polyps in the nasal cavity, pink to red in color, may be observed through an endoscope or otoscope. Growths may also occur outside the nasal cavity.
IV. Most polyps are soft and friable and bleed easily, but some are firm and verrucose in appearance. White specks may be seen in some polyps.
V. Reports of eye involvement in dogs have not been reported.

Diagnosis

I. The nasal discharge, if present, may be examined microscopically [in 10–20% potassium hydroxide (KOH) under the 10 × and 45 × objectives] for spores (7–9 μm) and possibly for spherules.
II. Polyps should be observed for whitish-gray specks, which are the spherules.
III. Polyps should be crushed and examined as above for spores and spherules. Spherules vary in size from 10 to 350 μm. Endospores are seen in mature spherules.
IV. Histopathologic sections of the polyps will also demonstrate the organism.
V. Attempts to culture the organism in vitro were unsuccessful until only quite recently.

Treatment

I. Complete, aggressive surgical removal of the polyps is the usual treatment. In humans a hot or cold snare has been used to avoid spreading infection to adjacent tissue.

II. Electrocoagulation or treatment with 1% iodine or 1% silver nitrate following surgery may prevent recurrence, which is commonly seen.

III. Dapsone (Avlosulfon, ICI) tid 1 mg/kg PO for 2 weeks, then decreasing to bid for several weeks, may be tried either alone, in combination with, or following surgery. It seems to inhibit growth of the polyps in some cases.

IV. Dapsone produces severe reactions in some dogs, including:
   A. Agranulocytosis
   B. Methemoglobinemia
   C. Hemolytic anemia
   D. Thrombocytopenia

V. Surgical removal of the polyps is preferred and may need to be repeated several times. Dapsone should be used in cases in which close monitoring of the dog is possible.

Public Health Considerations

Although it affects humans and animals, rhinosporidiosis is not a transmissible disease.

EUMYCOTIC MYCETOMA

Etiology

I. Eumycotic mycetoma (fungal tumor) in animals is caused by several fungi, most of which are dematiaceous. Mycetomas are characterized by a triad of signs: tumefaction, draining sinuses, and microcolonies or "grains" of the organism. It is the organization into grains that differentiates eumycotic mycetoma from phaeohyphomycosis (dark or hyaline hyphae in tissues) and from chromoblastomycosis (brown splitting bodies in tissues). In the human literature eumycotic mycetoma has been called *maduromycosis* or *madura foot* and can be caused by a number of agents. The term *eumycotic mycetoma* currently is reserved for those cases caused by true fungi in both humans and animals.

II. *Curvularia* and *Drechslera* spp. are frequently isolated from animals, and *Pseudallescheria boydii* (*Allescheria boydii*) has also been reported. These organisms are found worldwide and occur as saprophytes in the soil or on plants.

III. Entry into the subcutaneous tissues probably follows an injury. In two dogs with internal lesions there was a history of dehiscence following surgery.

IV. Most of the animal cases reported have occurred in the United States and have involved black microcolonies or grains, but cases with yellow and white grains have also been seen.

Clinical Signs

I. Tumefaction, draining tracts, and granules in the exudate are seen in typical mature lesions.

II. Swelling is not always evident, especially in early cases, and draining tracts may not be visible; however, grains can be found on biopsy.

III. Lesions can be found on any part of the body.

IV. Lameness is often present when lesions involve the foot.

V. The author has seen one case in a dog in which firm, dark granules were found only in the toe webs. Lameness was present.

Diagnosis

I. If the typical triad of signs is present, a tentative diagnosis can be made immediately.

II. The mycetoma and exudate should be examined carefully for grains, which may be dark or light in color. The grains should be crushed, placed in KOH, and observed microscopically for large, dark chlamydospores and true hyphae.

III. Culture is necessary to identify the specific causative organism. The grains can be washed vigorously in several changes of sterile water or saline, blotted dry with sterile fabric or paper, and placed on the surface of a Sabouraud dextrose agar plate (pH 7.0) that does *not* contain cycloheximide (most of the causative fungi are sensitive to this inhibitor). The plate is incubated at room temperature.

IV. Botryomycosis, a clinical condition similar to mycetoma, will have grains made of cocci or rods that are visible on a Gram stain.

V. Tissue sections also may be sent to a pathology laboratory for diagnosis.

Treatment

I. Complete surgical removal is recommended when the diagnosis is made early. The mycetoma may recur.

II. Amphotericin B (Fungizone, Squibb), 0.2 mg/kg every other day for at least 3 weeks, may be used in conjunction with surgery, especially if the tumor recurs.

III. The prognosis is fair to good when cases involve the skin and extremities and are treated early. However, some animals will fail to respond to surgery or amphotericin B.

IV. In advanced cases or in those involving internal organs the prognosis is unfavorable.

Public Health Considerations

Mycetoma has not been transmitted from animal to animal or from animal to human.

PHAEOHYPHOMYCOSIS

Etiology

I. *Phaeohyphomycosis* is the term applied to fungal infections caused by various dematiaceous fungi that form hyaline to dark-walled, septate hyphae in tissue. Brown pigmentation also is seen in fungal cultures isolated from these cases. Most of the causative organisms are soil saprophytes, plant pathogens, or laboratory contaminants and are found worldwide. Many are difficult to identify in the laboratory owing to the lack of sporulation.

II. *Drechslera spicifera, Exophiala jeanselmei, Phialophora verrucosa, Pseudomicrodochium suttonii*, and *Scolecobasidium humicola* are some of the dematiaceous fungi that have been isolated from cases of phaeohyphomycosis in animals.

III. Entry into the tissue is probably through a wound.

IV. Lesions usually consist of purulent centers surrounded by wide zones of epitheloid tissue, with hyphae dispersed singly or in small groups. Odd hyphal forms and round forms may be found. All the causative agents appear morphologically similar in tissue.

V. Infection has been reported in dogs, cats, horses, fish, and birds. More cases have been reported in cats than in other animals; often the infection is concurrent with squamous cell carcinoma, crypto-coccosis, or leukemia.

Clinical Signs

Various cutaneous and subcutaneous lesions, multiple or single, may be present on different parts of the body. They include the following:
  I. Abscesses, unopened or draining
 II. Shallow, raw ulcers or "punched-out" areas on the skin
III. Granulomas
IV. Firm cutaneous nodules
 V. Skin plaques

Diagnosis

  I. History of a lesion not responding to standard treatment should lead one to consider the possibility of a fungus infection.
 II. Pus, tissue scrapings, or biopsies should be examined for hyphae in KOH, under $10\times$ and $45\times$ magnification.
III. Many of the hyphal walls are dark brown while others are hyaline or colorless. Septations are present, hyaline or dark round forms may be found, and some forms appear to bud.
IV. In a few cases dark pigmentation of the hyphae may be lacking. Additional slides should be prepared and a careful search made for dark hyphae.
 V. Cultures should be made and a dematiaceous fungus should be recovered.
VI. To identify the specific organism specimens should be cultured at room temperature on modified Sabouraud dextrose agar without cycloheximide. If spores are present, identification may be made with the aid of a textbook on mycology.
VII. Many dematiaceous fungi are difficult to sporulate even when spor-ulation agar is used. These should be sent to a reference laboratory.
VIII. Histopathologic studies can be used to diagnose phaeohyphomy-cosis but will not identify the fungus. Hematoxylin and eosin will reveal dark hyphae; overstaining with methenamine silver should be avoided.

Treatment

I. Complete surgical excision is the preferred treatment in animals.
II. Lesions may recur if excision is not complete, necessitating additional surgery.
III. Antifungal therapy using amphotericin B, 0.2–0.25 mg/kg every other day for several weeks, may be used in addition to excision in dogs, although this usually is not necessary.

Public Health Considerations

Although humans and animals can be infected with similar organisms, transmission between human and animal or animal and animal has not been reported.

SPOROTRICHOSIS

Etiology

I. Sporotrichosis, caused by the dimorphic fungus *Sporothrix schenckii*, is a chronic infection of cutaneous and subcutaneous tissue but can also involve the lymphatics and internal organs.
II. *Sporothrix schenckii* occurs worldwide. It is found in soil and on plants and wood and has been isolated from water, sphagnum moss, humans, grasses, fleas, ants, and horsehair, and also from frankfurters in cold storage.
III. The saprophytic or mycelial form is found in nature, while the parasitic or yeast form is found in the host's tissue. Environmental temperature may affect the organism's ability to grow in nature and in the host.
IV. Severe winter weather and direct sunlight are harmful to the fungus but it appears to be fairly resistant to drying.
V. Entry into the body is gained through trauma, but the organism can also be inhaled or ingested.
VI. Sporotrichosis can be an occupational disease in florists, horticulturists, farmers, and gardeners.

VII. Animals in which the disease has been reported include dogs, cats, horses, mules, cattle, swine, mice, hamsters, camels, chimpanzees, and armadillos.

Clinical Signs

I. Lesions are confined primarily to the skin and subcutaneous tissue, but dissemination to the lungs and other internal organs can occur, especially in cats.

II. Cutaneous lesions in the form of raw, shallow ulcers, granulomas, nodules, abscesses, draining tracts, and various nonresponsive lesions are seen either on the extremities or in a random pattern over the body in dogs.

III. In addition to the lesions described for dogs, crusty, circular lesions and areas of necrosis may be present in cats. Some cats also test positive for feline leukemia virus.

IV. Wartlike lesions may occur.

V. Lesions on the extremities, some healing and some active, may follow along lymphatics, but visible lymphatic involvement generally is not present.

Diagnosis

I. The organism frequently cannot be demonstrated in either a stained smear or a wet mount. However, if pus is present, round to elongated yeast forms may sometimes be found.

II. Diagnosis by culture is the most reliable method and requires 5–14 days. Both the saprophytic and parasitic forms should be recovered to confirm the presence of *S. schenckii*. Culturettes containing a transport medium are satisfactory for submitting specimens to the laboratory.

III. The mycelial form is cultured on Sabouraud dextrose agar (with or without cycloheximide and chloramphenicol) at room temperature, while blood agar or brain-heart infusion agar incubated at 35°–37°C is used to recover the yeast form.

IV. Fluorescent antibody staining, not available commercially, can be performed at the Centers for Disease Control, Atlanta, Georgia. Staining is performed on direct smears of lesions or on paraffin-fixed sections.

V. An immunodiffusion test using nonhemolyzed serum is also available.

Treatment

I. The usual treatment in the dog involves inorganic iodides.

II. Successful results have been obtained with the following dosages:
   A. Sodium iodide: 1.0 ml of 20% NaI per 4.5 kg body weight PO bid
   B. Potassium iodide: 0.5 g KI in the feed daily for 6 weeks; 20–30 drops of saturated KI in the feed or orally bid for 4–5 weeks.

III. The above treatments should be continued for at least 1 month following disappearance of lesions to prevent relapse.

IV. Vomiting and diarrhea may occur in some dogs; the dosage may be decreased or treatment changed to amphotericin B or ketoconazole (Nizoral, Janssen Pharmaceutica). The dose for the latter in the dog is 10–30 mg/kg/day.

V. Most cats with localized lesions respond well to amphotericin B. When the infection is systemic, however, the prognosis is poor. Oral iodides are not well tolerated by cats.

VI. When treating cats with amphotericin B, the author has found the following method satisfactory:
   A. Dilute the dry amphotericin B powder with 20 ml of diluent. Dosage for an adult cat, regardless of weight, is:
      1. Dose 1: 0.2 mg in 10 ml of 5% dextrose in water (D5W)
      2. Dose 2: 0.4 mg in 10 ml D5W
      3. Dose 3: 0.6 mg in 10 ml D5W
      4. Remaining doses: 0.8 mg in 10 ml D5W
      5. The above is given IV every 3–4 days until the lesions are completely healed. The solution should be administered rapidly through a 25-gauge needle.
   B. If an elevated blood urea nitrogen occurs, it may be controlled with lactated Ringer's solution.

VII. The dosage for ketoconazole in the cat is 10 mg/kg/day for at least 30 days or until lesions disappear.

VIII. Surgical procedures on infected animals should be avoided.

IX. Iodine solutions may be applied directly to the lesions in conjunction with oral iodides.

Public Health Considerations

I. *Sporotrichosis is transmissible from animals to humans, especially from an infected cat.*

II. In some human cases there was no history of having been bitten or scratched by a cat.

III. Fomites may transmit the infection.

IV. Persons handling or treating infected animals should wear gloves.

V. Owners should be warned of the possibility of infection.

ZYGOMYCOSIS AND PYTHIOSIS

Etiology

I. Zygomycosis is an opportunistic infection caused by several species of fungi in the class *Zygomycetes*. Impaired immunologic defenses or some underlying condition may be predisposing factors to development of this disease.

II. The term *zygomycosis* is presently used instead of *phycomycosis* because the former class *Phycomycetes* was used to accommodate too many unrelated fungi.

III. Pythiosis is a chronic and progressive infection caused by *Pythium* spp. of the class *Oömycetes*, order Peronosporales.

IV. Broad, relatively nonseptate hyphae are produced in the tissues in both infections.

V. In zygomycosis members of the orders Mucorales (asexual spores produced in a sporangium) and Entomophthorales (asexual spores occurring as free conidiospores or as sporangiospores that are forcibly discharged) are involved.

 A. In the family Mucoracea species of the genera *Absidia, Mucor, Rhizomucor*, and *Rhizopus* are pathogenic.

 B. In other families, the species of *Cunninghamella, Mortierella, Saksenaea, Syncephalastrum*, and *Apophysomyces* are pathogenic.

 C. *Conidiobolus coronatus* and *Basidiobolus haptosporus* are the Entomophthorales species that are pathogenic.

VI. These organisms are found worldwide in soil and on plants. Entry into the body may follow trauma.

VII. *Pythium* spp. (asexual spores are motile zoospores) include aquatic, amphibious, and terrestrial organisms.

VIII. The sexual phase of the *Pythium* spp. (*Hyphomyces destruens*) causing disease in animals is unknown, so it has not been given a specific name.

   IX. Zygomycotic infections have been reported in dogs, cats, horses, cattle, swine, monkeys, a whale, rattlesnake, mink, okapi, and certain rodents.

    X. *Pythium* infections have occurred in horses, dogs, and cattle.

Clinical Signs

    I. Lesions often occur on the extremities but can be found on any part of the body and in the mouth. These lesions do not respond to standard treatments.

   II. Presenting lesions occur as swellings, draining tracts, ulcerated areas, and granulomas, sometimes with lymph node involvement. Bullae also can be seen.

 III. With systemic involvement there is anorexia, vomiting, diarrhea, and weight loss. Often an abdominal mass may be palpated.

 IV. Superficial lesions of pythiosis include granulomas, draining tracts, and ulcerated areas with or without dark areas of necrosis. These lesions progress rapidly.

  V. None of the lesions of canine pythiosis seen by the author has resembled the characteristic "leeches" or "kunkers" seen in horses.

Diagnosis

    I. Exudates, tissue, and tissue scrapings should be examined in 10–20% KOH for the large, broad, relatively nonseptate hyphae. Several slides should be examined.

   II. To determine the identity of the organism, it should be cultured on Sabouraud dextrose agar (without cycloheximide) at room temperature.

 III. If *Pseudomonas* or *Proteus* spp. are present in large numbers, recovery of the fungus is very difficult. The author has had success using V8 juice agar and Youssef's agar when this contamination has been a problem.

 IV. Refrigeration temperature is detrimental to some zygomycetes, and *Pythium* is killed by it. This should be kept in mind when sending tissues to the laboratory. A phone call to the laboratory prior to submitting specimens is recommended.

  V. When histopathologic studies are to be performed, fungal stains are recommended.

VI. A recently developed immunodiffusion test for pythiosis is both diagnostic and prognostic. It is not available commercially but is performed at the Centers for Disease Control, Atlanta, Georgia.

Treatment

I. Treatment is unsuccessful in most cases and the prognosis is poor.
II. Temporary improvement may be seen in dogs initially treated with amphotericin B, but flare-ups occur, usually within 10–14 days. If amphotericin B is used, the highest dose that can be tolerated by the patient should be given.
III. If the lesion is localized and limited to an extremity, complete surgical removal and extensive debridement may be successful, especially if an early diagnosis has been made. Amphotericin B may be used in addition to the surgery; freezing the area with liquid nitrogen may also be helpful.
IV. Amputation of the limb is necessary if the lesion is progressing rapidly. This frequently will save the dog's life if performed early.
V. Immunotherapy with autogenous preparations of the organism (especially *Pythium* spp.) is in the experimental stage and has shown promise in horses. A problem arises because of the rapid progression of the lesions and the time needed to grow and prepare the antigen (10–14 days).
VI. Lesions involving internal organs are often diagnosed at necropsy, but even when diagnosed earlier, treatment is usually unsuccessful.

Public Health Considerations

Zygomycosis and pythiosis are not transmissible to humans or animals.

SUGGESTED READINGS

Rhinosporidiosis

Allison N, Willard MD, Bentinck-Smith J, et al: Nasal rhinosporidiosis in two dogs. J Am Vet Med Assoc 188:869, 1986
Castellano MC, Idiart JR, Alcides AA: Rhinosporidiosis in a dog. Vet Med/Small Anim Clin 79:45, 1984

Lees GE, McKeever PJ, Ruth GR: Fatal thrombocytopenic hemorrhagic diathesis associated with dapsone administration to a dog. J Am Vet Med Assoc 175:49, 1979

Levy MG, Meuten DJ, Breitschwerdt EB: Cultivation of *Rhinosporidium seeberi* in vitro: interaction with epithelial cells. Science 234:474, 1986

Nair KK: Clinical trial of diaminodiphenylsulfone (DDS) in nasal and nasopharyngeal rhinosporidiosis. Laryngoscope 89:291, 1979

Rippon JW: Medical Mycology: The Pathogenic Fungi and the Pathogenic Actinomycetes. 2nd Ed. WB Saunders, Philadelphia, 1982

Stuart BP, O'Malley N: Rhinosporidiosis in a dog. J Am Vet Med Assoc 167:941, 1975

Eumycotic Mycetoma

Bridges CH: Maduromycotic mycetomas in animals. *Curvularia geniculata* as an etiologic agent. Am J Pathol 33:411, 1957

Brodey RJ, Schryver HF, Deubler MJ, et al: Mycetoma in a dog. J Am Vet Med Assoc 151:442, 1967

Jang SS, Popp JA: Eumycotic mycetoma in a dog caused by *Allescheria boydii*. J Am Vet Med Assoc 157:1071, 1970

Kurtz HJ, Finco DR, Perman V: Maduromycosis (*Allescheria boydii*) in a dog. J Am Vet Med Assoc 157:917, 1970

Rippon JW: Medical Mycology: The Pathogenic Fungi and the Pathogenic Actinomycetes. 2nd Ed. WB Saunders, Philadelphia, 1982

Phaeohyphomycosis

Ajello L, Padhye AA, Payne M: Phaeohyphomycosis in a dog caused by *Pseudomicrodochium suttonii* sp. nov. Mycotaxon 12:131, 1980

Ajello L: Phaeohyphomycosis: definition and etiology. p 126. In Mycoses: Sci Pub No 304, Proc 3rd Int Cong Mycoses. Pan Am Health Org, 1975

Ajello L, Georg LK, Steigbigel RT, et al: A case of phaeohyphomycosis caused by a new species of *Phialophora*. Mycologia 66:490, 1974

Bostock DE, Coloe PJ, Castellani A: Phaeohyphomycosis caused by *Exophiala jeanselmei* in a domestic cat. J Comp Pathol 92:479, 1982

Haschek WM, Kasali OB: A case of cutaneous feline phaeohyphomycosis caused by *Phialophora gougerotti*. Cornell Vet 67:467, 1977

Muller GH, Kaplan W, Ajello L, et al: Phaeohyphomycosis caused by *Drechslera spicifera* in a cat. J Am Vet Med Assoc 166:150, 1975

Pukay BP, Dion WM: Feline phaeohyphomycosis: treatment with ketoconazole and 5-fluorocytosine. Can Vet J 25:130, 1984

Rippon JW: Medical Mycology: the Pathogenic Fungi and the Pathogenic Actinomycetes. 2nd Ed. WB Saunders, Philadelphia, 1982

Sporotrichosis

Anderson NV, Ivoghli D, Moore WE, et al: Cutaneous sporotrichosis in a cat: a case report. J Am Anim Hosp Assoc 9:526, 1973

Dion WM, Speckmann G: Canine otitis externa caused by the fungus *Sporothrix schenkii*. Can Vet J 19:44, 1978

Dunstan RW, Reimann KA, Langham RF: Feline sporotrichosis. J Am Vet Med Assoc 189:880, 1986

Kier AB, Mann PC, Wagner JE: Disseminated sporotrichosis in a cat. J Am Vet Med Assoc 175:202, 1979

Koehne G, Powell HS, Hail RI: Sporotrichosis in a dog. J Am Vet Med Assoc 159:892, 1971

Rippon JW: Medical Mycology: the Pathogenic Fungi and the Pathogenic Actinomycetes. WB Saunders, Philadelphia, 1982

Zygomycosis and Pythiosis

Adler PL: Phycomycosis in fifteen dogs and two cats. J Am Vet Assoc 174:1216, 1979

Barsanti JA, Attleberger MH, Henderson RA: Phycomycosis in a dog. J Am Vet Assoc 167:293, 1975

Dawson CO, Wright NG, Aitken JP, et al: Canine phycomycosis: a case report. Vet Rec 84:633, 1969

Heller RA, Hobson HP, Gowing GM, et al: Three cases of phycomycosis in dogs. Vet Med/Small Anim Clin 66:472, 1971

Lucke VM, Morgan DG, English MP et al: Phycomycosis in a dog. Vet Rec 84:645, 1969

Mendoza L, Kaufman L, Standard PG: Immunodiffusion test for diagnosing and monitoring pythiosis in horses. J Clin Microbiol 23:813, 1986

Rudel JA: Gastric phycomycosis in a dog. Southwest Vet 27:274, 1974

33

Aspergillosis

Ralph E. Barrett

ETIOLOGY

I. Aspergillosis is an opportunistic fungal infection of many species, including the dog and cat.

II. Canine aspergillosis most commonly presents as a nasal and frontal sinus infection; however, uncommon cases of disseminated aspergillosis have been seen.

III. Ten cases of feline aspergillosis have been reported. Variable organ involvement has been seen, including: nasal, intestinal, pulmonary, combined intestinal and pulmonary, orbital cellulitis, and cystourethritis.

IV. *Aspergillus* is a genus of common mold containing over 600 species distributed worldwide. Only a few species have been reported to cause disease; these include *Aspergillus fumigatus* (most pathogenic), *Aspergillus clavatus, Aspergillus glaucus, Aspergillus nidulans, Aspergillus niger, Aspergillus flavus*, and *Aspergillus terreus.*

V. Conidiophores grow from foot cells. The swollen, vesicle-like end of each conidiophore produces stalks called *sterigmata*. Chains of spores arise from the tips of these sterigmata.

VI. Laboratory identification of medically significant species is by colony color, vesicle shape, and arrangement of sterigmata and spores.

VII. *Aspergillus* spp. are ubiquitous, common saprophytes in the environment. They grow in stables, flower beds, gardens, other soils, and dead vegetation. Spores are present in dust, hay, straw, and grass clippings.

VIII. Because *Aspergillus* spp. are common in the environment but only infrequently cause disease, other factors must be important in the pathogenesis of aspergillosis.

    A. A higher incidence of infection in farm dogs could indicate that inhalation of large numbers of spores may contribute to the onset of nasal aspergillosis.

B. Immune deficiency appears to be a major contributing factor. Cell-mediated immunodeficiency has been documented in cases of canine nasal aspergillosis. Chronic neoplasia and chronic renal disease have also been seen concurrently with canine aspergillosis and may have depressed the immune response.

C. Tissue damage from trauma, other nasal infections, neoplasia, or nasal foreign bodies may also contribute to the onset of localized canine nasal aspergillosis.

D. Seven of ten reported cases of feline aspergillosis were in cats with leukopenia and aplastic anemia from feline panleukopenia syndromes. Feline leukemia virus should always be investigated as a predisposing agent in cats.

E. Nasal aspergillosis has been reported more frequently in dolichocephalic breeds of dogs, especially collies and German shepherds. These breeds appear to be genetically or anatomically predisposed.

CLINICAL SIGNS

I. Aspergillosis is more common in the dog than in the cat. Clinical syndromes differ between the two.

II. Canine aspergillosis is most often a chronic rhinitis with a unilateral or bilateral nasal discharge.

A. The chronic nasal discharge is nonresponsive to antibiotic or corticosteroid therapy.

B. All ages and both sexes are affected.

C. Dolichocephalic breeds, especially collies and German shepherds, are more commonly affected.

D. Nasal discharge varies in character from serous to mucopurulent to hemorrhagic.

E. Nasal sinus swelling or pain are uncommon.

F. Central nervous system (CNS) signs of encephalitis, including seizures, behavioral changes, ataxia, circling, and multifocal neurologic deficits, can rarely be seen when the infection erodes the cribriform plate and enters the CNS.

G. Canine disseminated aspergillosis is rarely seen but has been reported to cause vertebral osteomyelitis, discospondylitis, listlessness, weight loss, spinal pain, bilateral uveitis, peripheral lymphadenopathy, and renal, splenic, and hepatic infection.

III. Feline aspergillosis may affect several different organ systems.

A. Pulmonary signs are most commonly seen.
B. Other organs reported to be individually affected have been the intestines, nasal passages, orbit, and urinary bladder/urethra.
C. Clinical signs vary with the organs affected and can include weight loss, depression, anorexia, general debility, diarrhea, sneezing, and coughing.

DIAGNOSIS

I. Several ancillary diagnostic aids are needed to establish a definitive diagnosis of canine nasal aspergillosis (Table 33-1). These include hematology, clinical chemistries, nasal cytology and culture via the external nares, nasal and frontal sinus radiography, nasal endoscopy, and nasal sinus exploratory surgery for cytology, culture, and histopathology.

II. Hematologic findings vary between cases. Most often a stress response with leukocytosis, neutrophilia, and lymphopenia is seen. Eosinophilia has been reported uncommonly.

III. Clinical chemistries are normal except in rare cases of disseminated aspergillosis. Organ system of involvement would determine the abnormalities encountered.

IV. Cats with aspergillosis may have signs of panleukopenia with a non-responding anemia and leukopenia due to feline panleukopenia syndromes. Feline leukemia virus tests may also be positive.

V. In the most common form of canine nasal aspergillosis, radiographs of the nasal and frontal sinuses often show an increased soft tissue density and decreased nasal turbinate density. Maxillary and frontal sinus densities may also be seen. Open-mouth nasal and skyline frontal sinus radiographs are recommended. Differential diagnoses would include neoplasia, nasal foreign body, and bacterial and fungal infections.

VI. Nasal swabs or flushes for cytologic evaluation and fungal culture are occasionally diagnostic; however, it is more often necessary to perform a nasal trephine or nasal flap exploratory surgery to obtain adequate samples for cytology, histology, and culture.

VII. Because fungal elements are usually not present in large numbers in exudates, cytologic evaluation of external nasal discharges usually is not helpful for establishing a diagnosis. Cytologic studies usually indicate a nonspecific mucopurulent or hemorrhagic exudate.

TABLE 33-1.   CLINICAL CHARACTERISTICS OF CANINE NASAL
ASPERGILLOSIS

Breed	All breeds More common in dolichocephalics (collies, German shepherds); less common in brachiocephalics
Age	All ages
Sex	Either sex
Duration of nasal discharge	Acute, but more often chronic
Hematology	Stress leukogram; occasionally eosinophilia
Nasal cytology via external nares by swab or flush	Nonspecific inflammation or infection; uncommon to see fungal elements
Nasal culture via external nares by swab or flush	Nonspecific bacteria; uncommon to culture fungus False negatives and false positives possible
Nasal endoscopy	Usually negative owing to the presence of exudate
Nasal and frontal sinus radiography	Increased soft-tissue density and/or decreased nasal turbinate density
Nasal flap exploration/trephination for biopsy	Yellow-green fungal growth, gray-black necrotic tissue debris Hyphae and spores seen histologically
Nasal flap exploration/trephination for culture	*Aspergillus* spp. cultured
Serology	Counterimmunoelectrophoresis reliable Double diffusion reliable ELISA not reliable

VIII. It is often difficult to visualize fungal elements or to obtain diagnostic samples using nasal endoscopy owing to the presence of ob-
scuring exudates.

   IX. On nasal flap exploration, a thick yellowish-green fungal growth is
often visualized. Cytologically, the organisms appear as septate hyphae, 4–6 μm wide. New methylene blue, 10–20% potassium hydroxide, or unstained wet mounts can be used.

    X. Histologic evaluation of suspicious nasal or frontal sinus tissue is
most likely to result in visualization of the organism. Hematoxylin
and eosin, Gridley's fungus stain, and Gomori's methenamine silver
stain are useful.

XI. *Aspergillus* spp. growing in the nasal or frontal sinus cavities exposed to air will develop spores; organisms growing in tissue will only develop septate mycelial hyphae.

XII. Nasal fungal cultures of aspergillosis can be either false positive or false negative.

    A. False positive cultures occur because *Aspergillus* spp. are common environmental contaminants. Positive cultures must be considered together with all other diagnostic test results.

    B. Because nasal exudates are often void of fungal elements, negative cultures can be obtained.

    C. *Aspergillus* spp. will grow on Sabouraud dextrose agar and on blood agar.

XIII. Fine-needle pulmonary aspiration biopsy may be required to diagnose canine or feline pulmonary or disseminated aspergillosis.

XIV. Recently, serologic tests have been employed to detect the systemic antibody response to *Aspergillus* spp. Both double diffusion and counterimmunoelectrophoresis in agarose gel provide reliable methods for testing. Neither method gives false positive reactions.

    A. Counterimmunoelectrophoresis appears to be better for the rapid detection of *A. fumigatus* precipitins.

    B. Serologic diagnosis of canine nasal aspergillosis is complicated by a lack of standardized methods for preparing antigens. Several different commercially prepared antigens of *A. fumigatus* should be used when testing canine sera to reduce the chance of obtaining false negative results.

    C. Enzyme-linked immunosorbent assay (ELISA) is a less reliable method for diagnosis of canine nasal aspergillosis. False negative and false positive results have been seen.

XV. Histologic examination of biopsy specimens in disseminated aspergillosis will demonstrate granulation tissue with necrosis, neutrophils, and hyphae.

TREATMENT

I. Numerous medical and surgical treatments have been attempted for canine nasal aspergillosis. No single therapy has proved totally effective, but some have more merit than others.

II. Surgical trephination of affected sinuses, removal of all sinus tissue, and implantation of drains for prolonged flushing, combined with medical therapy, have produced the best results. Medical and surgical treatments must be combined whenever possible.

III. For sinus flushing, a ¼-inch Silastic tube is placed into each frontal sinus. A forcep is passed through the frontal sinus into the nasal passage to ensure free communication. The skin is closed and the tube is fixed to the skin by sutures. A French latex T tube can be used to join the tubes from each frontal sinus, or else they can be flushed separately.

IV. Postoperatively the sinuses are flushed with 5–20 ml of a solution consisting of 10 ml povidone-iodine in 1L of physiologic saline three times daily for 7–14 days.

V. Systemic medications usually unsuccessful in treating canine nasal aspergillosis include amphotericin B, sodium iodide, thiabendazole, and nystatin.

VI. Two newer antifungal agents have met with some success in treating nasal aspergillosis, either alone or in combination with nasal curettage. These are 5-fluorocytosine (5-FC) (Ancobon, Hoffmann-La Roche) and ketoconazole (Nizoral, Janssen Pharmaceutica).

A. 5-Fluorocytosine possesses in vitro and in vivo activity against opportunistic mycotic diseases, including aspergillosis.

   1. It inhibits nucleic acid synthesis in susceptible fungi but is not metabolized by mammalian cells.

   2. Skin eruptions have been seen in the dog with this drug.

   3. Dosage for 5-FC is 175 mg/kg/day PO divided tid for 2–3 months.

B. Ketoconazole appears to be the most promising new antifungal drug for treating aspergillosis.

   1. It is an imidazole derivative that is systemically active following oral administration and has been shown to inhibit growth of *A. fumigatus*, both in vitro and in vivo, at concentrations that are nontoxic.

   2. Dosages of 60–80 mg/kg/day in dogs are toxic and can cause mortality.

   3. Dosages of 40 mg/kg/day in dogs have been associated with anorexia, hypoalbuminemia, and elevated serum alkaline phosphatase and alanine aminotransferase.

   4. Dosages of 30 mg/kg/day in dogs have not been associated with side effects.

C. Presently research is being conducted on two newer azole derivatives. Local intranasal infusion of enilconazole and systemic therapy with itraconazole are being investigated. These are multisite, potent fungal inhibitors that may destroy some resistant strains of *Aspergillus* spp.

PUBLIC HEALTH CONSIDERATIONS

There is no public health significance to aspergillosis because the disease does not spread directly from animal to human or from animal to animal.

SUGGESTED READINGS

Barrett RE, Hoffer RE, Schultz RD: Treatment and immunological evaluation of three cases of canine aspergillosis. J Am Anim Hosp Assoc 13:328, 1977

Barsanti JA: Opportunistic fungal infections. p. 728. In Greene CE (ed): Clinical Microbiology and Infectious Diseases of the Dog and Cat. Philadelphia, WB Saunders, 1984

Braude AI: The aspergilli. p. 592. In Braude AI, Davis CE, Fierer J (eds): Medical Microbiology and Infectious Diseases. 2nd Ed. WB Saunders, Philadelphia, 1986

Goodall SA, Lane JG, Warnock DW: The diagnosis and treatment of a case of nasal aspergillosis in a cat. J Small Anim Pract 25:627, 1984

Harvey CE: Nasal aspergillosis and penicilliosis in dogs: results of treatment with thiabendazole. J Am Vet Med Assoc 184:48, 1984

Jungerman PF, Schwartzman RM: Veterinary Medical Mycology. Philadelphia, Lea & Febiger, 1972

Richardson MD, Warnock DW: Antigen selection for optimal serological diagnosis of *Aspergillus fumigatus* infection of the nasal chambers of the dog. Vet Rec 114:354, 1984

Richardson MD, Warnock DW, Bovey SE, et al: Rapid serological diagnosis of *Aspergillus fumigatus* infection of the frontal sinuses and nasal chambers of the dog. Res Vet Sci 33:167, 1982

Sharp N, Burrell MH, Sullivan M, Cervantes-Olivares RA: Canine nasal aspergillosis: serology and treatment with ketoconazole. J Small Anim Pract 25:149, 1984

34

Blastomycosis

Joyce S. Knoll
Peter S. MacWilliams

ETIOLOGY

I. Blastomycosis is a systemic mycotic infection caused by *Blastomyces dermatitidis*. Other names for this disease are North American blastomycosis, Gilchrist's disease, and Chicago disease. *B. dermatitidis* is a dimorphic fungus and thus can occur in a yeast form (parasitic phase) and a mycelial form (saprophytic phase).

   A. In tissues and on blood agar at incubation temperatures of 37°C, the organism is a round, thick-walled yeast averaging 8–20 μm in diameter, with broad-based buds (Fig. 34-1).

   B. At room temperature on Sabouraud dextrose agar, the organism produces a white or tan mycelium with branching, septate hyphae. Oval or dumbbell-shaped microconidia are borne on the sides of hyphae or on tips of short lateral branches.

II. The dimorphism of the fungus, environmental factors, and the host's immune response are involved in the pathogenesis of blastomycosis.

   A. Although *B. dermatitidis* has been recovered only rarely from the soil or environment, growth of the saprophytic phase in decaying organic matter, with subsequent release of conidia, is believed to represent the major source of infection.

   B. The lung is the initial focus of infection. Inhaled conidia lodge within alveoli, convert to the yeast phase, and produce an inflammatory response. The initial pulmonary infection may then be limited or eliminated by the animal's immune response, with minimal evidence of clinical disease.

   C. The development of systemic disease depends upon the cell-mediated immune response of the host. Inadequate cellular immunity allows dissemination of the organism via lymphatics or bloodstream and the establishment of infection at metastatic sites. The organism incites an inflammatory response that can be suppurative, pyogranulomatous, or granulomatous.

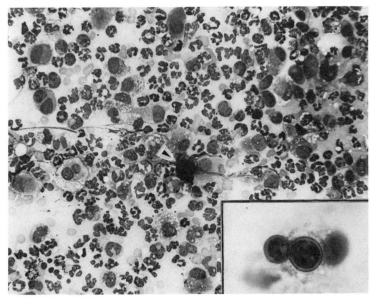

Fig. 34-1. *Blastomyces dermatitidis.* Smear of a lymph node aspirate, showing the inflammatory reaction (neutrophils, macrophages) and a single organism (arrow). (Wright's stain, × 250.) *Inset*: Enlargement of a thick-walled yeast cell, with a typical broad-based bud.

    D. The incubation period may be as long as 3 months in dogs and may be even longer if the initial respiratory signs are inapparent.

    E. Although the lung is the most frequent portal of entry, primary cutaneous infection can occur following skin trauma and inoculation.

    F. In usual situations blastomycosis is not contagious from animal to animal or from animal to human.

III. The occurrence of blastomycosis is affected by several factors.

    A. The disease is seen primarily in dogs. Approximately two-thirds of the cases occur in males of the larger breeds, with an age range of 2–5 years. Blastomycosis occurs rarely in cats; most cases have been reported in the Siamese breed.

    B. Occurrence of clinical cases is most frequent during June through September.

C. In North America blastomycosis is endemic in the regions bordering the Great Lakes and the Mississippi, Ohio, Missouri, and St. Lawrence river systems. Therefore the disease is encountered most frequently in the midwestern, middle Atlantic, and southeastern states, and along the southern borders of Manitoba, Ontario, and Quebec.

CLINICAL SIGNS

I. Blastomycosis begins as a pulmonary infection but usually spreads to other organs.
   A. Extrapulmonary sites frequently affected include hilar and peripheral lymph nodes (59%), eyes (41%), skin (26%), and bone (24%).
   B. Tissues affected less frequently (< 15%) include the subcutis, testes, prostate, central nervous system (CNS), and nasal cavity.
II. Presenting complaints and clinical signs vary with the scope and severity of organ involvement. The following is a composite of the clinical abnormalities.
   A. General symptoms are: gradual weight loss with emaciation in advanced cases; fever of 39.4°–40.7°C; depression.
   B. Respiratory signs are: cough, dyspnea, exercise intolerance, harsh bronchial sounds; regurgitation and vomiting due to esophogeal compression by enlarged hilar lymph nodes.
   C. Cutaneous: ulcerated skin lesion exuding a serosanguineous fluid
   D. Lymphatic: regional or generalized enlargement of peripheral lymph nodes, which may abscess and drain externally
   E. Ocular signs observed include epiphora, pain, swelling, corneal edema, uveitis, and iridocyclitis and, in advanced cases, panophthalmitis, secondary glaucoma, exophthalmos, and blindness.
   F. Lameness
III. Dogs or cats may be presented with apparent primary ocular or cutaneous blastomycosis without respiratory involvement. Traumatic inoculation represents a possible route of infection, but ocular and cutaneous lesions should be considered metastatic infections from the lungs until proved otherwise.
IV. The spectrum of clinical signs seen in cats is similar to that seen in humans and dogs. The pulmonary system is involved most frequently, but cases have been reported with cutaneous lesions, panophthalmitis, and involvement of the CNS.

DIAGNOSIS

I. History
   A. There usually is a history of having lived in or visited a geographic region in which blastomycosis is enzootic.
   B. Blastomycosis occurs most frequently in large-breed, male dogs 2–5 years of age.
   C. Frequent signs in affected animals include cough, fever, lymphadenopathy, and ulcerative skin lesions that persist and fail to respond to antibiotic therapy. A worsening of these conditions with corticosteroid or immunosuppressive drug therapy may be part of the history.

II. Radiographic findings
   A. The most common radiographic sign of blastomycosis is a diffuse, miliary or nodular interstitial lung pattern. The nodules have indefinite margins; some may coalesce to form patchy areas of consolidation.
      1. Enlargement of the hilar lymph nodes is a characteristic finding.
      2. Unlike the finding in histoplasmosis, mineralization of the lung lesions is not observed radiographically.
   B. Because skeletal lesions of blastomycosis tend to localize at the ends of tubular bone, they can easily be confused with primary bone neoplasms. The lesions are predominantly osteolytic, with reactive bone proliferation, a pronounced periosteal reaction, and an increased density of the adjacent soft tissue.

III. Clinical pathology
   A. Laboratory findings are consistent with changes induced by any chronic inflammatory disease.
      1. Frequent hematologic findings include a mild to moderate neutrophilic leukocytosis with a left shift, lymphopenia, monocytosis, and a mild nonregenerative anemia.
      2. Serum chemistries generally are unremarkable. Abnormalities such as hypoalbuminemia, hyperglobulinemia, decreased A/G ratio, decreased basal levels of T_3 and T_4, and hypercalemia have been reported but are not specific for blastomycosis.
   B. Direct microscopic visualization of the organism is the least expensive, most rapid, and most desirable method of obtaining a definitive diagnosis.
      1. Organisms usually are plentiful in affected tissue and can be identified in the following:

a) Impression smears of skin lesions, biopsy tissues, or excised lymph nodes
b) Needle aspirates of affected lymph nodes, skin lesions, lung lobes, or other tissues
c) Paracentesis fluid from the anterior or posterior chamber of the eye (organisms are found more frequently in the posterior chamber)
d) Sediments of tracheal washings or urine

2. Exudates are grayish yellow and viscid. Cytologic examination of infected tissues reveals pyogranulomatous inflammation with a mixture of neutrophils and macrophages and fewer numbers of lymphocytes, giant cells, and plasma cells (Fig. 34-1).
   a) Recognition of this pattern of inflammation necessitates a careful search for fungi, in repeated samplings if necessary.
   b) In addition to *Blastomyces, Histoplasma* and *Coccidioides* should be considered.

3. The yeast form of *Blastomyces* can be seen microscopically with or without staining.
   a) On air-dried smears the organisms can be seen with new methylene blue or Wright's stain.
   b) Without stain, a drop of exudate or a tissue fragment can be crushed between a slide and coverslip and examined under reduced light. Thick specimens may need to be cleared with a few drops of 10% potassium hydroxide.
   c) Yeast cells are as large as or slightly larger than the surrounding neutrophils; they may be free or phagocytized by macrophages or giant cells. The organisms are round to oval, with thick, refractile cell walls and singular, broad-based buds (Fig. 34-1).
   d) Unlike *Cryptococcus, Blastomyces* does not have a thick mucinous capsule.

IV. Special techniques
   A. Histologic examination of biopsy specimens or tissues from dead animals sometimes requires the use of stains such as periodic acid–Schiff (PAS), Gridley's, or Grocott's because the yeast forms can be difficult to see with hematoxylin and eosin.
   B. Serologic tests, which measure antibodies to *Blastomyces*, can be useful when clinical and radiographic findings strongly suggest blastomycosis but cytologic detection of the organism is not possible.
      1. Limitations of serologic tests include:

a) False positive reactions may result from past exposure, and false negative reactions may result from the host's inability to mount an antibody response. The latter situation often occurs in the terminal stages of the disease, when the animal's immune system is suppressed.

b) Cross-reactions between *Histoplasma* and *Blastomyces* are seen with some tests. Therefore simultaneous titers must be evaluated and the higher titer considered the more significant.

2. A rising titer in paired serum samples collected 2 weeks apart can indicate an active infection. Values for what constitutes a positive titer should be obtained from the laboratory performing the test.

3. Of the serologic tests available, counterimmunoelectrophoresis and agar gel immunodiffusion are currently considered the most reliable. Both are highly sensitive and specific; cross-reactions with *Histoplasma* or other fungi are rare. Counterimmunoelectrophoresis is the slightly more sensitive test and may be superior for early detection of disease.

C. Cultures of exudates or tissue samples are utilized when the organism cannot be seen cytologically or histologically. To confirm the diagnosis the organism should be grown in both the mycelial and the yeast phase.

1. The mycelial form grows well on Sabouraud dextrose agar at 30°C or at room temperature.

2. The yeast form grows on blood agar or yeast extract agar at 37°C.

3. Isolation by culture requires 10–14 days, but plates should be incubated for 6 weeks before a culture is considered negative. Treatment should not be delayed pending culture results if the organism has been identified by fine-needle aspiration or tissue biopsy.

V. Differential diagnosis

A. Blastomycosis must be differentiated from other granulomatous diseases such as cryptococcosis, coccidioidomycosis, and histoplasmosis in the dog and feline infectious peritonitis, toxoplasmosis, and cryptococcosis in the cat.

B. In addition bacterial, viral, or neoplastic diseases associated with pneumonia, ulcerative skin lesions, uveitis, lymphadenopathy, or skeletal lesions must be considered.

TREATMENT

I. Amphotericin B (Fungizone, Squibb) and ketoconazole (Nizoral, Janssen Pharmaceutica) have both been used for the treatment of blastomycosis.

   A. Amphotericin B is a polyene antibiotic, which binds to the fungal cell membrane and thereby causes leakage of cellular constituents and death of the fungus. It is poorly absorbed from the gut and does not penetrate the eye or CNS.

   B. Ketoconazole is a fungistatic imidazole, which inhibits the synthesis of fungal membrane lipids. The clinical response to ketoconazole is slower than that for amphotericin B because its activity depends on fungal growth rather than on direct killing. Ketoconazole is absorbed from the gut, especially from an acid environment.

II. Numerous dosage schedules using these drugs either singly or in combination have been described. A treatment regimen consisting of amphotericin B and ketoconazole given sequentially is used frequently.

   A. In dogs amphotericin B 0.5 mg/kg is given IV three times a week until a total dose of 4–6 mg/kg has been achieved. Once amphotericin therapy is complete, ketoconazole is given orally, 10–20 mg/kg once daily or divided bid, for 2–3 months. With neurologic, cutaneous, or ocular involvement, ketoconazole dosages of 30–40 mg/kg/day are necessary.

   B. In cats an initial dose of 0.1 mg/kg IV amphotericin B given three times a week is gradually increased to 0.5 mg/kg until a total dose of 4 mg/kg has been given. Ketoconazole is then given orally, 10 mg/kg once daily or divided bid, for 2–3 months. Some cats react adversely to ketoconazole and require alternate-day therapy at 20 mg/kg, given as a single or divided dose.

III. Amphotericin B in solution can be unstable and is a tissue irritant. The drug should be diluted in sterile water. Dilutions should not be made in electrolyte or acidic fluids or in solutions with preservatives because precipitation of the drug will occur.

   A. Amphotericin B is available in a 50-mg vial, the contents of which should be diluted in 10 ml of sterile water and mixed well. This concentrated solution can be stored for 24 hours at room temperature or at refrigerator temperatures for 1 week.

   B. The daily dose should be freshly diluted in 60–120 ml of 5 percent dextrose in water and given as a slow IV injection over a period of about 5 minutes. Solutions prepared for IV administration should be used promptly.

    C. Alternatively, the daily dose can be added to 500 ml of 5% dextrose in water and given as an IV infusion over 3–4 hours.

IV. Manifestations of adverse reactions or toxicity to these drugs include the following effects:

    A. Amphotericin B may cause shivering, vomiting, fever, diarrhea, cylindruria, phlebitis, hypokalemia, isosthenuria, and azotemia, and, as long-term effects, nonregenerative anemia and weight loss.

    B. Ketoconazole affects dogs and cats somewhat differently.

        1. In dogs anorexia, vomiting, pruritis, alopecia, reversible lightening of the haircoat, and reversible elevation of liver enzymes may occur.

        2. In cats the possible effects are anorexia, fever, depression, and diarrhea.

        3. Embryotoxicity and teratogenicity may occur in both species.

    C. Adverse reactions caused by amphotericin B are more severe and common. Nephrotoxicity, as evidenced by azotemia and isosthenuria, is the most significant complication.

        1. Blood urea nitrogen (BUN) and/or creatinine should be determined prior to each injection of amphotericin B; BUN values of 50–60 mg/dl or creatinine values higher than 3.0 mg/dl require interruption of treatment. Elevated values usually subside within a few days, after which therapy can be continued. Reducing the dosage or increasing the interval between infusions may be necessary to prevent recurrence.

        2. Isosthenuria usually abates 4–6 weeks after treatment ceases.

        3. Dogs with preexisting renal disease may tolerate amphotericin if it is administered along with 1 g/kg of mannitol (20% solution).

V. Treatment is continued until there is clinical improvement, failure to isolate or identify the organism, or resolution of radiographic signs in the lungs. Repeated serologic tests are not useful in monitoring the response to treatment.

    A. A decrease in antibody titer can occur while infection persists. Alternatively, clinical recovery can occur without a decrease in titer to normal limits.

    B. Interpretation of antibody titers in treated animals is further complicated by the frequent occurrence of normal or slightly increased titers in dogs with fulminant blastomycosis.

VI. Several factors influence the prognosis.

    A. Retrospective studies suggest that a poor prognosis should be given in clinical cases with one or more of the following characteristics:

1. Severe radiographic lung lesions
2. Nonsegmented neutrophil counts greater than 2,500/μl
3. Involvement of the CNS
3. Male gender

B. In animals with ocular involvement the prognosis for restoring eyesight is poor. Enucleation often is indicated.

PUBLIC HEALTH CONSIDERATIONS

Zoonotic transmission of blastomycosis from dog to human has not been reported; rather, a common environmental source of infection should be suspected when dogs and humans in the same household are affected.

I. Humans bitten by infected dogs have developed cutaneous blastomycosis.

II. Veterinarians should not take undue risks when handling exudates or ulcerated skin lesions because infection resulting from accidental inoculation has been reported.

III. Laboratory personnel should be especially careful while handling and examining cultures of the mycelial phase because conidia are infectious and may become airborne.

IV. The geographic distribution of canine blastomycosis is similar to that of the human disease. Because dogs have a 10-fold higher infection rate than humans, canine blastomycosis serves as an epidemiologic marker for the human disease.

SUGGESTED READINGS

Attleberger MH: Systemic mycoses. p. 1180. In Kirk RW (ed): Current Veterinary Therapy. Vol. 8. Small Animal Practice. WB Saunders, Philadelphia, 1983

Barsanti JA: Blastomycosis. p. 675. In Greene CE (ed): Clinical Microbiology and Infectious Diseases of the Dog and Cat. WB Saunders, Philadelphia, 1984

Barta O, Hubbert NL, Pier AC, Pourciau SS: Counterimmunoelectrophoresis (immunoelectroosmosis) and serum electrophoretic pattern in serologic diagnosis of canine blastomycosis. Am J Vet Res 44:218, 1983

Dunbar M, Pyle RL, Boring JG, McCoy CP: Treatment of canine blastomycosis with ketoconazole. J Am Vet Med Assoc 182:156, 1983

Legendre AM, Becker PU: Evaluation of the agar-gel immunodiffusion test in the diagnosis of canine blastomycosis. Am J Vet Res 41:2109, 1980

Legendre AM, Becker PU: Immunologic changes in acute canine blastomycosis. Am J Vet Res 43:2050, 1982

Legendre AM, Selcer BA, Edwards DF, Stevens R: Treatment of canine blastomycosis with amphotericin B and ketoconazole. J Am Vet Med Assoc 184:1249, 1984

Legendre AM, Walker M, Buyukmihci N, Stevens R: Canine blastomycosis: a review of 47 clinical cases. J Am Vet Med Assoc 178:1163, 1981

Moriello KA: Ketoconazole: clinical pharmacology and therapeutic recommendations. J Am Vet Med Assoc 188:303, 1986

Pyle RL, Dunbar M, Nelson PD, et al: Canine blastomycosis. Compend Cont Ed Pract Vet 3:963, 1981

Roudebush P: Mycotic pneumonias. Vet Clin North Am [Small Anim Pract] 15:949, 1985

Walker MA: Thoracic blastomycosis: a review of its radiographic manifestations in 40 dogs. Vet Radiol 22:22, 1981

35

Coccidioidomycosis

Alice M. Wolf

ETIOLOGY

I. The etiologic agent is *Coccidioides immitis*.
II. This fungus has a dimorphic life cycle.
   A. The mycelial phase is free-living in the soil of endemic areas. This form produces arthroconidia, which represent the infective phase of the organism.
   B. Once inside the mammalian host, the organism is transformed into the spherular phase, which proliferates and may disseminate to cause clinical disease.
III. The disease is usually contracted by inhalation of infective arthroconidia from the environment. A few cases have resulted from direct inoculation of arthroconidia through the skin.
IV. As in humans, many *C. immitis* infections in animals are probably subclinical. This makes determination of the true incidence of infection difficult. Cats rarely develop clinical coccidioidomycosis; dogs, however, may develop severe disease. Males are apparently more susceptible than females, and boxers and Doberman pinschers reportedly are more likely to develop severe disseminated disease. Young dogs (less than 4 years of age) are affected more frequently than older animals.
V. The environmental distribution of *Coccidioides immitis* is restricted to the lower Sonoran life zone. This area includes parts of California, Nevada, Utah, Arizona, New Mexico, and Texas. The organism is also widespread in Mexico and in Central and South America. Obtaining a detailed travel history is very important because the clinical signs of coccidioidomycosis may not appear for weeks to years following exposure to the organism.

VI. The mycelial phase of *C. immitis* can be inactivated with 3% formalin solution. The spherular phase of the organism is much more sensitive and can be destroyed by most commonly used disinfectants.

CLINICAL SIGNS

I. Primary pulmonary coccidioidomycosis
   A. This is the acute, pulmonary phase of the disease, which usually occurs 1–3 weeks following infection.
   B. Clinical signs may be absent or may include:
      1. Mild, nonproductive cough
      2. Fever
      3. Partial anorexia
      4. Weight loss
II. Disseminated pulmonary coccidioidomycosis
   A. If the immune system is not able to confine the organisms locally, the infection will generalize throughout the pulmonary tree and the intrathoracic lymphatic system.
   B. Clinical signs will be more severe and will include:
      1. Severe cough, which may be productive
      2. Dyspnea (usually only in the terminal stages)
      3. Fever
         a) Fluctuating or persistent
         b) Unresponsive to antibiotic treatment
      4. Depression and/or weakness
      5. Anorexia
      6. Weight loss
      7. Pleural effusion
III. Disseminated coccidioidomycosis
   A. Organisms may spread beyond the pulmonary system to affect any organ or system in the body.
   B. Dissemination may occur very early in the course of the disease. Although the respiratory tract is the original portal of entry for the fungus, clinical signs of respiratory infection may not be observed prior to the development of other organ system involvement.
   C. Bone is a common site for dissemination of *C. immitis*. Most coccidioidomycosis lesions occur in the long bones; the vertebrae and flat bones are less frequently affected. Patients with advanced disease frequently have multiple bone involvement. Intra-articular infection is rare.

      1. Clinical signs associated with coccidioidal osteomyelitis include:
        a) Lameness
        b) Soft tissue swelling and pain over affected bones
        c) Regional lymphadenopathy
        d) Superficial draining tracts over affected bones
        e) Fever (variably present)
      2. Coccidioidal osteomyelitis of the vertebrae may cause paresis or paralysis.
   D. Other, less common sites for *C. immitis* dissemination and associated clinical signs include:
      1. Heart
        a) Pericardial effusion, granulomatous/constrictive pericarditis, myocarditis
        b) Signs that include congestive heart failure (usually right-sided), cardiac arrhythmias, ascites
      2. Skin: draining cutaneous abscesses and tracts
      3. Eye: granulomatous retinitis, uveitis, and keratitis.
      4. Lymphatic system: peripheral lymphadenopathy
      5. Reproductive tract: epididymitis and orchitis
      6. Central nervous system: granulomatous encephalitis and meningitis, ataxia, seizures, and coma.
      7. Gastrointestinal system and liver: chronic diarrhea, vomiting, and icterus
      8. Kidney: uremia
IV. Primary cutaneous coccidioidomycosis
   A. This is an extremely rare disorder.
   B. Direct inoculation of arthroconidia into the skin results in a self-limiting regional lymphadenitis and lymphangitis.
   C. This form of coccidioidomycosis must be differentiated from cutaneous lesions associated with osseous or cutaneous dissemination. Patients with primary cutaneous coccidioidomycosis will not have radiographic evidence of bone involvement and will not have serologic titers compatible with disseminated disease.

DIAGNOSIS

I. Hematology
   A. Hematologic parameters may be normal or may show nonspecific changes.

  B. Hematologic abnormalities associated with coccidioidomycosis depend on the chronicity and severity of the disease. They may include:
   1. Mild, nonregenerative anemia
   2. Neutrophilic leukocytosis, usually mild to moderate sometimes with a left shift
   3. Increased erythrocyte sedimentation rate
 II. Serum biochemistry
  A. Hypoalbuminemia and hyperglobulinemia are the most consistent changes and are usually associated with chronic disease.
  B. Other abnormalities may reflect other organ system involvement.
 III. Radiography
  A. Pulmonary coccidioidomycosis
   1. Pulmonary parenchymal changes associated with coccidioidomycosis are quite variable. Interstitial and mixed interstitial and bronchovascular patterns occur most commonly. These changes may have a diffuse or miliary and/or nodular distribution. Alveolar involvement is unusual.
   2. Hilar lymphadenopathy is a prominent feature of pulmonary coccidioidomycosis.
   3. Sternal and mediastinal lymphadenopathy are uncommon and are suggestive of dissemination.
  B. Osseous coccidioidomycosis
   1. Bone lesions may be productive or destructive or may show evidence of both types of osseous change. The infection may involve the endosteal, cortical, and/or periosteal portions of the bone.
   2. There is no radiographic pattern of osseous change that is pathognomonic for coccidioidomycosis. Major differential diagnoses include other forms of osteomyelitis and osseous neoplasia.
  C. Other
   1. Pericardial or myocardial involvement is rare. Radiographic findings may include enlargement of the cardiac silhouette and/or evidence of congestive heart failure.
   2. Other radiographic examinations may reveal lymphadenopathy or organomegaly in cases of disseminated disease.
 IV. Histopathology
  A. General
   1. Regardless of the collection procedure, it may be difficult to recover *C. immitis* spherules. There are usually few organisms in affected tissues.

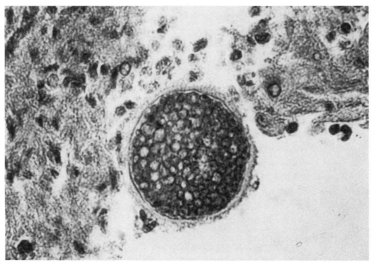

Fig. 35-1. *Coccidioides immitis.* A single large spherule containing numerous endospores is shown within a lymph node section. (Periodic acid–Schiff, × 480.) (Courtesy L. Ajello, Centers for Disease Control.)

    2. Recommended examination procedures and staining techniques include:
        a) Direct wet-mount examination is usually performed on aspirates or wash specimens with 10% potassium hydroxide. Organisms appear as refractile, double-walled spherules containing endospores (Fig. 35-1).
        b) Routine hematologic stains can also be used for aspirates and washes. Spherules are large and stain blue with a surrounding unstained capsule.
    3. Hematoxylin and eosin is used routinely and is generally satisfactory for examining biopsy specimens.
    4. Special stains for fungi include methenamine silver and periodic acid–Schiff (PAS). The use of these stains may improve detection when few fungal organisms are present.
  B. Exfoliative cytology
    1. Transtracheal and/or bronchial wash specimens may reveal evidence of granulomatous inflammation, but organisms usually are absent.

2. Fine-needle aspirates of the lung may be more likely to yield organisms, particularly if directed by radiographic localization of lung pathology.
3. Direct smears of exudates from draining cutaneous lesions frequently contain spherules of *C. immitis*.
4. Lymph node aspirates may be useful if regional or generalized lymphadenopathy is present.

C. Biopsy
1. Biopsy procedures *do not* appear to encourage spread of the fungal organisms.
2. Lung biopsy is occasionally needed to establish a diagnosis of coccidioidomycosis. Other tissues may be biopsied as indicated by clinical and laboratory findings.
3. It may be difficult to locate fungal organisms in bone biopsy specimens. Samples should be taken from several sites to improve diagnostic accuracy.

V. Fungal culture
A. *C. immitis* returns to the mycelial form and grows well on blood agar or fungal culture media incubated at room temperature. Colonies usually appear by the third day after inoculation and are cottony and white.
B. Because these fungal colonies are producing infectious arthroconidia, attempts to culture this organism in a routine practice setting are *not recommended*.

VI. Coccidioidomycosis serology
A. Tube precipitin test
1. The tube precipitin (TP) test detects the IgM antibody response, which develops early in the course of infection.
2. Antibodies to IgM are usually present within 2–4 weeks following *C. immitis* infection but wane rapidly, even if the disease becomes chronic.
3. A negative TP test may mean that there has been no infection or that the infection is early. Patients with chronic infections or fulminating and rapidly progressive acute infections may also test negative for precipitin antibodies. This test is usually negative in cases of primary cutaneous coccidioidomycosis.

B. Immunodiffusion test and complement fixation test
1. Complement-fixing (CF) antibodies of the IgG class develop more slowly following infection. The CF antibody titer increases with the severity and chronicity of the disease, which makes it a useful tool for assessing possible dissemination and for monitoring the response to treatment.

2. The agar-gel immunodiffusion (ID) test is usually used as a qualitative screening test for CF antibodies. If the ID test is positive, a quantitative CF test is performed.

3. Low CF titers (less than 1:16) may be found early in the course of acute disease or in a chronic, localized infection, or they may persist after the resolution of active disease.

4. Titers of CF antibodies above 1:16 to 1:32 are indicative of active, disseminated disease.

5. Patients with primary cutaneous disease should *not* develop CF antibodies.

6. Dog serum may have nonspecific anticomplementary activity, which can confuse interpretation of CF test results. This test should be performed only by a laboratory that is experienced in analyzing canine sera and that performs control studies to check for anticomplementary activity.

VII. Diagnosis summary

A. The diagnosis of coccidioidomycosis is usually based on a history of exposure to an endemic area, clinical signs, radiographic findings, and serologic data.

B. Routine hematologic and biochemical parameters may be normal or reveal nonspecific changes.

C. Biopsy and histopathologic examination may be required to confirm the diagnosis in some patients.

TREATMENT

I. Because of the danger of dissemination, systemic antifungal chemotherapy is recommended for all forms of coccidioidomycosis except primary cutaneous disease. Combined treatment with amphotericin B and ketoconazole appears to be the most efficacious regimen at this time.

II. Amphotericin B

A. This drug (Fungizone, Squibb) is fungistatic and has a rapid onset of action. Drawbacks include the necessity for IV administration and nephrotoxicity.

B. The recommended dosage is 0.25–1.0 mg/kg IV, two to three times a week until a total cumulative dose of 5–10 mg/kg has been achieved.

C. The drug is administered by adding the calculated daily dose to a suitable volume of 5% dextrose (500–1,000 ml) and giving it slowly IV over several hours.

    D. Adverse effects
       1. Nephrotoxicity
         a) This is a "normal" consequence of the use of amphotericin B. This drug should be used with caution in patients with preexisting renal insufficiency.
         b) The patient's blood urea nitrogen (BUN) levels must be monitored closely. If the BUN is below 40 mg/dl, treatment may continue; at 40–60 mg/dl, the veterinarian should watch for impending renal insufficiency; above 60 mg/dl amphotericin B should be discontinued and renal disease treated as necessary.
         c) The addition of 2.5% mannitol to the amphotericin B infusion will reduce the nephrotoxic effects of the drug.
         d) Experimental studies have shown that saline loading will also protect against amphotericin B nephrotoxicity, but no clinical trials using this technique have been reported.
       2. Thrombophlebitis
         a) This can be a significant problem owing to the irritative effects of the drug and the small size of the patients.
         b) Carefully placed IV catheters should be used and veins alternated frequently. If thrombophlebitis occurs, 25 mg prednisolone sodium succinate (Solu-Delta-Cortef, Upjohn) may be added to the infusion solution to decrease its inflammatory effects.
       3. Other adverse effects (fever, chills, anaphylaxis) have rarely been reported in animals.

III. Ketoconazole
    A. This drug (Nizoral, Janssen Pharmaceutica) is fungistatic at therapeutic dose levels and has a slow onset of action. The use of ketoconazole as a single agent has resulted in good rates of remission; however, some patients have relapsed when ketoconazole treatment was discontinued.
    B. Recommended dosage is 10 mg/kg PO bid. Treatment with this drug may be initiated concurrently with amphotericin B and should continue for at least 2 months following resolution of clinical disease in early cases and for 6–12 months in patients with disseminated disease. Radiographic and serologic studies should be performed to monitor the patient's progress. Some patients may require lifetime antifungal therapy. It may be possible to reduce the ketoconazole dosage to 5–10 mg/kg PO once daily and maintain remission in these chronic cases.
    C. Adverse effects

1. Inappetence and gastrointestinal disturbances are common effects of ketoconazole therapy. If these effects occur, administration should be discontinued for several days, and then reinstituted at 10 mg/kg once daily for 10–14 days. The dosage frequency can then usually be increased to bid without a recurrence of these problems.
2. Reported cutaneous effects include pruritus, alopecia, and lightening of the hair coat. These changes are reversible when drug therapy is discontinued.
3. Hepatic effects include transient elevations of liver enzyme values. These usually do not result in clinical signs severe enough to require termination of therapy.
4. Ketoconazole is teratogenic and embryotoxic. This drug *should not* be administered to pregnant animals.

IV. Itraconazole
   A. This is a second-generation imidazole in the same family as ketoconazole.
   B. Currently under investigational new drug status, it appears to have good efficacy against *C. immitis* and shows promise for the treatment of canine coccidioidomycosis.

PREVENTION

I. Experimental vaccines have been developed for use in humans and nonhuman primates. No products are available for companion animals.
II. It is not known whether companion animals develop solid, protective immunity following recovery from *C. immitis* infection or whether they are susceptible to reinfection if they remain in enzootic areas.
III. There is no practical way to protect animals residing in or passing through enzootic areas from exposure to *C. immitis*.

PUBLIC HEALTH CONSIDERATIONS

I. There is no known risk of direct transmission of coccidioidomycosis from animals to humans. However, humans residing in enzootic areas are likely to have the same risk of environmental exposure to infection as their pets.

II. Caution should be used in the care of animals with draining cutaneous wounds. Dressings should be changed frequently because fungal organisms present in the exudate may revert to the mycelial phase and produce infectious arthroconidia on the surface of the bandages.

III. If typical *C. immitis* fungal colonies are seen in culture, the plate or tube should be sealed tightly and disposed of as soon as possible. *Handling mycelial cultures is extremely dangerous.*

SUGGESTED READINGS

Armstrong PJ, DiBartola SP: Canine coccidioidomycosis: a literature review and report of eight cases. J Am Anim Hosp Assoc 19:937, 1983

Barsanti JA, Jeffery KL: Coccidioidomycosis. p. 710. In Greene CE (ed): Clinical Microbiology and Infectious Diseases of the Dog and Cat. WB Saunders, Philadelphia, 1984

Jackson JA, Mauldin RA, Bauman DS, George TJ: Treatment of canine coccidioidomycosis with ketoconazole: serological aspects of a case study. J Am Anim Hosp Assoc 21:572, 1985

Macy DW, Small E: Deep mycotic infections. p. 237. In Ettinger SJ (ed): Textbook of Veterinary Internal Medicine: Diseases of the Dog and Cat. 2nd Ed. WB Saunders, Philadelphia, 1983

Moriello KA: Ketoconazole: clinical pharmacology and therapeutic recommendations. J Am Vet Med Assoc 188:303, 1986

36

Cryptococcosis
George T. Wilkinson

ETIOLOGY

I. *Cryptococcus neoformans*, the causative organism of cryptococcosis, is a saprophytic, yeastlike fungus, which is widely distributed in the environment. The yeast is round in shape, is 4–6 μm in diameter, and in the tissues of an infected animal is surrounded by a wide polysaccharide capsule. This capsule constitutes a valuable diagnostic feature of the organism which can be seen in smears of exudate, in fine-needle aspirates, etc. Reproduction is by the formation of blastoconidia or buds, which can be distinguished from those of *Blastomyces* by their "pinched-off" or narrow-necked appearance. The most common and prolific source of the yeast in the environment is the excreta of pigeons and other birds. Clinical avian infection is rare, probably because of the protective effect of the bird's high body temperature, and their role in the epizootiology of cryptococcosis is probably a fortuitous one. The organism has also been isolated from a variety of other sources, including the oropharynx, gastrointestinal tract, and skin of healthy humans; soil; fruit juice, milk, and butter; grass; and several species of insects.

II. Humans and animals are thought to contract the infection from sources in the environment, but the conditions underlying the establishment of such infections are only poorly understood. Although the organism is ubiquitous and persistent in nature, cryptococcosis is relatively rare in both animals and humans. Infection is thought to occur only in animals whose cell-mediated immunity, the body's main line of defense against fungal infection, has been compromised by malnutrition, debility, intercurrent disease, immune deficiency, or immunosuppression. In cats the most frequently reported of such conditions is intercurrent infection with the feline leukemia virus. However in a considerable number of the 25 canine cases recorded in the literature, a similar predisposing factor has not been identified. It has been shown that experimental infection of cats with the organism is facilitated by debility or by the prior administration of corticosteroids.

III. Although the organism probably has a worldwide distribution—small animal infections having been reported from the United States, Australia, Japan, the United Kingdom, New Zealand, Canada, Papua New Guinea, France, Austria, Italy, South Africa, and Uruguay— it would seem that climatic factors have an important influence on the incidence of the disease. Like most fungal infections, cryptococcosis is more common and more florid in its clinical manifestations in tropical and subtropical regions with warm, humid climates.

IV. In the dog there is a tendency for the large breeds to be affected. It has been suggested that this may be due to the less sheltered existence generally enjoyed by these breeds, consequently with greater exposure to the organism in the environment.

V. The route of infection is not known, although it is thought to be via the respiratory tract following inhalation. In the dog, as in humans, the main portal of entry is believed to be in the lungs, despite the fact that pulmonary lesions are uncommon in both dogs and cats. It has been postulated that in many cases of human cryptococcosis the pulmonary infection is transitory and heals without any recognizable residual lesion. This could also be true of feline and canine infections. In the cat the primary site is most often found in the nasal passages, probably owing to the arrest of inhaled organisms in the turbinates. From these sites the organisms may be widely disseminated throughout the body via hematogenous or lymphogenous spread. However there is a decided predilection in cryptococcosis for the central nervous system (CNS), including the eyes, for the lymph nodes, and for the skin, the latter site being more frequently affected in the cat. Infection of the underlying bone following contamination of traumatized skin wounds has been reported in the dog.

VI. Transmission of the infection from animal to animal or from animal to human has not been reported, although it is relatively easy to infect laboratory animals by the injection of infective material or cultures of the organism.

VII. In view of the ubiquitous nature of the organism in the environment and the special requirements for infection to become established, disinfection procedures are not relevant.

CLINICAL SIGNS

I. In the dog the presence of the organism invokes a marked cellular reaction in the form of granulomatous inflammation. In the cat there is usually a relative lack of host tissue response except where secondary bacterial infection has occurred (e.g., in an ulcerated skin lesion). This lack of host response is seen most frequently in the CNS, where lesions may appear as large cystic masses containing cryptococcal organisms in virtually pure culture. These lesions produce their clinical effects by pressure necrosis of surrounding tissues, caused by the rapidly expanding mass of organisms.

II. The clinical signs can be divided into four main syndromes, combinations of which may be seen in the same animal.

A. *Respiratory syndrome.*

This constitutes the most common form of cryptococcosis in the cat, in which the clinical signs reflect infection of the nasal passages and sometimes of the frontal sinuses. Hence there are sneezing and snuffling, often associated with the presence of a chronic unilateral or bilateral mucopurulent, watery, or hemorrhagic nasal discharge. Small masses of granulation tissue may be evident at the entrance to one or both nostrils; on rare occasions these may occlude the nostrils and lead to mouth breathing. A common feature is the development of a firm, sometimes hard, almost bonelike swelling over the bridge of the nose, which imparts a rather "Roman nose" appearance to the cat's profile. Ulceration of the skin overlying the swelling may occur. The regional lymph nodes are usually enlarged, firm, and painless to palpation, and may be nodular. Coughing and other signs of lower respiratory tract involvement are rare in the cat but may occur in the dog.

B. *Neurologic syndrome.*

This constitutes the most frequent clinical manifestation of canine cryptococcosis and is also commonly seen in the cat. The clinical signs reflect involvement of the meninges, brain, and spinal cord in the disease process; thus signs that often occur, depending on the location of the lesions within the CNS, include disorientation, depression, neck pain/stiffness, circling, balancing difficulties, head pressing, anisocoria, pupillary dilation, blindness, deafness, loss of the sense of smell, ataxia and posterior paresis, paraplegia, and paralysis.

C. *Ocular syndrome.*

Cryptococcal infection of the eye usually manifests itself as anterior uveitis, posterior uveitis (chorioretinitis), and optic neuritis. Thus there may be photophobia, blepharospasm, corneal clouding, inflammatory edema of the iris with dullness of its surface (sometimes resulting in a change of eye color), haziness, hyphema and fibrin deposition in the anterior chamber, and posterior synechia. Examination of the retina may reveal cystic detachments, focal hemorrhages, papilledema, and exudation into the preretinal, retinal, and subretinal areas. There may be pupillary dilation, loss of the pupillary light reflex, and blindness due to optic nerve damage.

D. *Cutaneous syndrome.*

This form of cryptococcosis occurs most frequently in the cat, in which the predilection site is the skin of the head and neck. However, lesions may be distributed over much of the body surface, apparently as a result of hematogenous or lymphogenous dissemination of the organism. The lesions take the form of multiple, fairly rapidly growing, firm to hard, often flattened, painless nodules in the dermis and subcutis, ranging in diameter from 1 mm to 1 cm. The nodules have a tendency to ulcerate, exposing a raw, granular surface, which has a scanty serohemorrhagic exudate and which fails to heal. More rarely, there may be larger, primarily ulcerative lesions or large fungating masses, the latter showing a predilection for the extremities.

E. In most cases of systemic cryptococcosis the animal is in poor condition, and there may be a peripheral lymphadenopathy, particularly with the cutaneous form of the disease. In some canine cases the presenting sign has been lameness in one leg, owing to bone involvement following localized spread of infection from a traumatic skin wound.

DIAGNOSIS

I. Any dog or cat presented in poor bodily condition, with associated signs of upper respiratory infection, multifocal CNS involvement, uveitis/chorioretinitis, lymphadenopathy, or multiple skin nodules, should raise strong suspicions of cryptococcosis. However, the variety of clinical presentations frequently makes diagnosis of the condition difficult. Fortunately, the organisms usually are present in considerable numbers in smears of exudates, ulcerated skin lesions, cerebrospinal fluid (CSF), needle aspirates, etc. and can be detected by microscopic examination or by culture.

II. Smears obtained from lesions and the CSF may be stained as wet preparations by mixing with India ink or can be dried and stained with new methylene blue, Giemsa, or mucicarmine. Examination of such smears usually reveals large numbers of the characteristic budding yeasts surrounded by large, wide capsules, often with little evidence of an inflammatory cell response (Fig. 36-1).

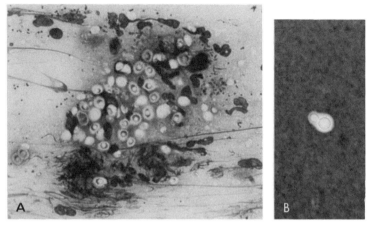

Fig. 36-1. *Cryptococcus neoformans.* (**A**) smear of ulcerated skin lesion from a cat, showing cryptococcal organisms contained primarily in macrophages. (Giemsa stain, × 400.) (**B**) India ink preparation (× 400).

III. In the CSF there is usually also a decrease in glucose concentration and a pleocytosis, frequently involving mononuclear cells but occasionally polymorphs as well.

IV. A latex agglutination test (Crypto-LA Test, International Biological Laboratories) is available. It is unusual among serologic tests in that it determines the amount of cryptococcal polysaccharide capsular antigen present in the serum of the affected animal rather than the antibody titer. Kits suitable for in-office use are available, but because they have a shelf life of only 1 year and contain 40 tests, they are uneconomical for use by most veterinary practitioners. However, most medical pathology laboratories will perform the test, and results obtained with animal sera appear to be comparable with those obtained with human sera. In addition to its use for diagnostic purposes, the latex agglutination test can be used to monitor the effectiveness of therapy because the titer falls as the organisms are eliminated from the body. The test can also be performed on CSF in cases with CNS involvement.

TREATMENT

I. The traditional treatment of cryptococcosis is IV administration of amphotericin B (Fungizone, Squibb). Because this drug is expensive and is also unstable once in solution, the following regime has been recommended for use in cats and can be adapted for canine patients.

A. The agent is supplied in vials containing 50 mg of the active constituent in powder form, to which is added 10 ml of sterile water for injection. The vial is protected from light and shaken gently until a clear solution results. This solution, which now contains 5 mg/ml, is divided into 1.5-ml aliquots, which are placed in individual vials and then stored at $-20°C$ until required. On the Monday of each week of treatment a vial is thawed and 0.5 ml of solution is withdrawn and diluted with 2.0 ml of 5% dextrose in water in a disposable plastic syringe. The dose is 0.3 mg/kg injected IV over a period of 5 seconds three times each week. The remaining 1 ml of amphotericin in the vial is protected from light and stored in a refrigerator (4°C), 0.5 ml being used for the Wednesday treatment and the remainder for the Friday dose. In the case of dogs weighing more than 8 kg the amount of the aliquot in each vial will need to be adjusted. With this regime the agent remains active in solution and there is little or no wastage.

B. Because amphotericin B is nephrotoxic, the blood urea nitrogen (BUN) concentration must be monitored each week. If the level rises above 50 mg per 100 ml (18 mmol/L), treatment should be suspended until the normal concentration is regained. Nephrotoxicity may be reduced by the subcutaneous injection of 100–150 ml of 5% dextrose in water prior to amphotericin administration.

C. Therapy with amphotericin B is prolonged, partly owing to the necessity of suspending treatment when the BUN level rises, and the course of injections may need to be extended to several weeks. The latex agglutination test should be used to monitor progress.

II. 5-Fluorocytosine (Ancobon, Ancotil, Roche) is an antimycotic agent that has been used successfully, both alone and in combination with amphotericin B, in the treatment of cryptococcosis in dogs and cats. It has the advantages that it is administered orally and is not nephrotoxic; however, because it is excreted almost entirely through the kidneys, the dosage must be reduced in patients with impaired renal function. The main disadvantages are that the agent is expensive and that *C. neoformans* soon becomes resistant to it. When it is used in conjunction with amphotericin B, there is a synergistic action and the dose of amphotericin can be reduced, sometimes by half, with a consequent reduction in its nephrotoxic effects. The recommended dosage rate for 5-fluorocytosine is 100 mg/kg divided qid; some authorities suggest that doses of 150–200 mg/kg daily should be used to delay or minimize the development of drug resistance. Signs of toxicity, which are rare in small animals, include oral or cutaneous ulceration, enterocolitis, leukopenia, and thrombocytopenia. The agent is marketed in 500-mg tablets.

III. A new antifungal agent, ketoconazole (Nizoral, Janssen Pharaceutica), has recently proved effective in the treatment of feline and canine cryptococcosis. Like 5-fluorocytosine, the drug is administered orally and is not nephrotoxic. The recommended dose is 10 mg/kg once or twice daily. The primary disadvantages of this agent are high cost (especially when the patient is a large dog) and hepatotoxicity, which has been reported in some cats. The drug is marketed in 200-mg tablets.

IV. Recently the author has successfully employed immunotherapy in some cases of feline cryptococcosis using an ethyl alcohol–killed autogenous *C. neoformans* vaccine, which is given in doses of 0.1 ml injected intradermally every 2 weeks in conjunction with either 5-fluorocytosine or ketoconazole therapy. The method of preparing the vaccine, which could be produced by any microbiological laboratory, is as follows: The organisms are grown on Sabouraud dextrose agar at 37°C for 4–6 days. The culture is then washed off the medium with absolute ethyl alcohol and dried in vacuo at 60°C. The dried fungi are suspended in 0.5% phenol saline to a dilution of 0.1%, and the vaccine tested for sterility.

PREVENTION

I. In view of the variable factors underlying the establishment of clinical cryptococcosis, it is difficult to suggest effective prophylactic measures. Obviously the chief sources of the organism in the environment, pigeons and other birds, should not be kept in close proximity to catteries or dog kennels, and wild birds should be discouraged from roosting near such establishments.

II. Dogs and cats should be maintained on a high plane of nutrition to encourage the development and maintenance of an effective level of immunity. Catteries should be free of feline leukemia virus.

PUBLIC HEALTH CONSIDERATIONS

Although transmission of cryptococcal infection from animal to human has never been reported, the comparative ease with which laboratory animals can be experimentally infected by the injection of infective material or cultures of the organism indicates that it would seem prudent for veterinarians and their nursing staff to take sensible precautions. These might include wearing masks and gloves when handling affected animals, particularly those with discharging or otherwise "open" lesions, and avoiding being scratched or bitten. Owners treating affected pets should be counseled similarly. Personnel in poor health or whose immune status may be questionable should not be allowed to come into contact infected animals.

SUGGESTED READINGS

Barrett RE, Scott DW: Treatment of feline cryptococcosis: literature review and case report. J Am Anim Hosp Assoc 11:511, 1975

Beemer AM, Davidson W, Kuttin ES, et al: Vaccine and mycostatin in treatment of cryptococcosis of the respiratory tract. Sabouraudia 14:171, 1976

Macy DW, Small E: Deep mycotic diseases. p. 237. In Ettinger SJ (ed): Textbook of Veterinary Internal Medicine: Diseases of the Dog and Cat. Vol. 1. 2nd Ed. WB Saunders, Philadelphia, 1983

Sutton RH: Cryptococcosis in dogs: a report on 6 cases. Aust Vet J 57:558, 1981

Wilkinson GT: Feline cryptococcosis: a review and seven case reports. J Small Anim Pract 20:749, 1979

37

Histoplasmosis
David J. Polzin

ETIOLOGY

I. Histoplasmosis is a systemic fungal disease caused by the dimorphic, saprophytic fungus *Histoplasma capsulatum*.
   A. The organism grows as a small, oval budding yeast in animal tissues and on blood agar at 30–37°C. It forms white, moist colonies when grown on blood agar.
   B. The fungus occurs in a mycelial phase in soil and on Sabouraud dextrose agar at room temperature. On Sabouraud agar it appears as a fluffy, white to brown mold. In the environment the organism is found primarily in moist soils with a high nitrogen content, particularly those enriched by decomposing wood or fecal droppings of birds or bats. Birds and bats do not generally serve as the source of the organism; instead, their excrement creates a soil environment that promotes growth of the fungus. *Histoplasma* does not infect birds but can infect bats.
II. *H. capsulatum* occurs in temperate and tropical climates around the world. In the United States histoplasmosis is enzootic in the central Mississippi River valley, in the Ohio River valley, and in areas along the Appalachian Mountains. States with the greatest incidence of histoplasmosis include Arkansas, Illinois, Indiana, Iowa, Kansas, Kentucky, Mississippi, Missouri, Ohio, Oklahoma, Tennessee, and Texas. Exposure to the organism and subclinical infection appear to be common in dogs and cats living in enzootic areas.
III. Infection usually follows inhalation of microconidia produced by the mycelial phase of *H. capsulatum*. Exposure to the organism typically occurs subsequent to aerosolization of spores by wind, digging, or other physical disruption of contaminated soil. The organism can often be cultured from soil at suspected exposure sites.

327

A. After inhalation, microconidia undergo conversion to the yeast phase, presumably in alveolar macrophages. Dissemination occurs when organism-laden macrophages enter lymphatic channels and are transported to the vascular system. Enteric histoplasmosis may result from dissemination from a pulmonary focus.

B. Although the preponderance of data supports the respiratory system as the portal of entry for *Histoplasma*, other routes of transmission have been proposed.

   1. Because some animals develop enteric histoplasmosis in the absence of pulmonary pathology, it has been hypothesized that infection may occur by ingestion of the organism. This route of infection remains unproved, however.

   2. It is unknown whether blood-sucking ectoparasites can transmit the infection; however, the organism has been found in ticks that fed on an infected dog.

IV. Histoplasmosis is usually a benign and self-limiting disease; animals developing clinical signs may have a defect in their immunologic responses.

A. Adequate cell-mediated immunity is essential for the control of mycotic diseases.

B. Concurrent debilitating conditions, such as parasitism, bacterial infection, or inadequate nutrition can adversely affect immune system capabilities and disease prognosis.

CLINICAL SIGNS

I. Clinical signs of histoplasmosis generally relate to the respiratory or gastrointestinal system. The most common signs are chronic cough and/or diarrhea unresponsive to previous therapy. The disease typically occurs in young dogs (those less than 4 years of age), particularly in sporting breeds and in hounds.

II. Respiratory signs can range from a mild cough to pneumonia with coughing and dyspnea.

A. Thoracic radiographs of dogs and cats with histoplasmosis commonly demonstrate interstitial pulmonary infiltrates and tracheobronchial lymphadenopathy. Tracheobronchial lymphadenopathy may cause coughing and dyspnea.

B. Pulmonary lesions of histoplasmosis heal by encapsulation and frequently calcify. Thoracic radiographs of dogs with previous pulmonary histoplasmosis may reveal the presence of calcified nodules, with or without hilar lymphadenopathy. These lesions are reported to be common in dogs living in enzootic areas. *His-*

toplasma may often be cultured from these lesions even though the infection itself is inactive.

III. Chronic diarrhea may be localized to the large or small bowel.
   A. Large bowel diarrhea (colitis), characterized by hematochezia, mucus, frequent defecation, and tenesmus, is common. Rectal granulomas may occur.
   B. Small bowel diarrhea, characterized by profuse, foul-smelling, watery feces, malabsorption, steatorrhea, and weight loss may also occur.
   C. Vomiting is an inconsistent clinical sign.
   D. Mesenteric lymphadenopathy often accompanies gastrointestinal involvement.

IV. Hepatomegaly and splenomegaly are both common in histoplasmosis. *Histoplasma*-induced hepatic granuloma formation may be manifested clinically by icterus, hypoalbuminemia, and ascites.

V. Nonlocalizing signs commonly observed in dogs and cats with chronic histoplasmosis include weight loss, anorexia, debility, pyrexia, normocytic normochromic anemia, and emaciation.

VI. Relatively uncommon clinical manifestations of histoplasmosis include peripheral lymphadenopathy, ocular lesions (aqueous flare, miosis, multifocal retinitis, papilledema), cutaneous lesions, oral ulcerations, central nervous system signs (ataxia, incoordination), and lameness (caused by skeletal involvement).

DIAGNOSIS

I. Tentative diagnosis of histoplasmosis and localization of the disease may be made on the basis of clinical signs and preliminary laboratory evaluation.
   A. Hematologic abnormalities may include neutrophilic leukocytosis (with or without a left shift), monocytosis, and normocytic normochromic anemia.
   B. Serum chemistry evaluations may indicate evidence of cholestatic hepatic disease, characterized by increased serum alkaline phosphatase activity and hyperbilirubinemia (direct bilirubin). Hypoalbuminemia and increased sulfobromophthalein retention may also be detected. Serum alanine aminotransferase levels are less commonly increased.

C. A diffuse interstitial pattern with linear to finely nodular opacities, hilar lymphadenopathy, and, occasionally, patchy or diffuse alveolar disease may be seen on thoracic radiographs. Abdominal radiographs may confirm hepatomegaly and splenomegaly.

II. The most rapid and definitive method of diagnosing histoplasmosis is cytologic identification of the organism in tissues.

   A. Selection of samples for cytologic examination is based on the physical, laboratory, and radiographic findings. Samples potentially useful for diagnostic purposes include:

      1. Transtracheal wash or fine-needle aspiration lung biopsies from patients with pulmonary involvement

      2. Colonic mucosal scrapings or biopsies (obtained with a colonoscope) from patients with colitis

      3. Fine-needle aspirates or percutaneous needle biopsy of the liver (obtained with a Menghini or other suitable biopsy needle) from patients with hepatomegaly.

      4. Fine-needle aspiration biopsy of enlarged peripheral or mesenteric lymph nodes

      5. Buffy coat smears of peripheral blood, which may reveal the organism in leukocytes

      6. Fine-needle aspiration biopsy of an enlarged spleen (*Caution*: Splenic biopsy may occasionally be associated with substantial hemorrhage.)

      7. Biopsies of unusual lesions (e.g., impression smears of skin lesions, aspirates from bone lesions, smears of abdominal or thoracic fluids) or bone marrow aspiration biopsies.

   B. Samples should be stained with Romanowsky stains (Wright's or Giemsa) or any rapid polychromatic stain (e.g., new methylene blue). The organism *cannot* be seen if wet mounts or potassium hydroxide (KOH) preparations are used.

   C. The yeast phase appears in tissues as a well-defined, achromatic, double-refractile capsule about 2–4 μm in diameter. The central region of the organism is basophilic and is surrounded by an unstained halo (Fig. 37-1).

      1. Organisms are usually found intracellularly, within monocytes, macrophages, or histiocytes; several organisms often occur together in a single cell.

      2. Occasionally organisms may be found in extracellular locations; these organisms are sometimes larger and less spherical in shape.

   D. The organism may be difficult to detect in some cases.

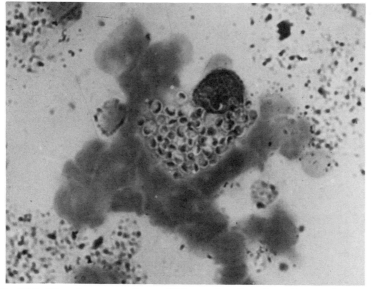

Fig. 37-1. *Histoplasma capsulatum.* Oil-immersion view of a canine rectal mucosa scraping, showing the small intracellular yeast forms within a macrophage. Note that each yeast cell contains a central dark-staining region surrounded by a clear halo. (Courtesy A. M. Wolf, Texas A & M University.)

      1. Sometimes the organism may be detected by biopsy of tissues unassociated with obvious clinical signs (e.g., hepatic aspirates in the absence of hepatomegaly or colonic mucosal scrapings in the absence of clinical evidence of colitis).

      2. Tissue biopsy samples may be used to diagnose histoplasmosis when cytologic methods fail. The organism stains poorly with standard hematoxylin and eosin (H & E), but special stains can be used to facilitate its identification.

      3. When the organism cannot be identified by cytology or histopathology, it may be necessary to make a tentative diagnosis based on immunologic testing.

III. Immunologic testing may be useful for developing a tentative diagnosis in difficult cases, but it is not sufficiently reliable for a definitive diagnosis. Serology does not detect the organism; rather it reflects the patient's response to the organism.

    A. Results of serologic tests lack specificity and sensitivity.

1. Other systemic mycotic agents cross-react in tests for *Histoplasma* antigens.
2. The levels of humoral immunity do not correlate well with the course of the disease. Animals with severe disease may have negative titers, and animals without disease may have positive titers.
3. A positive complement fixation titer of 1:16 or greater is reported to be strongly suggestive of histoplasmosis. Canine sera may be anticomplementary, however, making complement fixation impossible.
4. Agar gel immunodiffusion may also be used to detect antibodies.
5. Ideally, at least a fourfold increase in titers against *Histoplasma* should be documented, with paired samples used to confirm the diagnosis.

B. *Histoplasma* skin testing has been found to be unreliable for the diagnosis of histoplasmosis in dogs. Affected animals often have negative skin tests. Positive tests may indicate active infection or prior exposure.

IV. Because of the financial and time commitments required for successful therapy of histoplasmosis, a definitive diagnosis should be sought before initiating therapy.

TREATMENT

I. Severe pulmonary and disseminated histoplasmosis should be treated. Mild pulmonary histoplasmosis may or may not require antimycotic therapy.

II. Amphotericin B (AMB; Fungizone, Squibb) and ketoconazole (KC; Nizoral, Janssen Pharmaceutica) are both effective against histoplasmosis.

A. Nephrotoxicity and the need for IV administration are the principal disadvantages of AMB. Phlebitis consistently develops in peripheral veins used for administration of AMB; perivascular irritation will develop if extravasation occurs. In addition, humans treated with AMB may experience chills, fever, vomiting, and seizures. Dogs treated with AMB often develop a mild fever during the first treatment, which may persist for 24–36 hours posttherapy. Vomiting during or after treatment with AMB is occasionally seen in dogs.

B. Ketoconazole has the advantages of being less toxic than AMB and can be given orally, but the clinical response to KC is slower. Anorexia occasionally develops in dogs treated with KC. Other possible side effects include vomiting, hepatomegaly, elevated liver enzymes, lightening or graying of hair color, embryotoxicity, and teratogenicity.

III. Therapy for dogs and cats with severe pulmonary or disseminated histoplasmosis should be initiated with AMB.

A. In order to determine if preexisting renal dysfunction exists and to assess toxicity during therapy, the following determinations should be made: renal function (blood urea nitrogen (BUN) and serum creatinine concentrations and urinalysis); serum sodium, potassium, and chloride concentrations; packed cell volume; and total plasma protein concentration.

B. A flow sheet should be prepared for serially monitoring: BUN; serum creatinine concentration; body weight; serum electrolyte concentrations; packed cell volume; total plasma protein concentration; urinalysis results; cumulative AMB dose to date (milligrams per kilogram); and dose of AMB on the particular day of treatment.

C. Administration of 50 ml/kg of 0.9% saline IV over a period of 1–3 hours before administration of AMB should be considered in order to minimize nephrotoxic effects. However, the AMB solution should not be allowed to mix with the saline solution because this will cause the AMB to precipitate.

1. Dehydration and sodium depletion may promote AMB nephrotoxicity.

2. If IV saline loading is impractical, administration of supplemental oral sodium chloride (by salting the food) may be an alternative, although this is probably less effective.

D. Amphotericin B is best administered as a dilute solution given by slow infusion over several hours.

1. Proper reconstitution and handling of AMB are essential. It must be reconstituted with sterile water or with infusion solutions prepared with 5% dextrose in water, because acid solutions and electrolytes will cause the AMB to precipitate. In addition, the drug may be inactivated by prolonged exposure to light. Reconstituted AMB is stable for at least 1 week when stored at 4°C and protected from light.

2. Amphotericin B should be administered IV at a dose of 0.15–0.25 mg/kg for the first treatment and a dose of 0.5 mg/kg per treatment thereafter in dogs. A dose of 0.15 mg/kg per treatment is recommended for cats. However, susceptibility to AMB-induced nephrotoxicity is highly variable and may be dose-related. The dosage given per treatment may be modified within the range 0.1–1.0 mg/kg, depending on patient response and the severity of disease. Critically ill patients should be given higher doses if such doses are well tolerated.

3. The daily dose of AMB should be diluted in 500–1,000 ml of 5% dextrose in water (125–250 ml for small dogs) and infused IV over 4–6 hours. The bottle containing diluted AMB for infusion should be wrapped in aluminum foil to prevent exposure to light during the period of infusion. Alternatively, the daily dose of AMB may be diluted in 60–120 ml of 5% dextrose in water and administered IV over 2–10 minutes. Rapid administration may be associated with greater nephrotoxicity, however.

4. Amphotericin B is given on alternate days, 3 days per week, until the recommended total cumulative dose is achieved. The optimum total cumulative dose of AMB required for successful therapy of histoplasmosis has not been determined, but recommendations have been in the range 2–12 mg/kg.

   a) Treatment with AMB may be stopped when clinical improvement is apparent, the organism can no longer be detected cytologically, and radiographic findings indicate stabilization or improvement of the pulmonary lesions. A decrease in serologic titers may also support the decision to terminate AMB therapy.

   b) Total cumulative dose for AMB when used alone should probably be about 8–12 mg/kg. If AMB is combined with KC therapy, the total cumulative dose of AMB required may be reduced to 4–6 mg/kg.

5. Prior to each treatment BUN concentrations should be evaluated. Therapy with AMB should be stopped if the BUN exceeds 50 mg/dl. Therapy should then be withheld until the BUN is again below 50 mg/kg, at which time treatment may cautiously be resumed. Amphotericin B–induced nephrotoxicity is usually reversible upon termination of therapy. Dogs with primary renal failure are not good candidates for therapy with AMB; consideration should be given instead to using KC as the sole antimycotic agent in these animals.

      6. Amphotericin B therapy may be combined with KC therapy.
IV. Ketoconazole may be used to supplement AMB treatment or, in mild cases, as the sole therapeutic agent for histoplasmosis. Relapse of infection has been a problem with KC therapy.
- A. Ketoconazole is administered at a dose of 10–30 mg/kg/day PO in divided doses bid or tid. When KC is used as the sole therapeutic agent, treatment should be continued for 2–6 months. The decision to terminate treatment should be based on the same clinical considerations described for termination of AMB therapy.
- B. Ketoconazole probably is most effective when used in combination with AMB. Combination therapy takes advantage of both the rapid action of AMB and the low toxicity of KC. One suggested combination protocol is to treat with AMB to a total dose of 4 mg/kg, then continue therapy with KC at a dose of 10 mg/kg once daily for 2 additional months. For animals with very severe disease, AMB therapy may then be repeated to an additional total dose of 2–3 mg/kg followed by another month of therapy with KC.
- C. Because of the reported hepatic effects of KC, it has been recommended that liver enzymes be monitored monthly. If marked elevations are noted, consideration should be given to terminating KC therapy. Hepatic changes appear to be reversible upon termination of therapy.
V. Prognosis
- A. The prognosis for untreated severe pulmonary or disseminated histoplasmosis is very poor. Mild pulmonary histoplasmosis may be self-limiting but a persistent latent infection may result, with recrudescence of disease at some later time (endogenous reactivation).
- B. The prognosis for canine and feline histoplasmosis with treatment is guarded. Even when therapy appears to have been successful, a relapse or recrudescence of infection remains a possibility. Relapse may occur as long as 1 year or more after apparently successful therapy.

PREVENTION

I. No vaccines are available for prophylaxis of histoplasmosis.
II. Histoplasmosis is prevented by avoiding exposure to infected soil. This goal is best achieved by attempting to identify soils with high

concentrations of *H. capsulatum* associated with an outbreak. Areas reported to be of greatest risk include sites of previous chicken coops, old starling roosts, bat caves, or other areas with moist soils likely to have been enriched by avian or bat droppings. Infected soil can be treated with 3% formalin solutions to reduce numbers of organisms.

PUBLIC HEALTH CONSIDERATIONS

I. Canine and feline histoplasmosis present no significant public health risk. Infection results from inhalation of microconidia of the mycelial phase. The yeast phase that occurs in the infected dog or cat is not normally transmissible from animal to human or from animal to animal.

II. Concurrent infections may be seen in animals and their owners. Such instances reflect common exposure to the organism. Infections in dogs and cats may help identify possible sites of exposure and serve as a harbinger of disease in humans.

III. Accidental aerosolization of spores from mycelial cultures of *H. capsulatum* grown on Sabouraud dextrose agar at room temperature may serve as a means of infection. Such cultures should be considered dangerous and should be handled only by appropriate individuals.

SUGGESTED READINGS

Barsanti JA: Histoplasmosis. p. 687. In Greene CE (ed): Clinical Microbiology and Infectious Diseases of the Dog and Cat. WB Saunders Philadelphia, 1984

Breitschwerdt EB, Halliwell WH, Burk RL, et al: Feline histoplasmosis. J Am Anim Hosp Assoc 13:216, 1977

Ford RB: Canine histoplasmosis. Compend Cont Ed Pract Vet 2:637, 1980

Legendre AM: Systemic mycotic infections of dogs and cats. p. 29. In Scott FW (ed): Infectious Diseases. Contemporary Issues in Small Animal Practice. Vol. 3. Churchill Livingstone, New York, 1986

Rubin SI: Nephrotoxicity of amphotericin B. p. 1142. In Kirk RW (ed): Current Veterinary Therapy Vol. 9. WB Saunders, Philadelphia, 1986

38

Protothecosis*
George Migaki

ETIOLOGY

I. Protothecosis is a disease recognized only recently in dogs and cats. It is caused by a colorless (achloric) alga of the genus *Prototheca* and usually pursues a chronic, progressive course. In dogs the lesions are disseminated, with the intestine, eyes, brain, and kidneys being most commonly affected; in cats the lesions are apparently localized to the skin.

II. *Prototheca* is a genus of colorless or achlorophyllous unicellular microorganisms now considered to be mutants of the green algae in the genus *Chlorella*. One of the differences between the two genera is that the large cytoplasmic granules called chloroplasts are present in *Chlorella* but absent in *Prototheca*.

III. *Prototheca* reproduces by endosporulation (asexually by multiple fission), in which 2–20 or more endospores or daughter cells are formed within a mother cell. Rupture of the cell wall of the mother cell, which results from the enlarging endospores, releases daughter cells. Following the growth and maturity of the daughter cells the life cycle is repeated, resulting in large numbers of organisms.

IV. *Prototheca*, in culture or in tissue sections, is spherical to ovoid in shape, 1.3–13.4 μm in diameter, and 1.3–16.1 μm in length, the size depending upon the stage of development. The organism contains a thick (0.5-μm) hyaline cell wall, an abundant amount of granular eosinophilic cytoplasm, and a round to ovoid, centrally located nucleus.

---

* The opinions or assertions contained herein are the private views of the author and are not to be construed as official or as reflecting the views of the Department of the Army or the Department of Defense.

V. A ubiquitous organism, *Prototheca* has been isolated from the slime flux of trees, feces of various animals, potato skin, lake and marine water, acid stream water, sludge in waste stabilization ponds, and human fingernails.

VI. Two *Prototheca* species, *P. zopfii* and *P. wickerhamii,* have been incriminated as the cause of the disease in dogs and cats. Species identification can be accomplished by cultural studies (using sugar and alcohol assimilation tests) or by immunofluorescence.

VII. Little is known about the epizootiology of protothecosis. Infection is believed to be derived from the environment, and there is no evidence of transmission of the disease directly from animal to animal.

VIII. A relatively rare disease, protothecosis has been reported in 19 dogs, the first case being described in the literature in 1969. Three cases have been reported in cats, the first in 1976. The disease is geographically distributed, with cases reported from the United States, Great Britain, Africa, and Australia.

IX. Protothecosis has been reported in humans, cattle, a deer, and a fruit bat, in addition to dogs and cats.

CLINICAL SIGNS

I. Although the pathogenesis of protothecosis in dogs is not understood, it is suspected that the initial infection occurs in the intestine, most frequently in the colon, following ingestion of *Prototheca,* and that there is subsequent dissemination of the organism by blood and lymph vessels. *Prototheca* is considered to be an opportunistic organism. Whether alteration or suppression of the dog's immune system is necessary for infection to occur has not been determined. Preexisting disease may represent a predisposing factor. In cats the localized involvement of the skin suggests trauma at the site of the lesions.

II. Because the lesions are widely disseminated, clinical signs may vary depending upon the organs involved and the lesion severity.

III. Episodes of blood-stained feces or bloody diarrhea that fail to respond to antidiarrheal medication constitute the most common early clinical sign.

IV. Blindness, another relatively common clinical observation, is an indication of intraocular involvement.

   V. Neurologic disorders, including paralysis of the hindlimbs, ataxia,
      circling, incoordination, and tilting of the head are observed when
      the brain and spinal cord are affected.
  VI. Deafness, indicated by failure to respond to voice commands and
      sudden loud noises, occurs when the auditory apparatus is affected.
 VII. Urinary dysfunction, including polydipsia and polyuria, occurs
      when there is diffuse and severe involvement of the kidneys.
VIII. Vomiting results when the stomach is affected.
  IX. Progressive weight loss and debility occur, reflecting the chronic
      progressive nature of the disease and its effects on the general health
      of the animal.
   X. Crusty exudates and ulcers may be found when the skin is affected.
  XI. In cats lameness occurs, with infection of the foot pads. Constant
      sneezing is seen when the lesions are located at the mucocutaneous
      junction of the nose.

DIAGNOSIS

   I. Clinical Pathology
      A. The hemogram and biochemical profiles usually are normal ex-
         cept for occasional lymphopenia.
      B. Cerebrospinal fluid analysis in some cases may reveal a cloudy
         fluid characteristic of eosinophilic meningoencephalomyelitis.
      C. Fluid from the subneurosensory retinal space may yield pro-
         tothecal organisms.
      D. Barium enema radiographs confirm a shortened colon and de-
         creased lumen diameter due to thickened walls in dogs sus-
         pected of having chronic colitis.
      E. Examination of the exudate from cutaneous lesions may reveal
         protothecal organisms.
      F. Sediments of urine derived from affected kidneys may contain
         protothecal organisms.
  II. Microbiology
      A. Prototkecal organisms can be cultured on Sabouraud's dextrose
         agar without fungal inhibitors. The colonies are yeastlike and
         white to light tan in color.
      B. For direct microscopic examination, the cell walls and endo-
         spores can be readily demonstrated if the cultures are stained
         with Gram's iodine solution. Protothecal organisms have a
         thick, refractile, hyaline cellulose wall, granular basophilic cy-
         toplasm, and a single centrally located nucleus.

    C. Species of *Prototheca* can be differentiated by sugar and alcohol assimilation tests and by the fluorescent antibody technique. *P. zopfii* is most commonly isolated from disseminated cases and *P. wickerhamii* from cutaneous cases.

III. Pathology

    A. In dogs with disseminated protothecosis, numerous small, firm white nodules may be found diffusely scattered through the intestine, kidneys, lymph nodes, eyes, liver, heart, brain, and lungs. The mucosa and submucosa of the colon are severely affected, with resulting ulceration and necrosis.

    B. Histologically, the granulomatous inflammatory response contains necrotic areas wherein large aggregates of protothecal organisms have replaced most of the normal tissues. The presence of two or more daughter cells within a mother cell and the absence of chloroplasts are diagnostic features of *Prototheca*. The organisms may be found free in the tissue or may be phagocytosed by macrophages and multinucleated cells. Use of special histochemical stains such as Gomori methenamine-silver nitrate or periodic acid–Schiff (PAS) greatly enhances the demonstration of *Prototheca*. There is a moderate leukocytic response, composed mostly of lymphocytes, plasma cells, and macrophages; neutrophils generally are absent.

IV. Differential Diagnosis

    A. *Prototheca* is morphologically similar to *Chlorella*, but the two genera may be differentiated by the presence of chloroplasts in *Chlorella*, which impart a greenish color to gross lesions. Immunofluorescent staining of the organisms in culture and in tissue section can be used to differentiate the two organisms.

    B. *Prototheca* must be differentiated from yeastlike fungi. Pseudohyphae and hyphae are found with *Candida*, while budding forms are found with *Blastomyces* and *Cryptococcus*.

    C. *Prototheca* must be differentiated also from amoebas. The lack of daughter cells in the genus *Hartmanella* is useful in differentiating it from *Prototheca*.

TREATMENT

I. In dogs, chemotherapy has not been successful and the prognosis in disseminated cases is unfavorable.

II. Surgical excision has been successful, however, in the treatment of cutaneous lesions. In cats with such lesions, complete surgical excision of the infected tissue is recommended.

PREVENTION

Avoid contact with nonpotable water. This, at least, will lower the risk factor for infection.

ACKNOWLEDGMENT

This work was supported in part by Public Health Service grant RR00301-21 from the Division of Research Resources, National Institutes of Health, U.S. Department of Health and Human Services, under the auspices of Universities Associated for Research and Education in Pathology, Inc.

SUGGESTED READINGS

Chandler FW, Kaplan W, Callaway CS: Differentiation between *Prototheca* and morphologically similar green algae in tissue. Arch Pathol Lab Med 102:353, 1978

Cook JR, Tyler DE, Coulter DB, et al: Disseminated prototothecosis causing acute blindness and deafness in a dog. J Am Vet Med Assoc 184:1266, 1984

Finnie JW, Coloe PJ: Cutaneous prototothecosis in a cat. Aust Vet J 57:307, 1981

Gaunt SD, McGrath RK, Cox HU: Disseminated prototothecosis in a dog. J Am Vet Med Assoc 185:906, 1984

Imes GD, Lloyd JC, Brightman MP: Disseminated prototothecosis in a dog. Onderstepoort J Vet Res 44:1, 1977

Kaplan W, Chandler FW, Holzinger EA, et al: Prototothecosis in a cat: first recorded case. Sabouraudia 14:281, 1976

Merideth RE, Gwin RM, Samuelson DA, et al: Systemic prototothecosis with ocular manifestations in a dog. J Am Anim Hosp Assoc 20:153, 1984

Migaki G, Font RL, Sauer RM, et al: Canine prototothecosis: review of the literature and report of an additional case. J Am Vet Med Assoc 181:794, 1982

Sudman MS, Majka JA, Kaplan W: Primary mucocutaneous prototothecosis in a dog. J Am Vet Med Assoc 163:1372, 1973

Tyler DE, Lorenz MD, Blue JL, et al: Disseminated prototothecosis with central nervous system involvement in a dog. J Am Vet Med Assoc 176:987, 1980

Van Kruiningen HJ: Protothecal enterocolitis in a dog. J Am Vet Med Assoc 157:56, 1970

39

Leishmaniasis

Ralph G. Buckner

ETIOLOGY

I. Leishmaniasis is a sporadic, zoonotic granulomatous disease caused by protozoa of the genus *Leishmania*. The response to reticuloendothelial cell infection by these organisms in humans, dogs, some rodents, and (rarely) cats may be classified as mucocutaneous, disseminated cutaneous, or generalized visceral, depending upon the leishmanial species and the nature of the host response. Concurrent human and canine infections are common; however, canine infections also occur in the absence of human disease.

II. Multiplication of the organisms in the host or insect vector occurs by binary fission. Sandflies of the genera *Phlebotomus* (Old World) and *Lutzomyia* (New World) attack the mammalian hosts—dogs, humans, and, in some parts of the world, wild rodents—delivering the motile (flagellated) promastigote form during a blood meal. Development of the amastigote then occurs within wandering and fixed macrophages of the mammalian host. Infection may also be transmitted by direct contact with a discharging skin lesion or by smashing the fly on unbroken skin. The sandfly completes the life cycle of the protozoon by subsequently receiving from the mammalian host the nonmotile amastigote. This form moves to the midgut of the fly and develops into the motile promastigote, ready to be injected through the proboscis of the fly into another mammalian host. Recently it has been demonstrated that the brown dog tick, *Rhipicephalus sanguineus,* may also transmit *Leishmania*. Other reported vectors include mosquitoes, *Culicoides* spp., flies of the genus *Stomoxys,* and lice.

III. Leishmaniasis is endemic in Central and South America, Africa, southern Europe, Asia, and the Orient. An endemic focus exists in the United States in Oklahoma, and it has been suggested that another exists in Texas.

IV. Environmental conditions favoring reproduction of the sandfly vectors include:
   A. Altitudes below 2000 ft
   B. Humidity not less than 70%
   C. Temperature range 45°–100°F

CLINICAL SIGNS

I. The initial lesion is a small, almost unidentifiable erythematous papule, which is followed 6–14 months later by infection of the lymph nodes, liver, spleen, bone marrow, skin, and other internal organs. Depending upon the species and host resistance, clinical signs will vary with invasion and enlargement of the various organs.

II. Clinical signs vary, but those most frequently observed include:
   A. Intermittent lameness
   B. Anorexia, weight loss
   C. Dermatologic lesions, which appear as dry, scaly, focal areas of alopecia, erythema, and hyperpigmentation (Fig. 39-1)
   D. Pruritis (variably present)

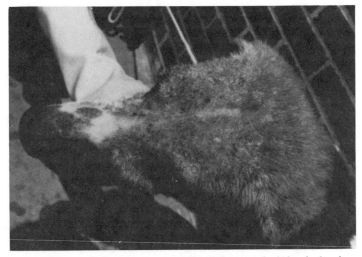

Fig. 39-1. Leishmaniasis. Dry, crusty, scaling lesion on a dog's head, showing evidence of alopecia, hyperpigmentation, and lichenification.

III. The most common signs found on clinical presentation include:
   A. Enlarged lymph nodes
   B. Splenomegaly and occasionally hepatomegaly
   C. Diarrhea, vomiting
   D. Epistaxis
IV. Demodicosis, scabies, staphylococcal hypersensitivity, and atopy must be differentiated as primary etiologic conditions.
 V. Clinical laboratory findings frequently include hyperglobulinemia, hypoalbuminemia, and nonregenerative anemia.

DIAGNOSIS

I. The diagnosis is best made by identifying (Giemsa- or Wright-stained preparations) the amastigote form of the organism in bone marrow biopsies or aspirates, lymph node aspirates, or biopsies of liver, spleen, or skin lesions. Scraping of the skin lesions may frequently be very rewarding. Figure 39-2 demonstrates the organism (amasti-

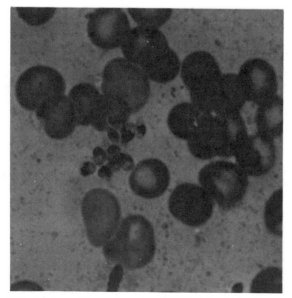

Fig. 39-2. Leishmanial organisms in a Wright-stained blood smear.

gote form) in macrophages of the peripheral blood. Amastigotes have also been demonstrated in synovial fluid.

II. Serologic testing can be accomplished by experienced laboratories equipped to perform the complement fixation, indirect immunofluorescence, or indirect hemagglutination tests. These tests detect the presence of antibodies but not necessarily active infection and disease.

III. Tissues obtained from suspected cases may be cultured on several different media. Experienced laboratory personnel are required to produce interpretable results.

TREATMENT

I. Response to therapy in the naturally occurring disease is difficult to assess. In vitro success does not always indicate that a satisfactory response will be obtained in vivo. Drugs that have shown some success in laboratory animals have not demonstrated efficacy in the dog.

II. Furthermore, drugs that have reportedly shown the greatest degree of response in dogs are not commercially available to the practicing veterinarian in the United States. These drugs include the pentavalent antimonials Pentostam (sodium stibogluconate, Wellcome) and Glucantime (meglumine antimonate, Rhodia).

III. To acquire these drugs for animal administration, the practicing veterinarian must initiate a request through his or her local state health department for transmission to the Parasitic Disease Services, Centers for Disease Control, Atlanta, Georgia. Reports recommend that the drugs be given either IV or IM at a dose of 30–50 mg/kg/day. A 14-day regimen of therapy is recommended, which often needs to be repeated before the possibility of a complete recovery can be contemplated. Other recommendations suggest injections every other day at the above dosage for a total of not less than 15 injections. Further controlled studies are needed, however, to adequately determine the efficacy of these drugs for treatment of canine leishmaniasis. Tolerance of the suggested dosages is acceptable in the dog, with minimal evidence of toxicity (e.g., hepatitis, nephritis, and cardiovascular signs).

IV. Other therapeutic agents suggested but without established laboratory or field results in the dog and cat include ketoconazole, amphotericin B (liposomal preparation), metronidazole, a combination of rifampin and isoniazid, trimethroprim and sulfamethoxazole, furazolidone, or a combination of chlorpromazine and quinacrine. Local heat therapy was reportedly successful in three human patients with diffuse cutaneous leishmaniasis.

PREVENTION

I. A vaccine for use in dogs is not available. Progress has been made, however, in development of a vaccine for humans, which employs the promastigote form of *Leishmania tropica*.
II. Prophylactic drugs have not been identified. Control depends on reducing populations of the recognized vectors.

PUBLIC HEALTH CONSIDERATIONS

I. For human infection to occur there must be a susceptible host population, an appropriate vector, and a reservoir of the infectious agent. In endemic areas humans and dogs are frequently found in close association.
II. Scrupulous sanitary procedures must be followed when handling an animal suspected of harboring *Leishmania* because directed infection from canine to human has been reported. Contamination of the skin by material from ulcers or other discharging cutaneous lesions thus must be avoided.

SUGGESTED READINGS

Anderson DC, Buckner RG, Glenn BL, et al: Endemic canine leishmaniasis. Vet Pathol 17:94, 1980

Chapman WL, Hanson WL: Leishmaniasis. p. 764. In Greene CE (ed): Clinical Microbiology and Infectious Diseases of the Dog and Cat. WB Saunders, Philadelphia, 1984

Giles RC, Hildebrandt PK, Becker RL, et al: Visceral leishmaniasis in a dog with bilateral endophthalmitis. J Am Anim Hosp Assoc 11:155, 1975

Lennox WJ, Smart ME, Little PB: Canine leishmaniasis in Canada. Can Vet J 13:188, 1972

Longstaffe JA, Jefferies AR, Kelly DF, et al: Leishmaniasis in imported dogs in the United Kingdom: a potential human health hazard. J Small Anim Pract 24:23, 1983

Yamaguchi RA, French TW, Simpson CF, et al: *Leishmania donovani* in the synovial fluid of a dog with visceral leishmaniasis. J Am Anim Hosp Assoc 19:723, 1983

40

American Trypanosomiasis (Chagas' Disease)

Jeffrey E. Barlough

ETIOLOGY

American trypanosomiasis, or Chagas' disease, is caused by the flagellate hemoprotozoon *Trypanosoma cruzi*. Two hosts are required for the completion of this organism's life cycle.

I. Hosts

    A. Mammalian

        Humans and a large number of wild and domestic animals, including dogs and cats

    B. Arthropod

        Winged hematophagous insects of the family Reduviidae, subfamily Triatominae (known as "cone-nose," "kissing," or "assassin" bugs), particularly of the genera *Triatoma, Eutriatoma, Rhodnius,* and *Panstrongylus* (Fig. 40-1).

II. Life cycle

    A. Infection of animals and humans

        Infection occurs when an infected triatomine insect defecates while feeding on a susceptible animal or human. Metacyclic trypomastigote forms passed in the insect's feces either are deposited in the bite wound itself or penetrate through the mucous membranes; irritation at the site of the bite may cause the victim to rub infected feces into the skin while scratching. The organisms infect local histiocytes and proliferate as amastigotes. Organisms then pass from the primary site to local lymph nodes and eventually to other areas of the body via lymphatic channels. The liver,

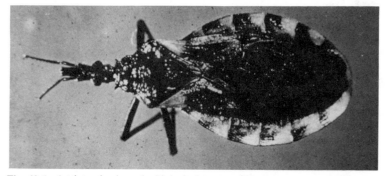

Fig. 40-1. A triatomine bug, the biological vector of *Trypanosoma cruzi*. (Courtesy T. M. Craig and T. S. Tippit, Texas A & M University.) (Tippit TS: Canine trypanosomiasis (Chagas' disease). Southwest Vet 31:97, 1978.)

lungs, spleen, bone marrow, smooth and cardiac muscle, and brain are commonly invaded. Large-scale rupture of host cells releases trypomastigote forms back into the bloodstream and is associated with the febrile response characteristic of the acute disease. There then can follow a prolonged, chronic stage of infection, during which progressive enlargement and denervation of the heart and segments of the smooth muscle of the gastrointestinal tract may occur, resulting in dilation (cardiomegaly, megaesophagus, megacolon). In humans the acute form of the disease is more common in children, while the chronic form is the usual manifestation in adults.
  B. Infection of the insect
     Triatomine insect vectors become infected by ingesting circulating trypomastigotes during a blood meal on a parasitemic vertebrate host. The trypomastigotes transform into epimastigotes within the midgut of the insect, multiply, and migrate to the hindgut to become metacyclic trypomastigotes, in which form they are excreted in the feces during subsequent bloodfeeding.
III. Epizootiology
  A. The geographic range of *T. cruzi* extends from South and Central America to the extreme southern and southwestern United States. Chagas' disease is a major human health concern in many countries, including Venezuela, Argentina, and Brazil, but is almost nonexistent as a health hazard in either humans or animals in the United States. However, fatal cases of canine Chagas' disease

have been reported from several states, including Texas, Louisiana, South Carolina, and Indiana.

B. Dogs and cats are important vertebrate hosts of *T. cruzi,* as are humans and many wild species (foxes, ferrets, skunks, opossums, armadillos, woodrats, raccoons).

C. The most efficient triatomine insect vectors are aggressive, nocturnal feeders that live in bedding, in cracks in the walls of buildings, and in woodpiles, generally in close physical proximity to their human and animal victims. They commonly feed on the thin skin around the eyes and lips, so that the infectious material is easily rubbed into the mucuous membranes.

D. Transmission occurs by contamination of bite wounds and abraded skin and mucous membranes by metacyclic trypomastigotes present in the feces of the insect vectors. Other, less common, means of infection in various animal species include ingestion of infected meat, congenital and transmammary transmission, and possibly contact with contaminated urine.

CLINICAL SIGNS

I. Physical signs

As in humans, the predominant clinical signs in dogs and cats with acute Chagas' disease are a reflection of cardiac dysfunction: tachycardia and other arrhythmias, pale mucous membranes, weak pulse and pulse deficits, lethargy, ascites, hepatomegaly, and pulmonary edema (usually without dyspnea). Neurologic signs may also be present, and Chagas' disease in dogs may mimic distemper: profound weakness, ataxia, and chorea, referable to meningoencephalitis, may develop. Additional signs indicative of systemic disease, such as anorexia, weight loss, diarrhea, lymphadenopathy, splenomegaly, and the nephrotic syndrome, may be seen in some animals. Sometimes however, unheralded collapse and death are the only signs of disease. Fever is usually seen during acute episodes but wanes as the disease gains chronicity. Chronically affected animals may have intermittent bouts of low-grade fever and cardiac arrhythmias. In general, younger individuals are more commonly affected than are older animals.

II. Radiographic and clinicopathological findings

Frequently thoracic radiography will reveal evidence of pleural effusion, pulmonary edema, and cardiomegaly. Hematologic findings may include leukocytosis with lymphocytosis and possibly eosinophilia; however, these are inconsistent. Serum enzyme levels may be elevated as a reflection of ongoing muscle and liver cell destruction.

DIAGNOSIS

I. Clinical
   A. Physical examination
      Diagnosis is based on clinical signs of cardiac dysfunction and possibly associated systemic signs, as detailed in the previous section.
   B. Radiography
      Signs of pleural effusion, pulmonary edema, and cardiomegaly may be evident.
   C. Electrocardiography
      Arrhythmias, low-amplitude QRS complexes, prolonged PR intervals, and ST segment variation may be seen. Of these, the first two abnormalities are considered to be the most common.
II. Geographic locality
    In the United States the vectors are most commonly found in the extreme southern and southwestern states: Texas, Louisiana, South Carolina, Arizona, New Mexico, California. The disease is enzootic, however, in many areas of Central and South America.
III. Identification of the organism
     This is most readily accomplished during the febrile (acute) stage of the disease.
     A. Blood film
        The simplest method involves a coverslip preparation of fresh heparinized blood, stained with Wright's or Giemsa, to look for trypomastigote forms (Fig. 40-2). Unfortunately, as the disease progresses, the number of organisms in the blood decreases, replenishing only during subsequent febrile episodes. More sensitive procedures for detecting the parasite include examination of tissue smears from lymph node biopsies (for amastigote forms) and buffy coat fractions of centrifuged blood samples. The presence of the kinetoplast is important in distinguishing amastigotes of *T. cruzi* in tissues from other parasitic forms.
     B. Culture
        The organism is difficult to grow in vitro and requires a special medium.
     C. Xenodiagnosis
        This is generally not a practical procedure in veterinary medicine. It involves feeding of *T. cruzi*–free triatomines on suspected patients or their blood and subsequent examination (7–10 days) of the insects for the development of parasitic forms in the gut.

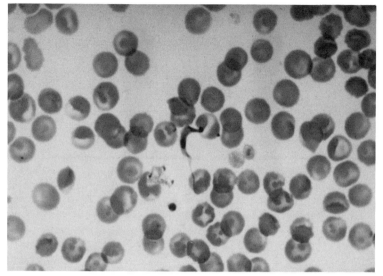

Fig. 40-2. Trypomastigote of *Trypanosoma cruzi* in the blood of an infected dog. (Courtesy T. M. Craig, Texas A & M University.)

D. Animal inoculation

Blood from a suspect case is inoculated into laboratory mice and the animals' blood subsequently examined in 2–4 weeks for the presence of parasites.

IV. Serology

Serologic tests (complement fixation, immunofluorescence, latex agglutination, hemagglutination) are available for detection of antibodies to *T. cruzi,* but the presence of these antibodies is not necessarily indicative of active clinical disease.

V. Necropsy findings

A. The principal gross lesions are found in the cardiovascular system: generalized cardiomegaly affecting particularly the right atrium and right ventricle; subendocardial hemorrhage; and fibrotic plaques on the inner and outer surfaces of the myocardium. Extracardiac lesions may include pulmonary edema, hepatomegaly, visceral lymphadenopathy, splenomegaly, and ascites.

B. The most consistent histologic lesion is a multifocal to diffuse, granulomatous myocarditis associated with the presence of pseudocysts containing amastigote forms of *T. cruzi,* with extensive necrosis and hydropic degeneration of myocardial fibers and infiltration by mononuclear inflammatory cells. There may also be lymphoid hyperplasia, nonsuppurative encephalitis, and granulomatous myositis of skeletal muscle and of the smooth muscle of the gastrointestinal tract.

TREATMENT

I. Of the hemoflagellate parasitisms, Chagas' disease is one of the least responsive to available chemotherapeutic modalities. Nevertheless, promising results have been reported for at least one investigational compound, nifurtimox (Lampit, Bayer), given orally at a dosage of 8–30 mg/kg/day for 3–5 months.

II. However, because the disease is frequently fatal and is also potentially transmissible to humans, treatment of confirmed cases in either dogs or cats must be strongly discouraged.

PREVENTION

I. The only method of prevention is avoidance of contact with infected triatomine insect vectors.

II. Infested premises should be treated thoroughly with residual insecticides such as benzene hexachloride. Spraying should be directed not only toward human habitations but also to animal shelters and stables, pigsties, chicken houses, woodpiles, and other places where insect vectors may be secreted. Repeated treatment at 1- to 5-month intervals is recommended.

III. Oral cythioate (Proban, Haver), given twice weekly to healthy animals at risk of *T. cruzi* infection (3 mg/kg for dogs and 1.5 mg/kg for cats) has been used to help control the insect vectors in certain domestic situations.

PUBLIC HEALTH CONSIDERATIONS

I. Chagas' disease is a major human health concern in the southern Americas, involving millions of infected humans and millions more at risk of infection.

II. Several species of triatomine vectors known to harbor *T. cruzi* are present in the southern and southwestern United States; however, cases of the disease in humans and domestic animals are relatively uncommon in this country. This may be because the insect vectors are less adapted to human habitations and close human and domestic animal contact than are those present in Central and South America.

III. Infections in wild and domestic animals nevertheless are known to occur in the United States, and the disease is considered to be enzootic in certain areas of central Texas.

IV. Chagas' disease in the dog is of considerable importance not only because of the severity of the clinical illness but also because of the possibility of vector transmission from infected dogs to humans or direct transmission through body fluids of infected dogs. Extreme caution must be advised in handling and caring for affected animals.

SUGGESTED READINGS

Barr S, Baker D, Markovits J: Trypanosomiasis and laryngeal paralysis in a dog. J Am Vet Med Assoc 188:1307, 1986

Chapman WL, Hanson WL: American trypanosomiasis. p. 757. In Greene CE (ed): Clinical Microbiology and Infectious Diseases of the Dog and Cat. WB Saunders, Philadelphia, 1984

Haberkorn A: Studies with Lampit in *Trypanosoma cruzi* infected dogs. p. 419. In Hejzlar M, Semonsky M, Masak S (eds): Advances in Antimicrobial and Antineoplastic Chemotherapy. Vol. I/1. University Park Press, Baltimore, 1972

Northway RB: Prevention of trypanosomiasis with cythioate. Mod Vet Pract 64:219, 1983

Snider TG, Yaeger RG, Dellucky J: Myocarditis caused by *Trypanosoma cruzi* in a native Louisiana dog. J Am Vet Med Assoc 177:247, 1980

Tippit, TS: Canine trypanosomiasis (Chagas' disease). Southwest Vet 31:97, 1978

Williams GD, Adams LG, Yaeger RG, et al: Naturally occurring trypanosomiasis (Chagas' disease) in dogs. J Am Vet Med Assoc 171:171, 1977

41

Giardiasis

Carl E. Kirkpatrick

ETIOLOGY

I. Giardiasis is an enteric disease of dogs, cats, and some other mammals as well as of humans, which is caused by parasitic protozoa of the genus *Giardia*. Several species of *Giardia* have been named, usually after the host species in which they were found; however, most *Giardia* spp. are superficially indistinguishable.

II. The causative agent occurs in two forms or stages. The trophozoite stage (Fig. 41-1), found predominantly in the upper portion of the small intestine of the dog and in the lower portion of this organ in the cat, is a motile, teardrop-shaped flagellate. Trophozoites multiply asexually by division. Nutrients are absorbed by the parasite through the outer membrane, and a large, ventral suction disk facilitates adherence to the intestinal epithelium. Invasion of the mucosa by *Giardia* trophozoites rarely occurs. The cyst form (Fig. 41-2) is a walled, dormant stage adapted for survival in the environment.

III. The life cycle does not involve an intermediate host. Following ingestion of cysts and their exposure to gastric and duodenal enzymes, trophozoites emerge and colonize the small intestine. Transition of the trophozoite to the cyst form occurs during passage from small to large intestine. Cysts, excreted in feces, are immediately infective for another, susceptible host; they may survive for several days, even weeks, in cool, moist conditions.

IV. Transmission among hosts occurs by the fecal-oral route. Direct contact with cyst-laden feces and ingestion of food or water contaminated with cysts are the likeliest modes of acquiring *Giardia* infection.

V. The prepatent period of infection is usually in the range of 1–2 weeks. The incubation period (time until clinical disease occurs) may be as short as 5 days.

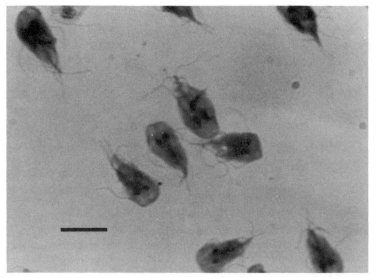

Fig. 41-1. *Giardia* trophozoites from culture. Note the presence of two nuclei, flagella, median bodies (the centrally situated, darkly staining bars) in some of the organisms, and axonemes (longitudinally arranged, slender rods). (Giemsa; bar = 10 μm.)

VI. Giardiasis has a worldwide distribution. The prevalence of infection varies depending on the population studied (e.g., stray vs. pet animals) and on the sensitivity of the diagnostic method used. Generally, approximately 4% of cats and 8% of dogs may be assumed to harbor *Giardia;* however, only a fraction of these animals may be expected to show clinical signs of giardiasis.

CLINICAL SIGNS

I. Signs of disease do not necessarily occur in all animals that become infected with *Giardia* (i.e., inapparent carriers are common).
II. Although the pathogenesis of giardiasis is incompletely understood, it appears to be multifactorial, involving both host- and parasite-related components. The underlying causes of clinical signs are maldigestion and malabsorption of certain nutrients; chief among these are fats, carbohydrates, and some vitamins.

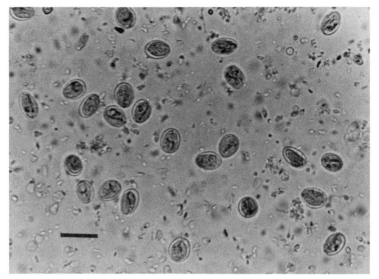

Fig. 41-2. *Giardia* cysts from a zinc sulfate flotation of a canine fecal specimen. A thin, transparent wall may be seen surrounding some of the cysts. (Iodine; bar = 20 μm.)

III. The clinical sign most commonly associated with giardiasis is chronic diarrhea. The diarrhea may be either continuous or intermittent, lasting for weeks, months, or, in unusual cases, years. In clinically affected animals stool consistency is usually semiformed or pasty. Often, feces are paler than normal, with an exceptionally foul odor. Steatorrhea is also likely to be present. Appetite may or may not be depressed, and infected animals may be lethargic. During prolonged bouts with giardiasis, fully grown animals may lose weight, and immature animals may fail to gain at the expected rate.

IV. Differential diagnoses include other infectious and noninfectious causes of diarrhea. In particular, other causes of intestinal malabsorption and maldigestion, such as pancreatic exocrine insufficiency, should be considered.

DIAGNOSIS

I. Because signs of giardiasis resemble those of many other causes of small-intestinal disease and because antigiardial drugs may affect certain other microbial enteropathogens, a definitive diagnosis of giardiasis requires identification of *Giardia* organisms.

II. The method of fecal analysis chosen for identification of *Giardia* organisms depends on the stage of the organism that is sought (i.e., trophozoites predominate in very loose or watery stools, whereas cysts predominate in formed to semiformed stools).

III. To detect trophozoites, a smear, in saline, of freshly passed feces is examined under 250–400 × magnification. Trophozoites (Fig. 41-1) measure approximately 15 μm long by 10 μm wide and on side view appear thin (about 3 μm) and crescent-shaped. They demonstrate a vigorous, tumbling, erratic motion. Because they are transparent, trophozoites may be difficult to detect if the microscope illumination is too bright or if the condenser diaphragm is opened too wide. Phase-contrast illumination is preferred to visualize both stages of the parasite. Alternatively, staining the preparation with a drop of Lugol's iodine (or the equivalent) makes the organisms and their internal structures more conspicuous; however, iodine renders trophozoites immotile.

IV. Cysts are best detected by concentration of a fecal specimen by the zinc sulfate centrifugal flotation method. Zinc sulfate solution, 33% w/v, specific gravity 1.18, is used. Sodium nitrate, sucrose, and salt (NaCl) solutions, commonly used for fecal parasite flotation in veterinary practice, will seldom result in identification of *Giardia* cysts. Centrifuge tubes (15 ml) made of polypropylene or siliconized glass are preferred to those made of polystyrene or plain glass because the latter seem to promote *Giardia* cyst adherence. Should the amount of fat in a fecal specimen make diagnosis by flotation difficult, the formalin–ethyl acetate sedimentation method may be used to detect cysts. Cysts are nonmotile, oval, and slightly smaller than trophozoites. As with trophozoites, iodine staining will improve the likelihood of detection and identification of cysts (Fig. 41-2).

V. Parasites usually are shed intermittently; thus at least three fecal specimens collected over a week's time should be checked before discounting the possibility of *Giardia* infection.

VI. In some cases even multiple fecal analyses may not reveal *Giardia* organisms. In infected dogs, duodenal aspiration using normal saline should recover trophozoites. Not only may trophozoites be found in the aspirate, but if an endoscope or flexible catheter is used to collect the aspirate, the duodenal mucus coating the end of the collection tube may also contain trophozoites.

VII. In fecal smears trophozoites of the flagellate protozoon *Pentatrichomonas* may be confused with *Giardia* trophozoites. *Pentatrichomonas* differs from *Giardia* in having an undulating membrane, a single nucleus (*Giardia* trophozoites have two), and progressive motility.

TREATMENT

I. For *Giardia*-infected dogs, quinacrine hydrochloride (Atabrine, Winthrop-Breon) tablets are effective at a dosage of 6.6 mg/kg bid for 5 days. Vomiting, pyrexia, anorexia, and lethargy are side effects that may be experienced by some dogs during quinacrine therapy, but these effects should disappear within a few days following cessation of therapy. Lower dosages may be effective, also.

II. Metronidazole tablets (Flagyl, Searle) at a dosage of 25 mg/kg for dogs and 10 mg/kg for cats may be given bid for 7 days. Tablets should not be crushed and suspended or placed in food because the drug has a bitter, unpleasant taste.

III. Furazolidone suspension (Furox, Smith Kline) may be given orally (via a syringe placed in the mouth) to cats at a dosage of 4 mg/kg bid for 7 days. Furazolidone has a sweet taste and is easily administered.

IV. In treating relatively large groups of dogs (e.g., in kennels) the addition of ipronidazole hydrochloride (Ipropran, Hoffman-La Roche) to drinking water (126 mg/L) for 7 days may be effective. Fresh ipronidazole should be made up daily.

V. Pregnant animals should not be treated with metronidazole, ipronidazole, or furazolidone unless absolutely necessary.

PREVENTION

I. Because contact with feces or surfaces contaminated with *Giardia* cysts is a likely mode of transmission, sanitation is an important aspect of giardiasis control.

II. Cysts are susceptible to dessication, surviving best under cool, wet conditions. Therefore, keeping kennel runs and cages clean and dry will inhibit cyst survival.

III. Disinfection of surfaces exposed to animal feces may be accomplished by application of Lysol or chlorine bleach.

IV. Removal of animal feces from yards and parks will limit environmental contamination with *Giardia* cysts.

PUBLIC HEALTH CONSIDERATIONS

The relatedness of *Giardia* spp. from various hosts, including human beings, has not been firmly established. Thus, the question of whether the *Giardia* spp. infecting dogs and cats are transmissible to humans is controversial. However, until it is proved that giardiasis is *not* a zoonosis, it is prudent to consider that a zoonotic potential for canine- and feline-source *Giardia* spp. exists. *Thus, treatment of clinically normal "carrier" cats and dogs should be undertaken.*

SUGGESTED READINGS

Abbitt B, Huey RL, Eugster AK, et al: Treatment of giardiasis in adult grey-hounds, using ipronidazole-medicated water. J Am Vet Med Assoc 188:67, 1986

Barlough JE: Canine giardiasis: a review. J Small Anim Pract 20:613, 1979

Gillon J: Giardiasis: review of epidemiology, pathogenetic mechanisms and host responses. Q J Med 53:29, 1984

Hewlett EL, Andrews JS, Ruffier J, et al: Experimental infection of mongrel dogs with *Giardia lamblia* cysts and cultured trophozoites. J Infect Dis 145:89, 1982

Jarroll EL, Hoff JC, Meyer EA: Resistance of cysts to disinfection agents. p. 311. In Erlandsen SL, Meyer EA (eds): *Giardia* and Giardiasis: Biology, Pathogenesis and Epidemiology. Plenum, New York, 1984

Kirkpatrick CE: Feline giardiasis: a review. J Small Anim Pract 27:69, 1986

Kirkpatrick CE, Farrell JP: Giardiasis. Compend Cont Ed Pract Vet 4:367, 1982

Pitts RP, Twedt DC, Mallie KA: Comparison of duodenal aspiration with fecal flotation for diagnosis of giardiasis in dogs. J Am Vet Med Assoc 182:1210, 1983

Roudebush P, Delivorias MH: Duodenal aspiration via flexible endoscope for diagnosis of giardiasis in a dog. J Am Vet Med Assoc 187:162, 1985

Smith PD: Pathophysiology and immunology of giardiasis. Annu Rev Med 36:295, 1985

Woo PTK, Paterson WB: *Giardia lamblia* in children in day-care centres in southern Ontario, Canada, and susceptibility of animals to *G. lamblia*. Trans R Soc Trop Med Hyg 80:56, 1986

Zimmer JF, Burrington DB: Comparison of four protocols for the treatment of canine giardiasis. J Am Anim Hosp Assoc 22:168, 1986

42

Amebiasis and Balantidiasis

Carl E. Kirkpatrick

ETIOLOGY

I. *Entamoeba histolytica,* the causative agent of amebiasis, is primarily a parasite of human beings and other primates; *Balantidium coli,* the agent of balantidiasis, is most commonly found as a commensal in swine. However, infection and colonic disease may be produced by both these protozoons in dogs, whereas only *E. histolytica* is known to infect cats. Because their pathogenic and clinical aspects are so similar, these two diseases will be discussed together in much of this chapter.

II. *E. histolytica* exists as a pleomorphic trophozoite (Fig. 42-1) within the colonic lumen, colonic wall, or, rarely, certain extraintestinal tissues. Trophozoites measure approximately 20–40 μm in diameter. They contain a single nucleus and variable numbers of cytoplasmic vacuoles and granules. The cyst form of *E. histolytica,* rarely seen in feces of animals other than primates, is spherical, measuring approximately 10–20 μm in diameter. The cyst is enveloped by a thin wall and contains one to four nuclei.

III. *Balantidium coli* also exists in two stages. Trophozoites (Fig. 42-2) are relatively large (approximately 35 × 60 μm), oval ciliates found within the colonic lumen or wall. Trophozoites possess a mouth and gullet, a large, bean-shaped macronucleus, an indistinct micronucleus, and many cytoplasmic vacuoles. Cysts are spherical and approximately 50 μm in diameter; they are surrounded by a relatively thick hyaline wall. The presence and arrangement of nuclei within the cyst are identical to those of the trophozoite stage.

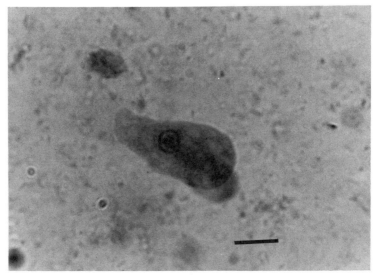

Fig. 42-1. *Entamoeba histolytica* trophozoite in a smear of human feces. Note the irregular outline and the single nucleus. (Iron-hematoxylin; bar = 10 μm.)

IV. The life histories of these two parasites are essentially similar. Infection begins by ingestion of the cyst form. Following excystation, emergent trophozoites colonize the lumen of the large intestine. Trophozoites divide asexually and also, in the case of *B. coli,* sexually by conjugation. Encystment occurs within the large intestine, and fully infective cysts are passed in the feces. No intermediate host is required for completion of either life cycle.

V. Transmission occurs by the fecal-oral route, either by direct contact with feces or by exposure to cyst-contaminated food or water.

VI. Although the extent of *E. histolytica* infection in dogs and cats is unknown, its prevalence in human beings is high in most tropical and subtropical areas of the world. Because the cyst is the infective stage and because infected dogs and cats normally excrete only trophozoites, cysts from human feces are the likeliest source of infection for dogs and cats. Thus, the occurrence of *E. histolytica* in these animals would be expected to parallel that in the human population of a particular region.

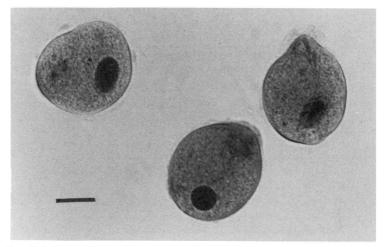

Fig. 42-2. *Balantidium coli* trophozoites. Note the large macronucleus within each organism. Cilia may be apparent on the surface of some of the trophozoites. At the conical end of the organism on the far right, the mouth and gullet are discernible. (Giemsa; bar = 20 μm.)

VII. The distribution of *B. coli* is worldwide, and like *E. histolytica,* this organism occurs predominantly in tropical regions. Usually found infecting the cecum and colon of pigs, in whom it seldom produces illness, *B. coli* rarely infects other animals. Infection due to *B. coli* in the cat is unknown.

CLINICAL SIGNS

I. Both *E. histolytica* and *B. coli* trophozoites may inhabit the large intestine without apparent harm to the host. The mechanisms by which these parasites invade the colonic mucosa are poorly understood, but both organisms are capable of secreting lytic enzymes. It is likely that tissue invasion occurs in conjunction with other, predisposing conditions, such as bacterial infections or depressed host resistance.

II. Colonic ulceration is produced by both parasite species owing to lytic activity of the trophozoites in the submucosa and to the accompanying host inflammatory reaction.

III. Chronic diarrhea, dysentery, weight loss, and anorexia are signs usually associated with *E. histolytica* and *B. coli* infections in susceptible hosts.

IV. Extraintestinal sites in the dog (e.g., lung, spleen, liver, and kidneys) may, on rare occasions, become infected with *E. histolytica* trophozoites.

DIAGNOSIS

I. Diagnosis of both diseases relies on identification of the organisms, either in feces or in biopsy specimens of colonic tissue.

II. In dogs and cats *E. histolytica* trophozoites may be observed in a direct saline smear of feces. Feces should be examined promptly following passage from the animal if the characteristic ameboid motility of the trophozoites is to be observed. Trophozoites have a single nucleus and may contain ingested erythrocytes, especially when passed from symptomatic individuals. Staining the direct smear with iodine or fixing and staining it with trichrome stain (a tedious process) are aids to identification.

III. Leukocytes, particularly macrophages (which may contain ingested erythrocytes), may be misidentified as *E. histolytica* trophozoites in feces.

IV. Because *E. histolytica* cysts are seldom excreted by dogs or cats, fecal flotation is a method of doubtful diagnostic utility.

V. Because *E. histolytica* trophozoites are often shed intermittently, sequential fecal specimens collected on different days may need to be examined.

VI. *Balantidium coli* cysts in feces may be detected by the zinc sulfate centrifugal flotation method. The motile, ciliated trophozoites of *B. coli* can be found by examination of a direct saline smear of freshly collected feces.

VII. Histologic examination of biopsy specimens of affected colonic tissue is the most reliable method of diagnosis for both types of infection.

VIII. Other, more likely causes of colitis must be considered in the differential diagnosis of either amebiasis or balantidiasis. In particular, in the dog infection with the whipworm (*Trichuris vulpis*) must be ruled out. Whipworm infection is frequently found in association with *B. coli* infection in dogs.

TREATMENT

I. Few reports of successful treatment of amebiasis or balantidiasis in dogs or cats have been made. A variety of drugs have been applied to the treatment of humans, but most of these have not been evaluated in animals.

II. Metronidazole (Flagyl, Searle), at an oral dosage of 25 mg/kg bid for 7–10 days, is likely to prove effective in the treatment of *E. histolytica* infections in dogs and cats and *B. coli* infection in dogs.

III. Furazolidone suspension (Furox, Smith Kline), given orally at a dosage of 2.2 mg/kg tid for 7 days, may be effective in curing dogs of *E. histolytica* infections.

PREVENTION

I. Sanitation and disinfection are important in limiting the transmission of both parasite species.

II. Isolating animals from contact with human feces (in the case of *E. histolytica*) and porcine feces (in the case of *B. coli*) will prevent infection.

III. To prevent *B. coli* infection, dogs should not be fed entrails of swine.

PUBLIC HEALTH CONSIDERATIONS

I. Humans are probably susceptible to *B. coli* infection from cysts passed in canine feces.

II. Amebiasis is potentially a serious disease of humans. However, because *E. histolytica* trophozoites do not survive for long once excreted and because they do not survive passage through the upper gastrointestinal tract if ingested, dogs and cats do not serve as reservoirs of amebiasis.

III. Because humans are the likeliest reservoirs of *E. histolytica*, the veterinarian, on discovering an *E. histolytica*–infected pet, should alert the owners to the possibility of infection in themselves.

SUGGESTED READINGS

Adam KMG, Paul J, Zaman V: Medical and Veterinary Protozoology. Rev. Ed. Churchill Livingstone, Edinburgh, 1979

Healy GR: Immunologic tools in the diagnosis of amebiasis: epidemiology in the United States. Rev Infect Dis 8:239, 1986

Kirkpatrick CE: Enteric protozoal infections. p. 806. In Greene CE (ed): Clinical Microbiology and Infectious Diseases of the Dog and Cat. WB Saunders, Philadelphia, 1984

Levine ND: Veterinary Protozoology. Iowa State Univ Press, Ames, 1985

Martínez-Palomo A: The Biology of *Entamoeba histolytica*. Research Studies Press, Chichester, England, 1982

Walsh JA: Problems in recognition and diagnosis of amebiasis: estimation of the global magnitude of morbidity and mortality. Rev Infect Dis 8:228, 1986

Wittnich C: *Entamoeba histolytica* infection in a German shepherd dog. Can Vet J 17:259, 1976

Zaman V: *Balantidium coli*. p. 633. In Kreier JP (ed): Parasitic Protozoa. Vol. 2. Academic Press, New York, 1978

43

Hepatozoonosis

Thomas M. Craig

ETIOLOGY

Canine hepatozoonosis is caused by the sporozoan protozoon *Hepatozoon canis*. The organism is related to *Plasmodium* spp., the cause of malaria in humans. As in malaria, two hosts are required for the completion of the life cycle.

I. Hosts
- A. Mammalian
  Dogs, coyotes, foxes, jackals, hyaenas, civets and various felines, such as the domestic cat, bobcat, ocelot, lion, and cheetah, have been identified as hosts.
- B. Arthropod
  The brown dog tick, *Rhipicephalus sanguineus,* is the principal arthropod host.
- C. Alternate arthropod hosts
  Hepatozoon species have been described in raccoons, mustelids, rodents, reptiles, and birds, with various mites and flies serving as vectors. Alternate arthropod hosts have not been implicated with *H. canis* infections, but epidemiologic investigations indicate that there is transmission in the apparent absence of *Rhipicephalus*.
- D. Direct transmission
  Transmission by the ingestion of infected prey has been documented with a reptilian *Hepatozoon* spp. but has not been proved in mammalian infections.

II. Life cycle
  The life cycle is typically coccidian:

A. Infection of dogs

Dogs become infected by ingesting infected ticks. The sporozoites are freed from the oocyst which is situated within the tick's
hemocele, and penetrate the gut of the dog. From there they are
presumably carried by the blood to various organs (bone marrow,
liver, spleen, lungs, and skeletal and cardiac muscle).

B. Merogony

Intracellular meronts are formed within various tissues. At maturity merozoites released from the meront either reenter tissue
cells to again form meronts or they become gamonts. The number
of generations of asexual (meront) reproduction is apparently un-
limited, at least until the host's immune system is able to limit
the parasite's reproduction.

C. Infection of the tick

Immature ticks become infected by feeding on dogs carrying
gamonts within circulating leukocytes. Within the gut of the tick
sexual union of gametes occurs. The resulting zygote, the ooki-
nete, penetrates the gut wall of the tick and develops into an
oocyst within the hemocele.

D. Development within the tick

After the immature tick is replete, sporulation of the oocyst
occurs off the dog while the tick molts to the next stage of its life
cycle. The sporulated oocyst contains hundreds of sporozoites.
After molting, the infected tick begins to feed on a susceptible
dog. For infection to occur the tick must be ingested by the dog,
because there is no mechanism for transfer of sporozoites through
the tick's mouthparts.

III. Geographic range

A. Western Hemisphere

In North America hepatozoonosis has been diagnosed in dogs
originating from Texas, Louisiana, and Oklahoma. The organism
has been identified in bobcats in California and Texas and in oce-
lots and coyotes from the Texas Gulf Coast. The infection has
been reported in dogs in Brazil, but its clinical manifestations in
that country are unknown at this time.

B. The infection is widespread throughout the Old World, where
Rhipicephalus is extant. In Europe, Asia, and Africa the organism
is generally accepted as a nonpathogenic agent, although there
are several references indicating its association with disease.

CLINICAL SIGNS

Despite the name *Hepatozoon,* the disease is one of the musculoskeletal system rather than of the liver. The meronts are found primarily in skeletal and cardiac muscle, and when located in other organs such as the intestine or lymph nodes, they are associated with muscle cells within those organs. Other species of *Hepatozoon* have been identified in the liver, and some reports indicate that the liver of the dog is occasionally infected.

I. Physical signs

   A. Fever

   The primary clinical sign is fever. Temperature fluctuations between 39.2°C (102.5°F) and 40.6°C (105°F) are common. The fever is unresponsive to antibiotics but may abate with anti-inflammatory drugs such as aspirin, corticosteroids, or other antipyretics. Many febrile dogs spontaneously undergo a clinical remission only to experience repeated episodes of fever.

   B. Musculoskeletal pain and wasting

   The dog may evidence pain on palpation, especially in the lumbar region. Hyperesthesia is manifest by a reluctance to move and by cervical and truncal rigidity. Infected dogs spend most of their time either lying down or assuming a "master's voice" posture. Owing to the disease and its accompanying inactivity, muscular atrophy develops rapidly. When forced to walk, some dogs place the hocks and plantar surfaces of the carpus on the ground in a plantigrade manner. Wasting is seen throughout the body but is especially evident in the temporal region.

   C. Oculonasal discharge

   A mucopurulent ocular and/or nasal discharge is commonly seen, especially early in the infection. The discharge seems to be more evident during febrile episodes.

   D. Bloody diarrhea

   A common sign is that of an intermittent, bloody diarrhea. The diarrhea may be the first clinical sign to be noted, especially in experimental infections. This diarrhea was often noted on the day following ingestion of ticks and frequently was the only sign observed in several experimentally infected dogs. In naturally infected dogs this sign is variably seen.

II. Radiographic signs

   More than half of the dogs with diagnosed cases have had periosteal new bone proliferation. Radiographic changes range from smooth to cauliflower-like periosteal lesions. The ilium, humerus, radius, ulna, femur, tibia, fibula, and vertebrae are most often involved. There may be one or more bones with lesions. A few dogs have had virtually the entire skeleton involved, except for the distal extremities. Dogs that have recovered from hepatozoonosis will show gradual improvement of the radiographic lesions.

III. Clinical pathologic findings

   A. Leukocytosis

   There is a leukocytosis in excess of 30,000/μl, and in some dogs in excess of 200,000/μl on occasion. The leukocytes are predominantly mature neutrophils, and there is occasionally a left shift.

   B. Anemia

   A mild regenerative anemia (packed cell volume of 26 to 35) is a consistent finding. Pale mucous membranes accompanied by a lack of energy and extreme fatigue are common.

   C. Serum chemistry

   Changes in serum biochemical constituents are variable. Serum alkaline phosphatase is elevated in approximately two-thirds of the cases, with levels exceeding 200 IU/L in half of these. Creatine phosphokinase tends to be in the high normal range. High neutrophil counts and utilization of glucose by these cells are thought to be the mechanism causing low blood glucose levels. Sodium fluoride should be utilized to prevent artifactually low glucose levels in suspected *H. canis*–infected dogs. Levels below 10 mg/dl were determined in several cases in which sodium ethylenediaminotetraacetate (EDTA) was used. Blood urea nitrogen levels are generally low early in the disease but become elevated shortly before death.

   D. The clinical, radiographic, and clinicopathologic changes are associated with microgranulomas throughout the tissues wherever meronts have ruptured. Not only will the space previously occupied by the meront be invaded by inflammatory cells, but muscle fasciculi surrounding the granuloma will often be separated by neutrophils.

DIAGNOSIS

I. Clinical

   A. Physical examination

   Diagnosis is based on clinical signs of fever, pain, plantigrade gait, wasting, mucopurulent oculonasal discharge, and bloody diarrhea.

B. Periosteal new bone proliferation where muscle attaches to bone

This lesion may be observed radiographically in approximately 50% of cases. Multiple or bilateral areas of periosteal new bone proliferation may be diagnostic in themselves.

C. Elevated white blood cell count

Dogs with white blood cell counts in excess of 30,000/μl, consisting predominantly of neutrophils, should be suspected of having hepatozoonosis.

II. Geographic locality

The disease is seen along Gulf Coast, although cases have been diagnosed in Illinois and New York in dogs originating from the Southwest. The disease may be spreading north and east, or else recognition of the disease process may be improving with development of better diagnostic tests. The vector is well adapted to much of North America, and the disease could reasonably be expected to be found wherever the vector occurs.

III. Identification of the organism

A. Blood film

The gamont utilizes monocytes and neutrophils as host cells. The parasitemia in most cases encountered in North America has been extremely low, in the range of 0.001–0.01%. Attempts to augment the low parasitemia by examination of buffy coats has been frustrating, probably because the gamont leaves the host cell in response to the drop in ambient temperature encountered outside the body.

B. Muscle biopsy

At this time skeletal muscle biopsy has been the most consistent method of diagnosis. Granulomas containing gamonts and/or merozoites, or cystic areas containing meronts, are of diagnostic significance.

IV. Serology

Attempts to develop a serologic test have been frustrated by the failure to identify a consistent and reliable source of target antigen.

TREATMENT

I. Specific therapy.

There is no specific therapy for hepatozoonosis at this time. Researchers in Africa have indicated that imidocarb (Wellcome) may be effective. The criterion for successful treatment was based on the loss of circulating parasitemia. However, loss of parasitemia is a part of the normal course of events in untreated infections in the United States. The only antiprotozoal that has shown promise is primaquine, a drug used to treat extra-erythrocytic malaria in humans. Several dogs treated (PO or IM) with 1 mg/kg primaquine phosphate (ICI Pharmaceuticals) gradually had an abatement of clinical signs. This should not be construed as evidence for success or failure of the treatment at this time, however.

II. Symptomatic therapy

Palliative treatment with nonsteroidal anti-inflammatory agents for the alleviation of pain has had some success in ameliorating clinical signs. Some dogs have spontaneously recovered from the disease with or without treatment. Corticosteroids may give considerable relief but cannot be recommended because they compromise the dog's resistance to the organism.

PREVENTION

I. Tick control

Control of the brown dog tick will prevent the infection unless alternate hosts are involved.

II. Concurrent disease

Many dogs with signs of hepatozoonosis also have concurrent ailments such as those caused by heartworm, distemper virus, parvovirus, or *Ehrlichia*. Attempts to reproduce the disease under controlled conditions indicate that immunologically compromised dogs are more susceptible to the organism. Therefore, the dog's immune status and freedom from concurrent disease may be major factors in determining whether or not clinical signs appear following *H. canis* infection.

SUGGESTED READINGS

Barton CL, Russo EA, Craig TM, Green RW: Canine hepatozoonosis: a retrospective study of 15 naturally occurring cases. J Am Anim Hosp Assoc 21:125, 1985

Craig TM, Smallwood JE, Knauer KW, McGrath JP: *Hepatozoon canis* infection in dogs: clinical, radiographic, and hematologic findings. J Am Vet Med Assoc 173:967, 1978

Craig TM, Jones LP, Nordgren RM: Diagnosis of *Hepatozoon canis* by muscle biopsy. J Am Anim Hosp Assoc 20:301, 1984

Craig TM: Hepatozoonosis. p. 771. In Green CE (ed): Clinical Microbiology and Infectious Diseases of the Dog and Cat. WB Saunders, Philadelphia, 1984

Davis DS, Robinson RM, Craig TM: Naturally occurring hepatozoonosis in a coyote. J Wildl Dis 14:244, 1978

Ezeokoli CD, Ogunkoya AB, Abdullahi R, et al: Clinical and epidemiological studies on canine hepatozoonosis in Zaria, Nigeria. J Small Anim Pract 24:455, 1983

Gaunt PS, Gaunt SD, Craig TM: Extreme neutrophilic leukocytosis in a dog with hepatozoonosis. J Am Vet Med Assoc 182:409, 1983

Gossett KA, Gaunt SD, Aja DS: Hepatozoonosis and ehrlichiosis in a dog. J Am Anim Hosp Assoc 21:265, 1985

Lane JR, Kocan AA: *Hepatozoon* sp. infection in bobcats. J Am Vet Med Assoc 183:1323, 1983

McCully RM, Basson PA, Bigalke RD, et al: Observations on naturally acquired hepatozoonosis of wild carnivores and dogs in the Republic of South Africa. Onderstepoort J Vet Res 42:117, 1975

Nordgren RM, Craig TM: Experimental transmission of the Texas strain of *Hepatozoon canis*. Vet Parasitol 16:207, 1984

Ogunkoya AB, Adeyanju JB, Aliu YO: Experiences with the use of Imizol in treating canine blood parasites in Nigeria. J Small Anim Pract 22:775, 1981

44

Coccidiosis

Kenneth S. Todd, Jr.
Allan J. Paul

Although toxoplasmosis is caused by a coccidium and there is an enteric form of the parasite in felids, there may also be a systemic infection. For this reason the information in this chapter is divided into sections, covering intestinal coccidiosis and toxoplasmosis separately.

INTESTINAL COCCIDIOSIS

Etiology

I. Canine coccidiosis has been attributed to the following species of *Isospora: I. burrowsi*, I. *bahiensis*, *I. canis*, *I. ohioensis*, and *I. neo-rivolta*. Two unnamed species of *Isospora* have also been reported from dogs. *Eimeria canis* and *Eimeria rayi* have been reported from dogs, but they are probably pseudoparasites. Dogs also serve as definitive hosts for the following species of *Sarcocystis: S. cruzi, S. tenella, S. miescheriana, S. bertrami, S. equicanis, S. fayeri, S. levinei, S. capricanis, S. horvathi, S. hemionilatrantis,* as well as two unnamed species. *Cryptosporidium* spp. have been reported infrequently from dogs.

II. Coccidia of the domestic cat are *Isospora felis* and *Isospora rivolta*. Several species of *Eimeria* have been reported from cats, but they are probably pseudoparasites. Cats are the definitive hosts for the following species of *Sarcocystis: S. hirsuta, S. gigantea, S. porcifelis, S. fusiformis, S. muris, S. leporum, S. cuniculi, S. cymruensis,* and three unnamed species. Cats have been reported to be intermediate hosts for *Sarcosystis* spp., but *Cryptosporidium* spp. have rarely been reported in cats. Cats also serve as the definitive hosts for *Besnoitia* spp.

III. The life cycle of these parasites may be summarized as follows:

    A. Ingested sporulated oocysts excyst in the small intestine.

    B. Sporozoites invade enterocytes.

    C. Asexual multiplication results in meronts containing merozoites.

    D. More than one generation of meronts occurs.

    E. Some merozoites may enter other organs and remain in an arrested state (hypnozoites).

    F. The last generation of merozoites enters enterocytes and forms gamonts.

    G. Merogony is absent in the intestinal stages of *Sarcocystis;* animals become infected by ingesting sarcocysts from infected intermediate hosts. Zoites initiate gamogony.

    H. Microgametes escape from microgametocytes and fertilize macrogametes.

    I. Resistant walls form around the zygotes to produce oocysts.

    J. Oocysts (*Isospora*) and sporulated sporocysts (*Sarcocystis*) pass in the feces.

    K. Oocysts sporulate to reach the infective stage.

 IV. Transmission in *Isospora* and *Cryptosporidium* is effected by ingestion of sporulated oocysts. Transmission in *Sarcocystis* (and also in some *Isospora*) is effected by ingestion of zoites from infected intermediate hosts.

  V. These parasites are cosmopolitan in distribution.

 VI. Oocysts are *resistant to all common disinfectants*. Oocysts and sporocysts are killed by boiling water or live steam. Sarcocysts are killed by thorough cooking of meat.

Clinical Signs

  I. There is some controversy concerning whether or not coccidia alone are pathogens. When the endogenous stages of the parasites leave infected cells, the cells are destroyed; this may lead to secondary bacterial infection. Subsequent diarrhea can lead to fluid and electrolyte loss. Hence clinical signs can include diarrhea, weight loss, decreased food and water intake, and dehydration.

 II. No clinical signs are seen in milder forms of the disease.

III. Coccidiosis is primarily a problem in young animals.

IV. No clinical signs are usually associated with *Sarcocystis* infection.

Diagnosis

The diagnosis is based on the history and clinical signs and on the finding of oocysts in feces by flotation.

Treatment

I. Secondary bacterial infections should be treated symptomatically.
II. Anticoccidial preparations
    A. Amprolium (Amprol, MSD AGVET)
        1. The canine dosage is 110–220 mg/kg of powder in the food for 7–12 days or, as a preventive, 1–2 tbsp of 9.6% solution in 1 gal of water. Should be given to the bitch 10 days prior to whelping as the only water source.
        2. Amprolium does not have FDA approval. Amprolium is a thiamine inhibitor; side effects after prolonged usage include vomiting, anorexia, diarrhea, and neurologic signs. Treatment should be stopped if these signs occur and animals should be treated with thiamine, calcium gluconate solution, and fluids.
        3. The drug is experimental; no contraindications are known.
    B. Sulfadimethoxine (Albon, Hoffman-LaRoche; Bactrovet, Pitman-Moore)
        1. The canine dosage is 55 mg/kg on day 1 and 27.5 mg/kg on days 2–4 or until asymptomatic.
        2. The drug does not have FDA approval. Supportive treatment is recommended.
        3. This is an experimental drug; no contraindications are known.
    C. Sulfadimethoxine-ormetoprim (Romet, Hoffman-LaRoche)
        1. The canine dosage is 55 mg/kg sulfadimethoxine and 11 mg/kg ormetoprim mixed with dry dog food for 23 days.
        2. This drug does not have FDA approval. It is used to prevent experimental coccidiosis.
        3. The drug is experimental; it has no known contraindications.
    D. Sulfadiazine-trimethroprim (Tribrissen, Coopers Animal Health)
        1. The canine and feline dosage is 15–30 mg/kg bid for 6 days. Animals weighing less than 4 kg should receive only one dose daily for 6 days.
        2. The drug does not have FDA approval.
        3. This is an experimental drug; it has no known contraindications.

Prevention

Prevention of intestinal coccidiosis should include measures for strict sanitation, treatment of carrier animals, and prevention of ingestion of infected intermediate hosts. Only thoroughly cooked meat should be fed.

Public Health Considerations

Human beings are not infected with most species of coccidia that infect dogs and cats, with the exception of *Cryptosporidium* spp. and, as described in the following section, *Toxoplasma*.

TOXOPLASMOSIS

Etiology

I. The causative agent is *Toxoplasma gondii*. The life cycle of this parasite in felids may be summarized as follows:
   A. Ingested sporulated oocysts excyst in the small intestine.
   B. Zoites released from the oocysts or zoites ingested from infected intermediate hosts penetrate intestinal epithelial cells and initiate asexual multiplication.
   C. Zoites later initiate a sexual cycle and form gamonts.
   D. Microgametes escape from microgametocytes and fertilize macrogametes.
   E. Resistant walls form around the zygotes to produce an oocyst.
   F. Oocysts pass in the feces and sporulate to reach the infective stage.
   G. Some zoites pass through intestinal cells and multiply in the lamina propria. These zoites then spread to extraintestinal cells via the lymphatic channels and bloodstream and initiate division.
   H. Infected cats usually become immune and recover; the parasites begin a resistant stage and form cysts in various organs.
   I. In immunosuppressed animals the encysted parasites may begin to multiply, resulting in clinical toxoplasmosis.
II. Transmission is effected by ingestion of oocysts in feces, by ingestion of zoites from infected intermediate hosts (e.g., rodents, uncooked meat), and by transplacental transfer.
III. This parasite is cosmopolitan in distribution.
IV. Oocysts are *resistant to most common disinfectants*. They can be killed, however, by exposure to 10% aqueous ammonia (the concentration found in most household ammonia preparations) for 30 minutes.

Clinical Signs

I. Most infections with *T. gondii* are asymptomatic.

II. When clinical toxoplasmosis occurs, signs seen can include fever, hepatitis, bilirubinemia, pneumonia, anemia, encephalitis, myositis, myocarditis, enteritis, and lymphadenitis.

Diagnosis

The diagnosis is based on the history and clinical signs; the presence of oocysts of *T. gondii* in the feces; and, in systemic infections, a rising antibody titer in paired serum samples.

Treatment

I. Systemic infections
  A. Sulfadiazine (Tribrissen, Coopers Animal Health) and pyrimethamine (Daraprim, Wellcome)
    1. The feline dosage is 60 mg/kg/day sulfadiazine divided into four to six daily doses, plus pyrimethamine at 0.5–1.0 mg/kg/day.
    2. These drugs do not have FDA approval. Sulfamerazine, sulfamethazine, sulfadoxine, or combinations may be substituted for sulfadiazine. Platelet and leukocyte counts are advised if treatment exceeds 2 weeks. When platelet or leukocyte counts drop to 25–50% of normal, drug antagonists (folic acid 1 mg/kg/day and baker's yeast 100 mg/kg/day) should be used with the treatment or prophylactically. Kidney and urinary tract disturbances may follow use. Side effects include anorexia, depression, hematuria, crystalluria, and elevated blood urea nitrogen.
II. Oocyst shedding phase
  A. Sulfadiazine and pyrimethamine
    1. The feline dosage is sulfadiazine 120 mg per 100 g in the diet, or 60 mg per 100 g plus 0.5 mg per 100 g pyrimethamine in the diet.
    2. The above comments on use of these drugs to treat systemic infections also apply here.

Prevention

I. Prevention of toxoplasmosis should include the following precautions:
   A. Feeding of raw or undercooked meat to cats should be avoided.
   B. Cats should not be allowed to roam freely and hunt.
   C. Litter boxes should be emptied and cleaned daily.

Public Health Considerations

I. Human infections usually result from ingestion of sporulated oocysts, ingestion of raw or undercooked meat, or transplacental transmission.
II. Ingestion of oocysts from contaminated cat feces may result in human infection.

SUGGESTED READINGS

Dubey JP: Toxoplasmosis in cats. Feline Pract 16(4):12, 1986

Dunbar MR, Foreyt WJ: Prevention of coccidiosis in domestic dogs and captive coyotes (*Canis latrans*) with sulfadimethoxine-ormetoprim combination. Am J Vet Res 46:1899, 1985

Jacobson RH: Toxoplasmosis—feline infections and their zoonotic potential. p. 1307. In Kirk RW (ed): Current Veterinary Therapy. Vol. 7. WB Saunders, Philadelphia, 1980

Levine ND: The coccidian parasites (Protozoa, Apicomplexa) of carnivores. Illinois Biol Monogr 51:1, 1981

Levine ND: Veterinary Protozoology. Iowa State University Press, Ames, 1983

Long PL: The Biology of the Coccidia. University Park Press, Baltimore, 1982

45

Babesiosis
David L. Huxsoll

ETIOLOGY

I. Babesiosis is an important, tick-transmitted hemoprotozoan infection characterized by the presence of the infectious agent in host erythrocytes. The disease is common in many tropical and subtropical areas of the world where the environment fosters development of the tick vectors.

II. Of the many species of *Babesia* identified in wild and domestic animals, at least two species are important in the dog and one in the cat.

A. *Babesia canis* is the more common and the larger of the two species infecting canines. It has been reported from all continents except Antarctica. In the United States it is most common in the South and the Southwest.

1. The primary vector is the brown dog tick, *Rhipicephalus sanguineus,* although *Haemaphysalis leachi, Hyalomma marginatum,* and *Dermacentor* spp. have also been reported to be vectors.

2. Transmission can also occur through blood transfusions from infected donors and by contaminated instruments and needles. Certain biting insects may serve as mechanical vectors.

3. *Babesia canis* is a pyriform (teardrop- or pear-shaped) organism measuring 5–7 μm in length and 2–4 μm in width. The organisms frequently occur in pairs in infected erythrocytes; 1–16 parasites have been noted in a single cell.

B. *Babesia gibsoni,* the smaller of the species infecting canines, has a more limited distribution than *B. canis.* It has been reported in Africa and Asia, and, more recently, in the United States in a dog that had never been outside the country (infections have been previously diagnosed in the United States in dogs brought from enzootic areas).

1. Both *Haemaphysalis bispinosa* and *R. sanguineus* transmit *B. gibsoni.* As with *B. canis,* transmission may occur by mechanical means or through blood from an infected donor.
2. *B. gibsoni* occurs in the form of rings measuring 1–3 μm in diameter. Unlike *B. canis,* the organism usually does not appear in pairs in infected cells.

C. *Babesia felis* occurs in the domestic cat and in certain wild Felidae in Africa and Asia. It is a small species, measuring 1–2 μm in diameter. Four daughter cells forming a typical "Maltese cross" are sometimes seen within an infected erythrocyte. The movement of humans and their pets from enzootic areas should alert the practitioner to the possibility of encountering *B. felis* in an unexpected geographic setting.

III. Babesial infections tend to be more severe in young animals, with the exception of the very young, which may have passive (maternal) immunity.

CLINICAL SIGNS

I. The clinical signs of babesiosis can be quite variable in nature, depending upon the strain of the infecting organism, the degree of parasitemia, the immune status of the host, and complications from concurrent infections. In enzootic regions many animals may have a subclinical infection and develop clinical signs only when stressed. The acute stage of the infection lasts for only a few days; during this stage the parasites usually can be detected in blood smears without difficulty.

II. Animals that survive the acute stage become carriers of *Babesia*. The carrier state results from an equilibrium between the organism and the defenses of the host. In most instances carrier animals cannot be distinguished clinically from normal, susceptible animals.

III. Disease occurs following invasion of the erythrocytes by the organism, which subsequently multiplies and destroys the host cells.

IV. Infections can be either acute, chronic, or inapparent.

V. *Babesia* infections in dogs, caused by either *B. canis* or *B. gibsoni,* result in similar clinical signs, which are related to development of hemolytic anemia.

A. The incubation period can vary considerably; for natural infections the range may be 7–21 days for *B. canis* and 14–28 days for *B. gibsoni*. Much longer incubation periods have been reported, however. The inoculation of dogs with blood from an acutely ill dog with significant parasitemia may result in the appearance of organisms in the erythrocytes of the recipient within 24–48 hours.

B. The acute disease is characterized by anemia, anorexia, depression, fever, hemoglobinuria, splenomegaly, hepatomegaly, lymphadenopathy, and, in some dogs, icterus. Dehydration and vomiting may also be observed. The oral mucous membranes may initially appear congested; they eventually become pale or nearly white in color. This form of the disease is frequently fatal. Peracute cases may be presented with extreme sudden onset and shock, followed by death. Heavy tick infestations are often associated with acute disease.

C. In chronic cases a mild anemia and icterus may be the only signs observed. In some cases these signs may be accompanied by anorexia, listlessness, and fever, which may fluctuate.

D. Although hematologic examinations may show various degrees of anemia, leukopenia, and thrombocytopenia, the findings usually are those of a regenerative anemia. Reticulocytosis and poikilocytosis are often evident. Erythrophagocytosis of normal and parasitized erythrocytes by mononuclear cells may be observed.

E. The carrier state can be readily broken by splenectomy. The spleen plays a key role in limiting spread of the infection during the acute state and controls the infection in carrier animals. Splenectomized animals (and humans) are highly susceptible to fulminating babesial infections.

F. Concurrent infections with *Ehrlichia canis* or *Hepatozoon canis* may result in complex signs of disease. In enzootic regions complications produced by dual infections should not be unexpected, because *R. sanguineus,* the brown dog tick, is a vector for both *B. canis* and *B. gibsoni,* as well as *E. canis* and *H. canis.*

IV. The disease caused by *B. felis* in cats differs in some respects from canine babesiosis.

A. In general, unstressed cats may show few clinical signs. In many instances the only sign observed is anemia, except in terminal cases, when extreme weakness is almost always observed.

B. Yellow feces are often noted, but clinical icterus is not frequently seen.

C. Fever is *not* characteristic of uncomplicated *B. felis* infection in cats.

DIAGNOSIS

I. In enzootic areas a presumptive diagnosis of babesiosis based on clinical signs is justified, especially when tick infestation is apparent. A confirmatory diagnosis is made by demonstrating the organism in the erythrocytes of affected animals. In acute stages of the disease, when parasitemia may be as high as 50% the organism may be readily identified. In chronic cases, however, it may be difficult to find the organism in routine blood films.

II. Certain procedures can facilitate identification of the organism in blood.

A. Of the common stains Giemsa is considered to be the stain of choice for detecting organisms in blood films.

B. Infected red cells have a lower specific gravity and tend to be larger than uninfected erythrocytes. These characteristics cause infected cells to concentrate in capillary blood. In preparing films, capillary blood from the ear should be collected, and the edge of the stained film should be examined closely for infected cells.

C. Because infected cells have a lower specific gravity, it is possible to concentrate them by centrifuging blood and collecting cells from the top of the column for the preparation of films.

D. The above techniques can be readily combined by filling a microhematocrit tube with blood collected by puncture at the periphery of the ear. Following centrifugation, a drop of blood collected from just beneath the buffy coat can be used to prepare the film.

III. Confirmatory diagnosis of a chronic infection can be made by inoculating a susceptible animal. In the case of suspected canine babesiosis, a splenectomized dog should be used for inoculation. If the infection is present, the splenectomized dog will develop clinical signs and the organism can be readily demonstrated.

IV. Serodiagnostic methods are available and have been used to confirm diagnoses, assess treatment, and develop enzootiologic data. These tests include complement fixation, indirect hemagglutination, capillary and slide agglutination, indirect fluorescent antibody (IFA), and precipitation tests and enzyme-linked immunosorbent assay. In most instances these tests are available only in research, diagnostic, or reference laboratories.

V. Dual infection with *E. canis* should be ruled out by a diligent search for the inclusion bodies, or *morulae,* of the rickettsial agent. This may be extremely difficult, even during acute ehrlichiosis. An IFA test for *E. canis* has been developed, however, and is useful in diagnosis of the infection.

TREATMENT

I. Several drugs have been shown to be effective in the treatment of canine babesiosis. Clinical relapses may occur, however, and appear to be more common with *B. gibsoni* infections.

II. Diminazene aceturate (Berenil, Farbwerke Hoechst; Ganaseg, Squibb) in a 7% solution, given as a single IM injection at a dose of 3.5 mg/kg, is effective in treating both *B. canis* and *B. gibsoni.* Doses as high as 7 mg/kg have been used, but this level should never be exceeded because single high or repeated doses may produce neurotoxic signs in dogs.

III. Phenamidine isethionate (Lomidine, May and Baker), administered as a single subcutaneous injection at a dose of 15 mg/kg, has been used effectively in treating canine babesiosis.

IV. A third drug, imidocarb dipropionate (Imizol, Wellcome), is highly effective at 5 mg/kg, given IM.

V. In reported studies the above compounds produced variable results in treating feline babesiosis caused by *B. felis.* In the case of *B. felis,* primaquine phosphate (ICI) was found to be the drug of choice. A single IM dose of 0.5 mg of primaquine base per kilogram is recommended.

VI. Supportive therapy of severely anemic animals is important and should include, where appropriate, blood transfusions, electrolyte solutions, and hematinics. Dehydrated animals must be given fluid therapy; lactated Ringer's solution is recommended.

VII. Broad-spectrum antibiotics of the tetracycline group are recommended if a dual infection with *E. canis* is suspected.

PREVENTION

I. Outbreaks of babesiosis and acute infections often have been associated with heavy tick infestations. Thus tick control is extremely important in preventing the disease. Control measures should be applied not only to the dog but to the premises as well. Impervious kennel floors and walls will reduce harborage of ticks and will enhance the efficacy of acaricides in controlling tick populations.

II. A vaccine for canine babesiosis has been developed and manufactured by Rhone Merieux of Lyon, France. This vaccine, marketed under the trade name Pirodog, consists of exoantigens from cultures of *B. canis*. Two cubcutaneous doses are given during the first year of immunization, followed by an annual booster. The vaccine is not commercially available in the United States.

PUBLIC HEALTH CONSIDERATIONS

I. Although *Babesia* spp. tend to be host-specific, a number of cases of human babesiosis caused by species normally found in animals have been reported. Among the species implicated in human infections are *Babesia, bovis, Babesia divergens,* and *Babesia microti*. Many of the cases have occurred in individuals who had been splenectomized; mortality has been substantial in these patients. The initial diagnosis in many of the human cases was malaria.

II. A particularly large number of human cases caused by *B. microti* have been identified on Nantucket Island, off the northeastern coast of the United States. The high incidence appears to be related to a recently described tick vector, *Ixodes dammini*. The adults of this species are commonly found on deer, and the larvae and nymphs feed on mice. Adult ticks have been reported to attach to humans.

SUGGESTED READINGS

Abdullahi SU, Sannusi A: Canine babesiosis. p. 1096. In Kirk RW (ed): Current Veterinary Therapy, Vol 9. WB Saunders, Philadelphia, 1986

Farwell GE, LeGrand EK, Cobb CC: Clinical observations on *Babesia gibsoni* and *Babesia canis* infections in dogs. J Am Vet Med Assoc 180:507, 1982

Futter GJ, Belonje PC: Studies on feline babesiosis. 2. Clinical observations. J S Afr Vet Assoc 51:143, 1980

Groves MG, Dennis GL: *Babesia gibsoni:* field and laboratory studies of canine infections. Exp Parasitol 31:153, 1972

Lewis GE, Huxsoll DL: Canine babesiosis. p. 1330. In Kirk RW (ed): Current Veterinary Therapy. Vol. 6. WB Saunders, Philadelphia, 1977

Potgieter FT: Chemotherapy of *Babesia felis* infection: efficacy of certain drugs. J S Afr Vet Assoc 52:289, 1981

Ristic M, Healy GR: Babesiosis. p. 151. In Steele JH (ed): CRC Handbook Series in Zoonoses, Section C, Vol. I. CRC Press, Boca Raton, 1982

Schalm OW, Jain NC, Carroll EJ: Veterinary Hematology, 3rd ed. p. 405. Lea & Febiger, Philadelphia, 1975

46

Cytauxzoonosis

Joseph E. Wagner
Ann B. Kier

ETIOLOGY

I. Feline cytauxzoonosis is a fatal hemoprotozoan disease of domestic cats caused by *Cytauxzoon felis,* a theileriid parasite. A great deal of interest surrounded the original report of this disease in 1976 because of suspicions that a foreign disease introduction was involved.

   A. The disease had many features of theileriasis, especially with regard to similarities in the piroplasms (intraerythrocytic phase of the parasite). Theileriasis is a disease of great economic significance to African livestock.

   B. Because of the fatal nature of the disease and its striking clinical presentation, characteristic lesions, and prominent histologic features, it was difficult to believe that it had gone unreported until 1976, prior to which time it had been reported only in wild African ruminants.

   C. Whether or not feline cytauxzoonosis represents the rather recent introduction of a foreign disease agent into the United States may never be determined.

II. Although initially reported in Missouri, it is now known that the disease is enzootic in the United States. It occurs primarily in the summer months, June through September, in the south central and southeastern states (southern Missouri, Oklahoma, eastern Texas, northern Arkansas, northern Louisiana, Mississippi, Georgia, and Florida).

III. Based on recent reports of piroplasms in the erythrocytes of bobcats (*Felis rufus*) and their subsequent transmission via ticks to domestic cats, it would appear that *C. felis* is a tick-transmitted parasite of the bobcat. It is likely that bobcats in the wild remain clinically unaffected, serving instead as reservoir hosts for the parasite. Subsequent transmission of *C. felis* to domestic cats by multiple-host ticks, such as the American dog tick (*Dermacentor variabilis*), then produces a fatal disease in this feline species.

CLINICAL SIGNS

 I. The early clinical signs of cytauxzoonosis are not particularly distinctive.
   A. The clinical signs may mimic those of acute haemobartonellosis. Because early clinical signs are subtle, veterinary attention frequently is not sought until the disease is quite advanced.
   B. The initial clinical signs are likely to include anorexia, weight loss, weakness, lassitude or depression, dehydration, pallor, and a body temperature rising to 41°C (106°F) or more over several days.
   C. Packed red blood cell volume and leukocyte counts may be subnormal. Anemia develops rapidly during the febrile period.
   D. The body temperature then drops over several days and becomes subnormal as the cat enters the terminal stages of the disease.
   E. The mesenteric lymph nodes may be palpably enlarged in the later stages of the disease.
   F. Icterus may develop late in the course of the disease.
   G. Affected cats may become dyspneic, recumbent, and moribund and may cry out or otherwise appear to be in pain during terminal stages.
   H. The course of the clinical illness is usually a week or less in duration.
 II. Cats of all ages are susceptible, but the disease is likely to occur more often in those animals with a greater tendency to roam (i.e., adult males).
   A. Cats with cytauxzoonosis are likely to be free-ranging animals presented during the summer months (i.e., the tick season) in the aforementioned regions or presented with a history of having visited such a region within the preceding 1–3 weeks. In one case involving a New York State family, the family cat became ill during a return trip from the Ozark region of southwestern Missouri, and veterinary attention was sought en route. The attending veterinarian, although not located in an area of enzootic cytauxzoonosis, astutely diagnosed the disease, but despite supportive therapy was unable to save the cat. The family had been camping for several weeks in a remote area of the Ozarks, during which time the cat

frequently explored in the woods and was noted to have acquired a few ticks. Interestingly, the family had spotted a bobcat while camping.
   B. Ticks may or may not be found on an affected cat during the clinical (or necropsy) examination.

DIAGNOSIS

The season of the year (tick season), geographic location, and patient environment and habits should all be considered while formulating a diagnosis. Clinical signs of dehydration, pallor, anemia, icterus, fever, and lethargy are important findings; nevertheless, cytauxzoonosis is rather difficult to diagnose in its early stages. The disease progresses rapidly and is diagnosed more readily as additional signs and lesions become manifest.
   I. Clinical pathology
      A. The most characteristic antemortem diagnostic feature is the appearance of piroplasms in peripheral red blood cells. Parasitized erythrocytes are likely to be found more frequently at the edges and feathered extremity of a blood smear. They can be detected by examination of such smears stained with Giemsa or other Romanowsky stains. The piroplasms appear within erythrocytes as small, rounded to slightly ovoid, signet-ring or oval bipolar "safety-pin" bodies 0.5–2 μm in diameter. The ring-shaped bodies, although small, are quite distinct and characteristic. The peripherally located nuclear chromatin (the signet of the ring) stains densely, appearing either deep blue or reddish purple in color, depending on the stain used. The darker bluish band of the ring surrounds the pale blue–staining cytoplasm of the piroplasm.
      B. Unfortunately, parasitemia may not appear until late in the course of the disease, and its extent is highly variable, ranging from 0 to 50% of erythrocytes parasitized. Usually less than 5% of erythrocytes are parasitized, however.
      C. Occasionally, large reticuloendothelial cells packed with schizonts (tissue phase of the organism) may be seen in stained peripheral blood smears collected late in the course of the disease. Typically, schizonts are seen only in these large reticuloendothelial cells, which may be seen in histologic sections lining vessels in many organs.
      D. An indirect fluorescent antibody test has been described but is not generally available to the practitioner.

E. Identification of *C. felis* within erythrocytes is greatly enhanced by examination of a well-prepared and well-stained blood film with a quality microscope.

F. If piroplasms are not seen initially, sequential blood smears should be made on consecutive days and examined.

II. Necropsy examination

A. Necropsy examination typically reveals a minimal amount of ingesta throughout the digestive tract, moderate to marked splenic enlargement, and petechial or ecchymotic hemorrhages in many areas, including the mucosa of the urinary bladder and beneath the serosal surfaces of the pleura, lungs, and epicardium.

B. Major veins of the abdominal cavity are distended and engorged with blood, including the posterior vena cava and the mesenteric, splenic, renal, and uterine veins.

C. The lungs are dense, edematous, and diffusely reddened. An excessive amount of fluid, sometimes straw-colored, may be found in the pericardial, peritoneal, and pleural cavities.

D. Lymph nodes generally are enlarged and edematous and appear hyperemic, with or without associated hemorrhage.

E. Some animals may have generalized icterus. There may be serous atrophy of fat depots, as in the pericardial fat. In cases running a longer course, the liver may be orange-brown in color and friable.

III. Histology

A. Histologically the lungs are usually edematous and congested. Erythrophagia may be seen in the lymph nodes and spleen. Hemorrhage may be found in almost any organ, and increased bile pigmentation may be observed in the liver. There may be thrombi in small blood vessels and fibrinoid necrosis of lymphoid follicles.

B. The characteristic lesion of cytauxzoonosis is the presence of numerous large, histiocytic macrophages, which contain intracytoplasmic schizonts and are filled either with a foamy-appearing material or with small, granular cytomeres and merozoites in various stages of development.

1. These large macrophages characteristically are associated with the endothelial lining of venous channels in major organs, especially those in the alveolar septa of the lungs, peritrabecular sinusoids of the spleen, and venules and sinusoids of the liver; in lymph nodes, myocardium, and bone marrow; and in renal glomeruli and the renal cortex. In many cases the accumulation of large macrophages in vessels is so extensive as to appear to occlude the vessel lumen.

2. The genus *Cytauxzoon* of the family Theileriidae is distinguished from the genus *Theileria* by the occurrence of schizonts in macrophages (schizonts of *Theileria* are found in lymphocytes).

IV. Differential diagnosis

A. The differential diagnosis must include *Haemobartonella felis* infection (feline infectious anemia), which produces similar clinical signs. Morphologically, *H. felis* differs substantially from *C. felis;* it is smaller, denser, and more monomorphic and tends to occur singly or in short chains on the surface or periphery of affected erythrocytes. By contrast, the slightly oval signet-ring piroplasm of *C. felis* usually occurs singly within the parasite. While stain precipitates and other artifacts may be confused with *H. felis,* this should not be the case with *C. felis*. In addition, the ring forms of *H. felis* are uniform, circular structures and lack the eccentric chromatin of *C. felis*.

B. Typical feline Howell-Jolly bodies (nuclear remnants in young erythrocytes), normally seen in up to 1% of erythrocytes, appear as circular, homogeneous, dark purple inclusions of variable diameter. Because of their uniform circular shape and tinctorial properties, occasional Howell-Jolly bodies with irregular staining should not be confused with *C. felis*.

C. On Romanowsky-stained blood smears Heinz bodies or erythrocyte refractile granules (denatured globin) have tinctorial properties nearly identical to those of normal hemoglobin and thus should not be confused with *C. felis*. The latter appear refractile when slightly out of focus.

D. Erythrocytes with basophilic stippling and siderocytes are recognized by the fine or irregular granular appearance of the inclusions.

TREATMENT

I. Virtually all naturally occurring and experimentally induced cases of feline cytauxzoonosis in domestic cats have been fatal. The rapid course of the disease, as well as the marked severity and generalized nature of the histologic lesions, suggests that an effective treatment modality will be difficult to devise.

A. In general, treatment with fluids, antibiotics, and other supportive therapies may prolong life for several days, but the outcome is predictably fatal.

B. Once the disease has been diagnosed, it may be appropriate to suggest euthanasia for animals in the terminal stages, at least until a more satisfactory treatment has been developed.

C. The few reported attempts at treatment with antimalarial drugs and antibiotics appear to have failed.

II. One ray of hope comes from the work of Uilenberg (personal communication, 1986) in the Netherlands, who successfully treated one experimentally inoculated cat with the drug parvaquone (Clexon, Cooper's Animal Health Ltd., England), which has been used for the treatment of bovine theileriasis. The cat was treated with 10 mg/kg, given IM, on day 11 postinoculation, when fever first appeared, and again with 16.5 mg/kg IM on day 13. Although severely ill, the cat began to recover on day 19 and proved solidly immune when subsequently challenged, although a persistent parasitemia had developed. However, another cat died following similar treatment. In another report researchers appear to have immunized a single cat with an inoculum of *C. felis* grown in tissue culture.

PREVENTION

Preventive measures should include restricted contact with tick vectors, which might necessitate confinement during the tick season. The disease is *not* transmitted by direct cat to cat contact. Similarly, it has not been possible to transmit the disease by intragastric inoculation. On one occasion the disease was transmitted by accidental injection of a cat with a contaminated needle. The disease appears to be transmitted only by parenteral inoculation or through the bite of a vector, presumably an infected tick.

PUBLIC HEALTH CONSIDERATIONS

No human cases of cytauxzoonosis have been reported. On the other hand, there are no reports of experimental inoculations of human or other anthropoid subjects to test susceptibility to cytauxzoonosis. Because relatively little is known about this disease and because of its extreme lethality in cats, caution while handling infected animals is recommended.

SUGGESTED READINGS

Bendele RA, Schwartz WL, Jones LP: Cytauxzoonosis-like disease in Texas cats. Southwest Vet 29:244, 1976

Blouin EF, Kocan AA, Glenn BL, Hair JA: Transmission of *Cytauxzoon felis* (Kier, 1979) from bobcats, *Felis rufus* (Schreber), to domestic cats by *Dermacentor variabilis* (Say). J Wildl Dis 20:241, 1984

Ferris DH: A progress report on the status of a new disease of American cats: cytauxzoonosis. Comp Immunol Microbiol Infect Dis 1:269, 1979

Glenn BL, Stair EL: Cytauxzoonosis in domestic cats: report of two cases in Oklahoma, with a review and discussion of the disease. J Am Vet Med Assoc 184:822, 1984

Glenn BL, Rolley RE, Kocan AA: *Cytauxzoon*-like piroplasms in erythrocytes of wild-trapped bobcats in Oklahoma. J Am Vet Med Assoc 181:1251, 1982

Hauck WN, Snider TG, III, Lawrence JE: Cytauxzoonosis in a native Louisiana cat. J Am Vet Med Assoc 180:1472, 1982

Kier AB, Wagner JE, Morehouse LG: Experimental transmission of *Cytauxzoon felis* from bobcats (*Lynx rufus*) to domestic cats (*Felis domesticus*). Am J Vet Res 43:97, 1982

Kier AB, Wightman SF, Wagner JE: Interspecies transmission of *Cytauxzoon felis*. Am J Vet Res 43:102, 1982

Shindel N, Dardiri AH, Ferris DH: An indirect fluorescent antibody test for the detection of *Cytauxzoon*-like organisms in experimentally infected cats. Can J Comp Med 42:460, 1978

Simpson CF, Harvey JW, Carlisle JW: Ultrastructure of an intraerythrocytic stage of *Cytauxzoon felis*. Am J Vet Res 46:1178, 1985

Simpson CF, Harvey JW, Lawman MJP, et al: Ultrastructure of schizonts in the liver of cats with experimentally induced cytauxzoonosis. Am J Vet Res 46:384, 1985

Wagner JE: A fatal cytauxzoonosis-like disease in cats. J Am Vet Med Assoc 168:585, 1976

Wagner JE, Ferris DH, Kier AB, et al: Experimentally induced cytauxzoonosis-like disease in domestic cats. Vet Parasitol 6:305, 1980

Wightman SR, Kier AB, Wagner JE: Feline cytauxzoonosis: clinical features of a newly described blood parasite disease. Feline Pract 7(3):23, 1977

47

Encephalitozoonosis

Karen Regan
John A. Shadduck
W. S. Botha

ETIOLOGY

I. Encephalitozoonosis is a protozoan disease involving a number of homeothermic species, including rabbits, mice, guinea pigs, blue foxes, and nonhuman primates, as well as dogs and cats.

II. The causative agent, *Encephalitozoon cuniculi*, is an obligate intracellular parasite belonging to the order Microsporidia.

   A. Parasite entry into the host cell may occur via direct penetration of the cell membrane by the polar filament of the organism. Alternatively, entry may be facilitated through phagocytosis of the spore or its sporoplasm by the host cell.

   B. Once inside the host cell, the parasite localizes within a parasitophorous vacuole in the cell cytoplasm.

   C. Parasite development progresses through two proliferative stages, during which division takes place by binary fission.

   D. During the final stages of development the proliferative forms mature into infective spores.

   E. Spores are released by rupture of the host cell.

III. The mode of natural transmission of the parasite is uncertain, but the predominant route is postulated to be horizontal, via ingestion or inhalation of spores. Infective spores are present in the tissues of affected animals and are also shed in the urine. Susceptible hosts become infected by ingesting the tissues of affected animals or by ingesting or inhaling material contaminated with their urine.

IV. Vertical transmission of *E. cuniculi* has also been postulated, and supportive evidence for this has been documented in blue foxes, rabbits, and mice. Results of investigations regarding vertical transmission in rabbits and dogs have been conflicting, however, and this point remains to be established.

   V. Natural outbreaks of encephalitozoonosis in carnivores have been reported most frequently in South Africa; in Pretoria, 18% of the canine population has anti-*Encephalitozoon* antibody titers of 1:20 or greater.

   VI. Sporadic cases of canine and feline infections with *E. cuniculi* have occurred in Europe and England. There have been three reported occurrences of the disease in the United States to date.

   VII. The geographic distribution does not suggest that climate limits the spread of the disease.

  VIII. The organism is resistant to mild changes in temperature and may retain infectivity at 4°C and 20°C for up to 13 weeks. Temperatures above 37°C but below 100°C significantly reduce infectivity, but some spores may survive for up to 2 weeks. Boiling or autoclaving for 10 minutes successfully eliminates infectious organisms.

   IX. Freezing alone or rapid freezing and thawing do not appreciably affect organism viability, nor does drying adversely affect infectivity.

   X. *E. cuniculi* spores are susceptible to many chemical disinfectants. Infectious *E. cuniculi* organisms are effectively eliminated by 30-minute exposures to Lysol, 1% (vol/vol) formalin, 70% (vol/vol) ethyl alcohol, 0.5% iodophor compounds, 1% hydrogen peroxide, or 1% sodium hydroxide. Quaternary ammonium compounds at recommended working dilutions do not consistently kill the organism and therefore should not be the disinfectant of choice.

CLINICAL SIGNS

   I. Encephalitozoonosis in carnivores occurs sporadically, and the clinical course is often progressive and insidious.

   II. The disease has been clinically apparent only in neonatal puppies and kittens, but adults of other species (blue foxes and suricates) have been affected, and the possibility that adult dogs and cats may develop clinical disease exists.

  III. The pathogenesis of the infection in carnivores has not been established. Histologically, the parasite is consistently found within endothelial cells and arteriolar smooth muscle cells, which suggests that a parasitemia is present at some stage of the infection. Subsequent dissemination to other body tissues can then occur.

IV. In addition to arteries, tissues frequently parasitized include the brain, kidneys, and liver; less frequently, the heart, lungs, spinal cord, and eyes are affected. Clinical signs reflect invasion and destruction of these tissues by the parasite, or possibly destruction of the tissue resulting from thrombosis of the vessels and subsequent infarction.

V. Initially, several puppies in a litter or individual dogs (from 2 weeks of age) develop nervous signs, which may include any combination of the following: muscle tremors, chorea-like spasms, hyperesthesia, unsteady gait, dysmetria, ataxia of the hind limbs, circling, aggressiveness, and epileptiform seizures. Periodic outbursts of low- and high-frequency howling are common in puppies.

VI. Signs of acute nephritis may be present in the acute and subacute stages of encephalitozoonosis. These include pain over the dorsal lumbar area and palpably enlarged kidneys.

VII. In rare instances sudden death occurs with fulminating infections in which large numbers of *Encephalitozoon* spores are disseminated to many tissues.

VIII. Intermittent or permanent partial to complete blindness occurs in some dogs. Amaurosis is the usual type of blindness encountered, but keratitis, uveitis, and focal retinitis may also occur in a small percentage of cases.

IX. Depression, general unthriftiness, anorexia, failure to gain weight, and a stunted appearance are common but nonspecific findings. Fever is rarely seen.

X. Some animals may recover from the initial nervous symptoms with supportive care, only to develop signs of acute or chronic nephritis.

XI. Chronic nephritis with uremia and poor growth rate may develop beginning at approximately 5 months of age in dogs infected neonatally. Enlarged lymph nodes may also be palpable.

XII. In kittens severe muscle spasms, depression, paralysis, and death occur in natural cases. Superficial keratitis is an unusual finding.

DIAGNOSIS

I. Hematology
A. Normocytic normochromic anemia is a consistent finding.
B. Reduced hemoglobin levels, erythrocyte numbers, and hematocrit values are found.

C. Early in the course of the disease there may be lymphocytosis and monocytosis. Lymphocytosis and neutrophilia occur in the agonal stages.

II. Biochemistry

    A. Mild increases in serum alanine aminotransferase and alkaline phosphatase activities can be expected when hepatic replication occurs during the acute phase of the disease.

    B. Serum creatinine and urea nitrogen levels are increased when subacute to chronic renal failure occurs; an increased retention of phenolsulfonphthalein is also seen.

    C. Total serum proteins are increased during the initial stages of the disease but are maintained at a high normal level in the subacute to chronic stage.

    D. Analysis of cerebrospinal fluid (CSF) may reveal an increase in protein or in mononuclear cells, indicating an ongoing encephalitis.

    E. Urinalysis is essential for elucidation of occult chronic renal disease. A low specific gravity, isosthenuria, and persistent proteinuria are indications of chronic nephritis.

III. Cytology

    A. Demonstration of *Encephalitozoon* spores by light microscopy and/or by scanning or transmission electron microscopy is the most accurate and reliable diagnostic approach.

    B. Cysts of organisms, individual spores, and phagocytized spores can best be demonstrated by routine Gram staining of urine sediment. Demonstration of spores, either free or within macrophages, in the CSF is also possible.

        1. Urine or other fluid is centrifuged at least 1,000 g for 15–30 minutes.

        2. The supernatant is discarded by carefully decanting or pipetting without disturbing the pellet.

        3. Resuspend the pellet in several drops of water or saline.

        4. Smears of the sediment are air-dried and Gram-stained. The specimens are best viewed under high dry or oil immersion.

            a) Mature spores of *E. cuniculi* are gram-positive, ovoid, and occasionally slightly curved; they have blunt ends and measure $1–1.5 \times 2.5$ μm. They have a large polar vacuole and a thick spore coat (Fig. 47-1).

            b) Immature or proliferative forms may be present. These usually are slightly larger than the mature spores and are gram-negative but will stain with Giemsa.

IV. Serology

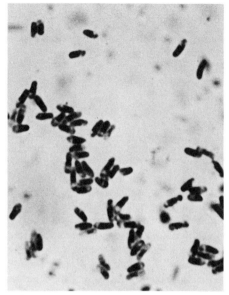

Fig. 47-1. Spores of *Encephalitozoon cuniculi* grown in rabbit embryo fibroblast culture and viewed under oil immersion. Note polar vacuole and the ellipsoid to slightly curved shape. (Gram stain.)

    A. The indirect fluorescent antibody (IFA) test is the most commonly used diagnostic method for serologic confirmation of canine and feline encephalitozoonosis. Puppies demonstrate a very rapid rise in antibody titer, which can be detected several days postinfection. Kittens, however, do not develop a significant titer until 4 weeks postinfection.

    B. The IFA titer at which an animal can be considered to harbor *Encephalitozoon* is 20–40 +, depending on the specific laboratory.

    C. Breeding bitches can seroconvert without showing clinical signs of disease.

  V. Isolation

    A. Successful tissue culture isolation of *Encephalitozoon* from urine has been reported in the rabbit but not in the dog.

    B. Primary and continuous kidney cell cultures can be used when animals are sacrificed.

 VI. Gross necropsy findings

   A. Dogs and cats dying of *E. cuniculi* infection may have no significant gross lesions at necropsy.

   B. If lesions are present, they most consistently occur in the kidney. The kidneys often will be pale and firm and may have an irregular subcapsular surface studded with small cysts. The cut surface may contain pale, grayish-white streaks extending from the cortex to the medulla.

   C. Other gross findings can include splenomegaly, petechiae, hydrocephalus, focal brain cysts, and hemorrhagic cystitis.

TREATMENT

   I. There is at present no specific treatment for encephalitozoonosis. In vitro antibiotic trials using gentamicin, penicillin, streptomycin, oxytetracycline, chloramphenicol, sulfonamides, and sulfadoxine-trimethoprim at recommended therapeutic doses only partially inhibited growth of *E. cuniculi*. Fumagillin is effective in inhibiting the replication of the parasite in vitro but is not safe in its present formulation for use in animals.

   II. Supportive therapy is indicated; if necessary, sedatives may be used.

   III. Because of the progressive nature of the disease, treatment is usually futile once clinical signs are apparent.

PREVENTION

   I. For pets kept in homes in which routine household sanitation methods are practiced, the disease is usually not a problem.

   II. Encephalitozoonosis is seen more frequently in kennels, where many dogs and/or cats are housed together in close confinement and where proper sanitation is difficult or not routinely practiced.

   III. Surfaces can be cleaned and organisms killed by any of the effective disinfectants previously mentioned.

   IV. In cases in which several animals from a kennel have been positively diagnosed as harboring *E. cuniculi,* either by serum IFA testing or by direct visualization of the parasite in urine or tissues, isolation of the affected animals and serologic testing of the rest of the animals in the kennel are warranted. Animals with positive titers, even in the absence of clinical signs, should be considered infected and may be potential reservoirs of infection for other animals.

PUBLIC HEALTH CONSIDERATIONS

I. Cases of human microsporidiosis have been reported. However, in most of these cases the causative organism was subsequently determined to be not identical to *E. cuniculi* on the basis of morphologic criteria. In the remaining reported cases, the identity of the causative organism as *E. cuniculi* is questionable.

II. There have been two confirmed cases of *E. cuniculi* infection in humans. In both cases the patients were children with clinical signs of neurologic disease. Both children recovered from the infection.

III. Serologic studies in Sweden indicate a high prevalence (33%) of serum antibody titers to *E. cuniculi* in homosexual men who have visited tropical countries. High serum titers have also been found in Sweden in patients with malaria (38%) and Chagas' disease (14.8%). These studies may indicate human microsporidiosis in immune-suppressed patients without development of clinical disease. The specificity of the immunofluorescence test in differentiating *E. cuniculi* from other microsporidian parasites has not been definitively established.

IV. *E. cuniculi* should be considered as a potential human pathogen, especially in immunocompromised individuals.

SUGGESTED READINGS

Bergquist R, Morfeldt-Mansson L, Pehrson PO, et al: Antibody against *Encephalitozoon cuniculi* in Swedish homosexual men. Scand J Infect Dis 16:389, 1984

Botha WS, Van Dellen AF, Stewart CG: Canine encephalitozoonosis in South Africa. J S Afr Vet Med Assoc 50:135, 1979

Bywater JEC: Is encephalitozoonosis a zoonosis? Lab Anim 13:149, 1979

Cole JR, Sangster LT, Sulzer CR, et al: Infections with *Encephalitozoon cuniculi* and *Leptospira interrogans,* serovars *grippotyphosa* and *ballum,* in a kennel of foxhounds. J Am Vet Med Assoc 180:435, 1982

Mohn SF, Nordstoga K, Krogsrud J, et al: Transplacental transmission of *Nosema cuniculi* in the blue fox (*Alopex lagopus*). Acta Pathol Microbiol Scand [B] 82:299, 1974

Nordstoga K: Nosematosis in blue foxes. Nord Vet Med 24:21, 1972

Pye D, Cox JC: Isolation of *Encephalitozoon cuniculi* from urine samples. Lab Anim 11:233, 1977

Shadduck JA, Bendele R, Robinson GT: Isolation of the causative organism of canine encephalitozoonosis. Vet Pathol 15:449, 1978

Shadduck JA, Pakes SP: Encephalitozoonosis (nosematosis) and toxoplasmosis. Am J Pathol 64:657, 1971

Shadduck JA, Polley MB: Some factors influencing the in vitro infectivity and replication of *Encephalitozoon cuniculi*. J Protozool 25:491, 1978

Stewart CG, Botha WS, Van Dellen AF: The prevalence of *Encephalitozoon* antibodies in dogs and an evaluation of the indirect fluorescent antibody test. J S Afr Vet Med Assoc 50:169, 1979

Szabo JR, Pang V, Shadduck JA: Encephalitozoonosis. p. 781. In Greene CE (ed): Clinical Microbiology and Infectious Disease of the Dog and Cat. WB Saunders, Philadelphia, 1984

Van Rensburg IBJ, du Plessis JL: Nosematosis in a cat: a case report. J S Afr Vet Med Assoc 42:327, 1971

Waller T: Sensitivity of *Encephalitozoon cuniculi* to various temperatures, disinfectants and drugs. Lab Anim 13:227, 1979

48

Pneumocystosis
Brian R. H. Farrow

ETIOLOGY

I. The precise taxonomy of the organism that causes pneumocystosis is uncertain. *Pneumocystis carinii* has been generally accepted as a protozoon, but certain ultrastructural and staining characteristics have suggested that there is a closer relationship to fungi of the class Ascomycetes, subclass Hemiascomycetidae. The organism has been found in the lungs of many species of animals, including humans, but it is not known whether *P. carinii* isolated from humans and from other animals are identical.

II. The most ubiquitous form of the organism is the trophozoite, which may divide to form other trophozoites. Alternatively, it may develop into a cystic structure, producing up to eight intracystic cells, which on rupture of the cyst wall are released as trophozoites. The cysts may be as large as 8 μm in diameter and the trophozoites are 1–2 μm in diameter. The cyst form can be readily identified with Gomori methenamine-silver or toluidine blue stains, while the trophozoites are best studied with polychrome stains such as Giemsa.

III. Although the organism has been found in normal lungs from many species of animals, where it may exist as a commensal, it only produces disease in immune-deficient individuals. In this context the disease has become a focus of attention in humans suffering from acquired immune deficiency syndrome (AIDS). It also occurs in individuals who have been immunocompromised by cancer, drug therapy, organ transplantation, or congenital immune deficiency disorders.

IV. The infection is acquired by the airborne route, and animal to animal transmission occurs. A remarkable feature of *P. carinii* is that the organism and the disease it causes remain (with rare exceptions) localized to the lungs, even in the most severely immunocompromised host.

CLINICAL SIGNS

I. Reports of naturally occurring pneumocystosis in animals other than humans are rare. The disease has been recorded in dogs but not in cats. Although isolated reports of the disease in dogs have emerged from a number of countries, the most detailed documentation has come from a series of miniature dachshunds seen in Australia. The predisposing factor in these cases has been shown to be a combined immunodeficiency. With the increasing use of immunosuppressive drugs in the management of certain disease conditions, clinicians should be mindful of the nature of this disease.

II. With congenital immune deficiency the disease will usually appear within the first year of life; with acquired immune deficiency onset will occur later. Animals are presented with signs related to the respiratory system: reduced exercise tolerance with occasional periods of cyanosis, coughing, and mouth breathing.

III. On physical examination affected individuals usually are alert, thin, and afebrile, although fever may be present and is a feature of most human cases. Dyspnea varies in intensity but is usually severe and characterized by tachypnea. Auscultation of the thorax reveals normal heart sounds with increased intensity on the right side. Rales may be heard. Abnormal physical findings resulting from this disease are confined to the thorax.

IV. Radiographs of the thorax reveal diffuse bilateral alveolar disease involving all of the lung parenchyma. Bronchi may be well defined in the pattern of an air bronchogram. There usually is tracheal elevation, with right cardiac enlargement and an enlarged pulmonary artery segment.

DIAGNOSIS

I. A definitive diagnosis requires the demonstration of *P. carinii* in lung tissue. The most dependable technique for obtaining such tissue is open lung biopsy. Because of the diffuse nature and severity of the lung disease, there are risks associated with this procedure and it should not be undertaken without considerable surgical skill and anesthetic expertise. At thoracotomy the lungs show a yellowish discoloration.

II. Transbronchial biopsy, endobronchial brushing, bronchopulmonary lavage, percutaneous needle biopsy, and percutaneous needle aspiration have met with varying degrees of success. Sometimes, *P. carinii* can be identified in stained preparations of sputum, swab specimens from the pharynx, and tracheal aspirates. Some practitioners achieve consistent and reliable identification of the organism in smears from bronchial washes without lung tissue biopsy. A small volume (2–5 ml) of sterile normal saline is introduced into a bronchus via a tracheal catheter; this is followed by aspiration of as much of the washing as possible. Two to five instillations may be necessary to collect an adequate sample. An equal volume of 50% ethyl alcohol should be added to the collected specimen before sending it to the cytology laboratory. Evaluation by a pathologist experienced in the identification of *P. carinii* facilitates diagnosis.

III. Giemsa-stained impression smears of biopsy material reveal numerous trophozoite and cyst forms of the organism. Preparations stained with Gomori methenamine–silver nitrate highlight the argyrophilic cystic bodies (about 8 μm in diameter).

IV. The histopathologic features of *P. carinii* pneumonia are predominantly related to the alveolar spaces. Hematoxylin and eosin-stained sections reveal foamy, weakly eosinophilic material filling the alveolar spaces. There is a slight thickening of the alveolar septa owing to edema and mononuculear cell infiltration. Gomori stain reveals numerous argyrophilic cystlike bodies scattered throughout this foamy material. Toluidine blue staining may also be used to demonstrate cysts and trophozoites in the alveolar spaces. Electron microscopic examination shows the foamy material to consist of tightly packed trophozoites and scattered precystic and cystic stages of the organism. Phagocytosis by alveolar macrophages is also apparent.

V. Hematologic examination usually reveals a leukocytosis consisting of neutrophilia and monocytosis, with lymphocyte numbers generally in the normal range. The blood picture is likely to vary according to the underlying cause of the immune suppression. Electrophoretic examination of plasma proteins in the cases examined has revealed a hypogammaglobulinemia.

VI. In humans with this disorder, the blood gas profile is a most useful laboratory study. Hypoxia with low arterial oxygen is observed, and the arterial pH is usually increased. These findings have not been documented in animals, although they are probably present.

VII. Serology has not been helpful as a diagnostic aid in humans because a majority of normal individuals acquire antibodies at an early age. In addition, because of the immune deficiency underlying the disease, antibody titers may be low despite an established and severe infection. Most infections are insignificant, and it is likely that the development of pneumocystosis represents activation of a latent infection in an immune-compromised host. In the absence of obvious explanations for immunosuppression, assessment of immune system function should follow a diagnosis of *Pneumocystis* pneumonia.

TREATMENT

I. Two preparations, trimethoprim-sulfamethoxazole (Septra, Wellcome; Bactrim, Roche) and pentamidine isethionate (Pentam, LyphoMed) are available for treatment, and demonstrate equal efficacy. Trimethoprim-sulfamethoxazole is the drug of choice because of its ready availability, ease of administration, and low toxicity. The recommended dose is 20 mg of trimethoprim and 100 mg of sulfamethoxazole per kilogram PO divided qid. A 14-day course of treatment is recommended.

II. Pentamidine isethionate is administered IM at a dosage of 4 mg/kg daily for 14 days. The injection is painful, and injection site reactions can be severe. Other signs of toxicity have been recorded in humans, including nephrotoxicity, hepatotoxicity, and blood and bone marrow changes.

III. There appears to be no advantage in treating with these two regimes simultaneously.

IV. Limited studies in the dog indicate that without treatment the disease appears to be as uniformly fatal as it is in humans. Treatment is associated with a good clinical response and disappearance of the organism from the lungs. Infection may recur because the underlying immune deficiency mitigates against production of effective immunity.

PREVENTION

In highly susceptible humans, such as those experiencing severe immunosuppression, observations suggest that the disease can be prevented by administration of trimethoprim-sulfamethoxazole. A dosage of 5 mg trimethoprim and 25 mg sulfamethoxazole per kilogram PO divided bid has been successful in humans.

PUBLIC HEALTH CONSIDERATIONS

The vast majority of infections are asymptomatic or insignificant, and the disease is only expressed in immune-compromised individuals. It appears that the organism is a commensal and that it only produces disease when normal immune surveillance mechanisms are severely depressed.

SUGGESTED READINGS

Farrow BRH, Watson ADJ, Hartley WJ, Huxtable CRR: Pneumocystis pneumonia in the dog. J Comp Pathol 82:447, 1972

Hughes WT: *Pneumocystis carinii* pneumonitis. Chest 85:810, 1984

Rorat E, Garcia RL, Skolom J: Diagnosis of *Pneumocysts carinii* pneumonia by cytologic examination of bronchial washings JAMA 254:1950, 1985

INDEX